PEDIATRICS AROUND THE BLOCK

The Journey From Country Doc To World
Renowned Pediatric Researcher/Opinion Leader

A Memoir by

Stan L. Block, M.D., F.A.A.P.

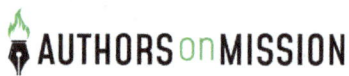

Tables and Figures

Figures

Tables

Foreword

As of 2025, I have known Stan since his arrival in Bardstown, KY, over 40 years ago. He has become a leader of a unique, vital pediatric group that provides excellent medical care and a medical home for the children in a three-county area in Central Kentucky. He also leads this group's prolific research efforts, which have added important data that have helped move the needle in pediatric care to the potential benefit of all children. He has become an excellent teacher for families and peers alike. He has become what we in academics call a "quadruple threat," excelling in the clinical, community service, teaching, and research areas, while working in a private pediatric practice. This, to me, deserves recognition for the enormous effort and energy that Stan has given to these endeavors.

First, Stan's dedication and skills in clinical pediatrics are without question. He and his partners have developed a unique clinical practice in which patients receive state-of-the-art pediatric care in a "medical home". The rigorous principles that we associate with the academic practice of medicine have been blended well in a seamless fashion into this community-based practice.

Secondly, Stan is highly regarded in his community and has been a contributing member on many levels. For example, he was the football team physician for the local high school for over 20 years. He has been a frequent speaker at local elementary, middle, and high schools regarding health matters, as well as at the local Lamaze classes. He served as a founding member of the Bardstown Foundation for Excellence in Public Education, which is a philanthropic group devoted to funding special projects in the public school system.

Thirdly, Stan has demonstrated a consistent commitment to teaching over the years. He regularly teaches and mentors medical students as well as Pediatric and Family Practice residents who rotate through his practice from both Kentucky universities. In addition, he actively contributes to the Continuing Medical Education (CME) of physicians, having delivered over 50 academic regional "Grand Rounds," and 2-3 lectures per month to physicians in various communities across and outside Kentucky. He draws on both his clinical experience and the original data generated during research in which he participated or was a leader. These lectures often cover important topics such as antibiotic resistance, otitis media, and the newest vaccines. Sizable portions of the data presented in the lectures derive from his/his group's research. He has also helped analyze and publish these data in peer-reviewed medical journals. This positions him as a credible and respected voice among fellow practitioners, who appreciate receiving practical, evidence-based information from a peer who understands their challenges, and he frames the information in language relatable to primary care providers. This teaching style encourages audience engagement, often sparking meaningful dialogue with practitioners seeking advice or insight into specific clinical problems.

Fourthly, I have been impressed by Stan's scientific productivity, particularly considering the demanding schedule he has maintained in both community service and clinical practice over the past decades. He has been an author of numerous publications in nationally recognized medical journals, frequently as the lead author. Further, he continues to generate impactful data. His work has earned him invitations to present as a physician-researcher at national and international conferences—opportunities resulting directly from the projects he has helped to design, implement, and analyze. He has also served on several important educational executive committees for the American Academy of Pediatrics and on many national vaccine advisory boards.

Stan embodies a balance of academic rigor, hands-on patient care, and community involvement. His high ethical standards and strong local reputation make him an exemplary role model for aspiring physicians. Therefore, I recommend you share in recounting his life's journey. In my experience, few private pediatricians have been able to blend compassionate, evidence-based medicine with teaching, prolific research, and multi-faceted service and connection to his community.

Sincerely,
Christopher J. Harrison, M.D. Professor of Pediatrics
Division of Pediatric Infectious Diseases,
Kansas City Children's Hospital

Table of Contents

A Personal Note: A Rube? Or Ruby in the Rough?

Among all the medical disciplines, pediatrics is a true art form using the fibers of medical science, compassion, life-long learning, and typically requiring several human interactions during each visit. To be proficient, **one must rely on one's intuitive sixth sense along with all 5 other senses**, as the patients are often non- or limited- verbal (babies, children, the disabled, and many reticent or immature children/teenagers). It is not only a profession, but also a vocation, and it requires that its practitioners be healers, teachers, child advocates, and, critically, trustworthy professionals.

Like all medical specialties, the path to becoming a pediatrician is characterized by intense educational efforts along with significant personal and financial sacrifices. But pediatrics requires that we have a strong desire to make a positive impact on the lives of each developing youngster. In this book, I will explore many personal experiences during that journey, what I learned, and how it blossomed into my current devotion to pediatric medicine, which eventually exploded exponentially to a monumental level, way beyond what you or I could have imagined at the start with just two everyday community general pediatricians! Or, simple country docs? Now our office has had 12 providers, 15 full-time research nurses and associates, and arguably the largest outpatient pediatric research group in the U.S.

And I still love my regular job. (Most days.) *Joie de vivre*!

I will recount a few of the stories from my formative years, from childhood memories, family customs, and important friends. Underneath the facade of being a "big dumb jock," the seeds of pediatric empathy were planted in these earlier years, along with my core principles of **compassion, delayed gratification, intellectual curiosity, and underdog advocacy.**

During my educational experience, I thrived on new challenges and discoveries at every stage. Much like my experience in the chaotic halls of high school, in the stimulating classrooms of a university, in the intense crucible of medical school, and in the demanding rotations of residency, these processes shaped not only my clinical acumen but also my character. During these years, the dichotomy of medicine was realized: the conflict between science and soul, between data and bedside manner, between humanity's godliness (like an amazing childbirth) and occasional malevolence (like horrific child abuse).

My path to becoming a pediatrician was mostly self-motivated (which I excelled at), coupled with many other influential and supportive persons and mentors. Along the way, I learned from my successes and disappointments. Patients of all ages taught me lessons that no textbook could ever impart. My late wife, a superb and beloved nurse and mother, became an essential partner in this journey. She was a confidante and a safe harbor from all the stress for over four decades, when some days I just wanted to yell in frustration, when some days I just needed a hug—like a big baby.

Upon entering my final occupational phase, my first goal was to establish myself in this special two-person pediatric and newly established adolescent practice in rural Kentucky. My commitment was both professional and personal. The pediatric needs in the community were high, the prior resources low, and the rewards priceless. You will also read here that my second, later, loftier goal was to establish and make sacrifices toward a world-class juggernaut in pediatric and adolescent research, which would supersede this routine office microcosm in this tiny hamlet. We would no longer just read about the medical news. Our work and research would now **be the medical news!**

And my third goal was to successfully raise four self-sufficient, highly educated, compassionate, and well-adjusted young daughters, to emulate their momma—my toughest, favorite job of all. I love my girls.

This memoir is a somewhat chronological account, along with some introspection and humor, involving milestones that marked a career and my personal and professional family. It also gives one a brief, insightful glimpse into the evolving nature of childhood diseases and vaccines, and into a few heart-wrenching ethical concerns that all pediatricians must deal with. It is also a reason to celebrate my many minor and major medical triumphs, such as lifting a teenage girl's personal black cloud, enabling a parent to understand their child's school frustration, and amazingly delivering to our patients the first-in-the-world morbidity-sparing and mortality-saving vaccines such as HPV4/9, Prevnar 7/13/20, Rotavirus5, and meningococcal vaccines, etc.

Pediatrics is a very future-oriented discipline. It is a specialty that is based on resilience, preventative medicine, physical/emotional growth, and enabling a child's full potential. And to avoid getting baby-whizzed on? In recounting this story, I would like to provide more than a personal narrative. I would also like to shed light on many common truths and misconceptions in pediatric medicine. I encourage those who might take up this field to do so with integrity, curiosity and a heart. But you had better be extremely smart, perceptive, love to learn, and have some "thick skin" at all levels. Your patients need you too much to ever perseverate on perceived shortcomings or on your becoming a victim of "impostor syndrome."

These pages will also take you through clinical puzzles and even some doubts. A few key topics and illnesses, which are typically very misunderstood, will thus be more thorough and heavier on the science. Move on if you wish to. More fun and clever insights are around the corner within a few pages.

And whatever category you fall into, whether medical student, practicing pediatrician, trainee, health professional, parent, or curious reader, I would like you to join me in pondering what it means to receive the sacred trust of **"Pediatrics Around the Block,"** whether in small-town Kentucky or throughout the U.S.

(In most cases, races, names, genders, dates, families, and, rarely, diagnoses may have been changed for privacy reasons.)

CHAPTER 1

Early Life and Educational Years

My Early Childhood

My momma said I was not a very pretty baby, as she teased me late in life. But, as my mother, she could still unconditionally love me. No argument from me. I saw the photograph.

I was born and raised in Louisville, KY, residing in a small suburban neighborhood surrounded by farmland at that time. Although small by today's standards, our house was the biggest in the neighborhood—and the rowdiest. Being the fifth boy by birth order in a family of seven children, I truly understood what it meant to be the underdog and the lowliest chicken in the pecking order of a large family. By necessity, I learned how to maneuver around four lumbering hulks of male aggression, my brothers, each two years apart in age. As older brothers often do, they took great pleasure in torturing, tormenting, and pummeling me for the most minuscule peccadillos, mostly just for their sheer delight. It was all in the name of brotherly love, which we all shared. And teasing in good faith. Over time, I quickly learned how to avoid these daily "froggings" of the deltoid muscle, and I learned the importance of having a mother's skirt to shield me. But I must be honest, in retribution, I used to sneak in an occasional retaliatory hit-and-run approach to get some payback for all these incidents. But we still love each other to this day.

Three of my four brothers were super-jocks, all-state in baseball and track, and talented in basketball. One brother (Mike) was even all-state in basketball—a monster, 6'5" tall and 230 pounds of muscle. They each thought they were Mario Andretti, many times on the interstate highway, occasionally paying the price for this speeding indiscretion in court fees, as I was told later by my parents. Hardly a day went by when we weren't playing basketball, baseball, or football in our backyard, often with my dad, who sold life insurance. (He could sell snowshoes to Carribbeans, my brother said.) He had also been a semi-professional baseball player in Brooklyn, NY. Weirdly, he was so talented that he played for the House of David, a semi-professional Jewish, long-bearded, baseball team in the area, who rode on donkeys when they batted. They were probably the original vaudeville-like, minor league "Savannah Bananas." I still cannot fathom how the donkeys worked, but my mother kept his old uniform for decades, as proof, I suppose, of this great talent.

He attended as many sporting events for his sons and daughters as humanly possible. No all-star or regular baseball game or basketball event was ever too far away for him. When he attended my own high school basketball games, he could be heard in the stands yelling, "Pop it, Chipper!" fairly frequently, which mortified me at the time.

I had become a skilled player by my high school junior year and was the team's leading rebounder and scorer in basketball during my senior year on a mediocre team. Kind of like Pat Conroy's *A Losing Season*.

Academically, I performed well in grade school and subsequently received a scholarship to one of the local all-boys Catholic high schools, Trinity High School (the paradox was that my dad had been raised in a Jewish family in NYC). Dress code: wear a tie every day. I can still tie a Windsor knot in my sleep. Yes, freshmen were occasionally hazed and stuffed in their lockers.

There, I excelled academically and in my basketball skills, even being selected for the Louisville "All 7th Region" honors. We are talking about a hotbed for really good basketball players. I was elected as the "Mr. Basketball" of my high school in my senior year. Yet I fouled out of most basketball games, after brazenly drawing two or three offensive charges.

"Hey, they were supposed to get out of the way, weren't they? Not my fault." Nonetheless, I averaged 16 PPG and 10 rebounds per game in my senior year.

Being a small center (6'2") on the basketball court and having had to negotiate my way through larger, lumbering, and taller males at home most days on our own basketball court provided me with the background to overcome similar difficulties on the high school basketball court despite my smaller size. One fine winter night during the season, I was competing against three huge opponent basketball players, 6'5", 6'7", and 6'8" from the number 1 team in the state, Male High School. I was able to use my slick hook shot in the first half, scoring quite well. However, in the second half, they decided to put the monstrous, 250-pound, 6'5" senior hulk (H. Husky) on me defensively, and this smothering ended my scoring run for the evening.

Thus, the motto for the opposing basketball teams in Louisville was: *If you stop Block, you stop Trinity*. Like in Pat Conroy's book *Losing Season*, it was another long, arduous basketball season for me, with our record barely breaking .500.

I was generally a robust, healthy, and very athletic teenager. But one evening during my junior year, playing basketball against our all-boys archrival, St. Xavier, in January, while standing on the foul line in the third quarter, I became very short of breath and pale. That night, I had insisted on playing after suffering from several days of the influenza virus. My friend on the opposing team (many of us played streetball together during the summer months and had a respect for each other's skill sets) asked me if I was OK. I responded by slowly heading to the bench, sitting down, and hyperventilating. Dang, I felt bad.

My parents brought me to the emergency room, where the ER doctor uncovered a loud cardiac murmur. Two medical visits later, I was in the cardiothoracic surgeon's office, being told that I had a patent ductus arteriosus (PDA) lesion that needed to be repaired that summer. I was told I needed to quit the basketball season for fear that I might go into heart failure or an arrhythmia due to the enormous physical stress of playing high-powered basketball. Well, we all know where that went as a teenage boy! I would take my chances and finish the season. After all, we had made it into the regional games past the district tournament, and I wasn't going to miss my chance for the "big stage."

By the third quarter of each subsequent game, I was fairly fatigued, and I labored to finish up the fourth quarter. I still got in my offensive charging fouls, by the way.

When we arrived at the big stage of the regional tournament, my sarcastic high school friends took up the chant: "Murmur, murmur, murmur," before the game, and each time I scored, to honor my cardiac predicament. Quite a novel cheer. Thanks, boys!

A PDA is a normal in utero blood vessel connection between the pulmonary artery and the aorta, which allows blood to bypass the lungs in utero when they are not receiving oxygen. After birth, this blood vessel connector is supposed to close up when exposed to oxygen during regular newborn respirations. But not in me. Dang. Typically, if this PDA remains open, it will be heard during normal newborn examinations or even during illness in the first few months, or at least by one year (I know this well, as I am a general pediatrician myself, listening to thousands of hearts over the decades). Not in me. Dang. No physician had auscultated this peculiar, distinct murmur until I had that episode during a flu illness at age 16. So, I was now scheduled to "undergo the knife" upon my 17th birthday to repair this defect.

The days before this major surgery, my reactive and introspective depression were quite pronounced. I was in terror. I finally realized that without surgery, I would be in heart failure within a decade and become cardiac disabled due to the continuous volume overload of blood extraneously pumping into the right side of my heart.

Back then, open-heart surgery through the posterior left lateral rib cage was the only way to repair it. This involved a 15-inch-long incision up my posterior thorax, spreading the ribs apart (OW!), then completely ligating the blood connector, and finally inserting a chest tube for drainage, to add to the fun.

Currently, we slickly repair this neonatal congenital defect by inserting a catheter up the groin and inserting a coil into the blood vessel to clot it off, making it almost an outpatient procedure. Not for me. An additional seven painful days in the hospital and a lot of morphine were what I received back then. But the sweet nurses did baby me a bit. I ate that up.

Now, there was another major cardiac trouble happening simultaneously as the murmur fiasco. I had fallen in love with a brilliant, lovely, talented red-headed girl from a nearby public school during that winter. But she had dumped me that spring just before my surgery, leading to a "true" and even more painful "broken heart." Quite the doldrums ensued for a sensitive, forlorn, and addled teenage boy. Several lessons were learned that summer:

Physical and emotional broken hearts are real and upsetting, with the latter problem being much more prolonged and debilitating. And post-operative pain from rib-spreading utensils is awful.

In Elementary School

I grew up in suburban Louisville, which at that time was mostly farmland, littered with orchards, cornfields, pastures, and creeks, all of which needed to be explored. I attended Catholic grade school for the first eight years of my education. However, when I was enrolled in kindergarten earlier, the teacher thought I was, quote-unquote, "a slow learner" after the first day of enrollment. I apparently did not realize that my formal birth name of "Stanley" was going to be used in my new school. The only name I knew at that point in my life was "Chip." Chip was a leftover name because my humorous Jewish father had named me Stanley Jr., and as such, I was literally a "chip off the old block." Haha. He had run out of surnames for his fifth boy. I had to somehow overcome this academic labelling during the first few years of my elementary school life, just like the first two years of medical school. They did not bother teaching me like the rest of the class, as I was often left alone. What did I care?

In late middle school, I was not much enthralled with the classic fiction books available to me, such as *Treasure Island* and *Huckleberry Finn*. Instead, I became deeply engrossed in aviation books about the British Royal Air Force, the Luftwaffe, the Mustang, the Spitfire, and the Russian MiG. I was a fan of naval stories about the frigate, *Old Ironsides* (*USS Constitution*), and other historical genres, particularly those about the Revolutionary War and the Civil War between the states, like *The Red Badge of Courage*. As a true nerd, I even occasionally perused the *World Book Encyclopedia* for nuggets of knowledge. The *Encyclopedia Britannica* was too erudite for me.

Yet, I spent as much time as I could roaming the corn fields, streams, and dirt piles in my developing neighborhood on Tanglewood Trail. Along with my buddies, we practiced our skills in playing chess, all versions of poker, bridge, and billiards (the pool table in my basement was a big draw and money maker for hustling). When I was 12, I even learned how to smoke Salem cigarettes that we pilfered from our neighbor's mother. But I found this to be most unpleasant and not worth the effort or the smell. Stupid boy.

My brothers and I, along with the neighborhood boys and some of the girls, were constantly into sports, playing wiffle ball, softball, basketball, kickball, "guns and knives" (to this day, I have never fired anything higher caliber than a pellet gun), and football. I even tried summertime tennis and golf in my teen years. Every summer, we spent most of our time at the swimming pool, even at some rock quarry lakes, roughhousing and wrestling with each other. There were times when we would walk onto several community golf courses, pick up a ball and some clubs from home, and start playing on different holes scattered throughout the city's golf courses. Of course, my large family couldn't afford country club membership, so this was a sheer delight for me to practice this wonderful skill, even though I was not very gifted at golf.

To summarize my family dynamics, my parents rarely knew where I was or what I was doing with my free time, and similarly, later on, with my life decisions. They trusted me implicitly throughout my schooling and my playtime. They knew that I was studying a lot at our kitchen table with our bustling, distracting household of four other rambunctious boys. They never had any complaints about my academics or grades. I was, however, close to being suspended from my freshman year of high school under Trinity's 10 demerits (suspension) and 15 demerits (expulsion) policy. All infractions were due to bad jokes and running our mouths too much. Nothing malicious, as I was also playing basketball full-time on the high school team, sharpening my basketball skills.

Heck, I was even one of eight freshman scholarship recipients due to my high scores on the Catholic high school admission test. I could even recognize my own name by then, eh? I would continue to be an excellent test taker throughout my life. As far as where I wanted to attend college, career choice, med school choice, pediatric residency choice, and summer job choice, I was similarly totally self-directed. One time, I even dared to ask my busy mom what she thought about my 4.0 grades one semester in high school. Response: "That's nice," as if I had taken my first baby step. Like I said: self-directed.

I just continued being driven by my own self-satisfaction about my academic grades. Two months before I graduated high school, I uncovered an amazing observation—that the school was actually keeping track of our class ranking. Who knew??? Certainly not me. That church-mousey guy, Joe Mattingly, was the only student ranked higher, and he never spoke a word in class. Never. But some people (wonder who?) spoke way too much in class. Oops. I had to spend the entire second half of my freshman year with a muzzle on my mouth to prevent that 10th demerit. I succeeded, and my parents never knew about my dilemma. I just thought that a boy was supposed to make all these jokes and wisecracks on his own. I was even smart enough **not** to join a high school drinking fraternity as well, despite intense peer pressure. I protested that "my dad would kill me," hyperbolically, and they left me alone. He was actually a gentle man. Now, don't get me wrong, my mom and dad were supportive, loving, and superb parents, and I think they knew that we boys were basically good kids, and very capable of making excellent choices. And I found out during my mom's last years that she was actually quite proud of me and my accomplishments. But she only once recognized that I finally hit the "big time" when the prestigious "scientific" magazine, *Good Housekeeping,* quoted me on some vaccine issue.

The Path to a Pediatrician

In order to enter the world of the rewarding, privileged status of a board-certified pediatrician, let me tell you about my path as an example.

Delayed gratification is essential. While everyone else, intelligent and non-medical, is entering the paying workforce, one must sacrifice inordinate time and energy, must pay whopping tuitions, and forgo income, with only zero to meager income to get there. Incessant, eternal student loans are key. One must also learn to be very efficient when studying, have an excellent memory, and have a zest to learn, especially esoteric scientific matters.

High School (4 Years)

Good grades are essential. No stupid mistakes. Avoid: drugs, chronic alcohol use, pregnancy (for both genders: child support, eh?), and bad decisions. The academics at Trinity High School were superb and challenging. Great school. I even passed out of my first semester in college with AP classes. Only one downside: unwisely, I tried to negotiate with some of my buddies who were the all-state, talented football jocks. They sometimes teasingly badgered and belittled my more introverted, nerdy academic high school friends. After all, we nerdy guys spent much of the day in a room for "independent study" of English and social studies, which they teased as "nerd-land." Most of us took little offense at that toying, testosterone-laden aspersion, but I occasionally intervened diplomatically for my friends. I was big enough, but I sorely lacked any necessary aggression, martial arts, or fighting skills. Probably stupid on my part, as any of my buddies could have overtaken me. But I was good at poker—and bluffing. And I tried to avoid bullies.

In addition, I did learn quite well how to accept the tirades of a yelling basketball coach who tried to emulate Indiana University's Bobby Knight or University of Kentucky's John Calipari. "Say 'yes, sir,' move on, and take nothing personally." This philosophy would truly help with raising my four teenage daughters and in my encounters with some of the more difficult mentors in my career. To assuage bees, honey is better than vinegar, and I always remembered the following axiom with my girls: "This too shall pass." (Harlan Coben).

University Undergraduate (4 years)

One needs four years of full university study with stellar grades (3.5 GPA or better). This science-heavy curriculum must include calculus math courses and all the sciences—biology, physics, chemistry—and especially the very difficult organic chemistry for two semesters. This is a course intended to weed out the less dedicated and those not meant for the rigorous sciences to come. In contrast, I dedicated many of my elective college courses to English, literature, and history, which helped me maintain my reading and writing skills, often overlooked in the sciences. What's not to love about Shakespeare and Modern English poetry? "Forsooth," "Readiness is all," and "Out, damn spot!" And stories of Kilgore Trout (Kurt Vonnegut)—so cool. "When have we not preferred some going round/To going straight to where we are?" said British-

American poet W. H. Auden about time and clocks. Think about it. Again, the 1970s era's atmosphere for me was perfectly depicted by Pat Conroy's other book, *South of Broad*.

Awarded a Rector academic scholarship, I attended my first two years at DePauw University in Greencastle, Indiana, an excellent liberal arts college. I made some delightful, memorable, forever friends in my fraternity there. The teachers were warm and welcoming.

I also played collegiate basketball my freshman year there, but I mostly rode the bench. I was nonetheless assigned the brutal task of guarding (maybe mugging?) the varsity all-conference senior center, Pittinger. Some folks called me "hacksaw," but my four older, bruising brother jocks had helped me refine my "defensive" skills. "No blood. No foul," eh? In fact, I heard my freshman coach say to the team, "That Block is no diamond in the rough. He is just rough!" Perhaps, "a ruby in the rough?"

So, I received my workouts, except on game days, and I learned patience. Yet, all the away game bus travel, fatigue, and the rigors of my science courses led me to realize that I couldn't balance collegiate basketball with the demanding high level of these academic courses. Plus, I was taking challenging liberal arts courses with term papers. I excelled in my science courses, earning As in physics and organic chemistry, which I weirdly enjoyed for its problem-solving and "detective work" aspect. This would be good for my eventual career. All my friends were taking junior semesters abroad. Instead, I transferred after two years because I wanted to experience a bigger campus and a warmer, southern atmosphere. More like *Wanderlust*, perhaps? And perhaps, in part, also due to a breakup and a broken heart (again) from one of the lovely, brighter, and older coeds, Jaimie, on campus? How much can a boy's heart stand?

During my sophomore year at DePauw, I saved my first life—one of many life-threatening cases destined for my future. My roommate, Tom Mote, a premed student and eventual future full-fledged MD anesthesiologist, was riding his bike in the "Little 500" race. He was accidentally knocked off his bike and sustained a mild concussion, or so he thought. When he returned to our dorm room in the fraternity house for a few hours, he looked extremely pale, with intermittent confusion and mumbling word salad.

I intuitively knew this was abnormal, so I called in a few upperclassmen, and we rushed him to the college doctor's office. He quickly called an ambulance. With the upperclassman, articulate Stuart Walker, riding along, Tom was on his way to Indiana University's emergency department for a burr hole and a metal plate in his skull to alleviate the blood clot on his brain, a condition known as an epidural hematoma. This is one of the most feared and deadliest head trauma complications in the emergency department. An hour or more delay, and we would be attending his funeral instead. Quixotically, Stuart, an enigmatic, rebellious type of guy, showed his true heart and remained with Tom at his hospital bedside for days, while he was in a prolonged coma. This act of selflessness still amazes me to this day, over 50 years later.

Junior Year at UNC Chapel Hill

For my upcoming junior semester, I had applied for a transfer to the University of North Carolina at Chapel Hill. I was encouraged by my high school best friend, Mike McCarthy, a real smart guy, a high school tennis superstar, who was now attending Duke University. He was studying to be a "sin-buster" (preacher). He was number five out of 281 in the high school class, while I was the class salutatorian. I could never afford Duke tuition. But he told me about this academic gem with lower tuition costs than DePauw, even on my scholarship. Little did I know, this UNC Chapel Hill school was a "suicide application" (a habit I had of submitting only one application to an extremely competitive academic acceptance process). They accepted only three junior-level out-of-state transfers annually! Who knew? I was one of three—whew. Sight unseen, my dad and I drove down the mountainous Appalachian roads (Norris Dam, before Interstate 40) to

Chapel Hill for my first day of classes. He dropped me off at the steps of the oldest public university dormitory in the U.S., my new home, Old East Dorm. Some true nostalgia here, though "wasted" on me then.

Speaking of "wasted," my roommate was a brilliant Morehead scholarship student who smoked a marijuana bong every day while I was his roommate the first semester at UNC. Thus, I spent most of my evenings studying in the library. I never smoked the stuff, but I figured this was part of my real-world pharmaceutical education for my premed inklings. In fact, my other dormitory neighbor showed and explained to me the drug world items that he was peddling on campus: "shrooms" (peyote seeds or psilocybin) and "Mr. Natural" (tiny paper stamps of LSD). Nice guy though.

One bright, warm autumn day, as I was walking to my dorm room, I spotted a tiny furry fluff ball in the bushes, squeaking, barely audible. It was a few-day-old baby squirrel, whose eyes were still fused. I took him up to my dorm room and thought that I would nurture and feed him since he was abandoned by his momma. On a trip to the drugstore, I then purchased some syringes and infant formula milk to feed him via an eye dropper. After a few days, he opened his eyes and he saw—Me! I was then "imprinted" as his momma. I took care of my baby every day, feeding and playing with him. Boy, was he fast, but really amazingly affectionate. He would wake up every morning, nudging me and licking my face at 7 a.m., like clockwork, for me to feed him. My roommate only complained about his little brown "presents" that he left around my books. One day, Scurry rummaged through my neighbor's garbage can and found a used pork chop to gnaw on. He only vomited a few times that night. Ugh.

Eventually, Scurry was ready to gain some "book knowledge" beyond acorns and dogs. So, I took him to my Modern Poetry class where he rode in my shirt pocket, sticking his head out periodically to understand the poetry works of W. B. Yeats. Professor Armitage spotted him, I think, but never remarked about it until I received a phone call from him, asking if his 15-year-old son could visit little Scurry later that afternoon. *Well, of course.*

Scurry was very friendly after a few minutes with people, so the two played some hide and seek outside. Like usual, he climbed his way up his legs with those sharp little claws. I had also trained Scurry to return for food by jiggling an empty Coke can with a penny in it. He would hop off the tree and onto my outstretched arm and jump right back into my pocket, poking his little fuzzy head out. This worked for about four more months.

Scurry's letter to the *Daily Tar Heel* newspaper at UNC Chapel Hill, 1974:

What have you been drinking? You must have the mind of a minnow! Squirrels act squirrelly. How can you hold something against somebody when they won't even let you near him? You don't. Yet you may look at a squirrel like me and, in a rather uppity tone, say, "That is a squirrelly squirrel." And that's the way it should be.

You people consider yourselves broad-minded and educated. You are really like a box of rocks. It's such a different story with squirrelly people. So would you please give your acorns and nuts to me, and not to those other danged people "squirrels." If you thought you could help feed hungry kids, look at me, the leaner and hungrier one.

Signed, scurrilously,
Mr. Scurry

On another evening, Scurry even went on a lark road trip to Miami, Ohio, with my female friend Lizzy and me in the middle of the night. He just ran circles around the steering wheel for hours while I was driving on the back roads of West Virginia, before finally dozing off in my pocket. But there was another time when he really misbehaved. Imagine that from a wild squirrel? One sunny spring day, I was sitting in my Modern American History class, learning about fascism from Hannah Arendt's book, when he popped out of my pocket, jumped out, and ran up and down the aisles of the classroom. Oh boy. The coeds were screaming bloody murder and jumping up on top of their desks, shouting, "There is a wild squirrel in the classroom!" Scurry couldn't care less about wild squirrels, eh? Finally, with the Coke can containing a penny and a treat, I coaxed him back into my shirt pocket. Close call. The professor never figured out what happened. Oh, and BTW, when encountering dogs, when you must grab him by the tail to save his little "behind," do not put your hand near his mouth while holding his tail. He will bite you out of instinct. Ouch.

Finally, after months of letting him play during the day in the large oak trees in the quadrangle of the dormitory, the Coke can trick became less appealing to him, and he would wander off for longer periods. Soon enough, he did not return. I suppose he found himself a girlfriend. Carolina squirrels are pretty. He already had me ghostwrite his biography, too.

UNC Senior Year and Then On to Medical School

"We are all here on earth to help others; what on earth the others are here for I don't know." —**W. H. Auden**

At the start of senior year, I applied to the University of Kentucky College of Medicine in August for early admission (another "suicide" single-site application). I was accepted by October and should have coasted into my collegiate retirement. By then, I was enamored with the singing and lyrical prowess of Jimmy Buffett—"A Pirate Looks at 40." But being a true nerd, I obtained a 4.0 GPA that semester and even passed a music appreciation course. Mozart and Vivaldi, here I come, with the original, real *Four Seasons* music. Jimmy Buffett would have to wait a semester. My final GPA at Chapel Hill earned me Phi Beta Kappa status. Maybe the streaker story later? Read the sequel!

In Louisville, it was a humid, warm summer night at the end of my junior year at UNC. I had just finished playing 2 hours of pickup basketball with

2 of my competitive high school friends on a random basketball court in Louisville. But, Dave and Ricky knew a girl from high school (what boy does not know a girl from high school?) who was having a party on the other side of town near the Ohio River. Dave was playing scholarship basketball for Ole Miss University, and Ricky was a gifted, all-state, muscular athlete in both basketball and football who was working at a local factory. We had already competed well in the top-notch, 3-man league "Dirt Bowl" in downtown Louisville, Shawnee Park, the week before. We had almost disproved the infamous movie axiom that "white men can't jump," starring Louisville native and famous rap singer, Jack Harlow. Although I must confess, my friend Ricky was Black.

Romance: Buffoon Style

So, we guys hopped in my trusted 4-door Chevy and traipsed across town. It was a homey party, and the booze was plentiful. I noticed across the room that a short, brunette, scintillating young lady of my age was flitting around the apartment. Not only was she beautiful, but she also possessed a distinct aura that captivated my eye. I had to meet her. Well, 3 hours later, after intermittently noticing her and sipping some Maker's Mark bourbon, this ole introverted Carolina Tar Heel mustered up enough courage to strike up a conversation. Far short of suave or brilliant, I managed to eventually acquire her phone number and mutteringly ask her if she would like to go out on a date.

I am sure she thought: *Who is this peculiar loser college boy? He is a bit inebriated, too.* But her sister, Suzie, whom I had just met, was also at the party and had encouraged me to talk with her. So, I did, with tremendous social anxiety.

One of the best decisions I ever made in my life—but that poor girl, eh?

Our first date was to the downtown riverside Kingfish restaurant, followed shortly by a most romantic??? trip to the Kentucky State Fair, to see the prize pigs and to look at her father's prize bantam chickens, which were on display there as well. As I looked at myself in the rear-view mirror, I recalled that axiom, "You just cannot make a silk purse out of a sow's ear."

OMG, I was in love as soon as I picked her up at her farmhouse on the Ohio River. That night, I think I jabbered on about my many esoteric philosophies and future plans. I did insert into the conversation somehow that I was planning something productive—applying to medical school. Importantly, she later told her mother this part.

Two more generic dates with her over the next two weeks, and the summer was over. As I was departing her apartment for the last time, she wrote down her phone number, handed it to me, and said, "Give me a call when you get back in town." As I walked to my car, I tore up that paper, tossed it on the sidewalk, and I thought: *She is not interested in me. Best to take your losses and move on.* As singer Kenny Rogers laments in a song about poker and about love: "Know when to hold 'em, know when to fold 'em." I am a realist most of the time. Fold 'em.

I had returned home for the Thanksgiving holiday to visit my folks when I received that fateful phone call. It was her—Melinda. What the heck? She wanted to see me again. Her prescient mother (yes, her mother!) had told her to call that nice-looking, strange, smart college boy from the East End. We talked a bit, and we shockingly arranged for a date for when I returned home in a few weeks during Christmas break. Who knew?

As the gods above would seriously toy with me again, guess what? Nancy, my old high school, lovely ginger flame, who broke my heart at the time of my heart surgery, happened to call me two hours later that night. She was attending prestigious Stanford University. WOW! Smart. She was now inquiring as to whether I would like to visit her in California next month, paying for my trip as well. Her parents were quite affluent. And they liked me and my boyish style.

Decision time!!!

The Choice: A girl unimpressed by my simpleton debonair nature, who had _touched_ my heart but only in a one-sided way? Or a previous love interest who had _torched_ my heart? Both were nice, gorgeous, and smart, probably smarter than me.

So, I told Nancy that at this point I had already committed to a date with an enchanting brunette here in town. The only reason I could think of on the fly. However, I would call Nancy if plans fell through. _So sorry, dear._ The unknown versus the known quantity. My gamble.

When December break arrived, so did the best 40+ year decision of my life. My soulmate. I was lucky enough to find mine, the daughter of a chicken farmer and grocery store manager. Seven months later, we would be married.

At this stage in life, we were both poor; we qualified for food stamps. I had no job but loads of debt. That was a true gamble on her part as well. She was giving up her decent job in Louisville to join me in Lexington for my medical school matriculation. But I had also convinced her to start her path to her own dream job—nursing school. No one in her family had ever attended college, not even on their radar. And she would work part-time as a nurse assistant at the hospital while schooling. Lucky her? Poverty did not scare her off. She was one of the bravest women I would ever know.

Marriage

No doubt, the most important person in my life was my wife, Melinda. We were married for 45 years, but for the last five years, my accomplished, magnificent wife had become a **cognitive ghost** with Alzheimer's. I had to care for her every basic need completely. A price I was more than willing to pay, and that I will talk about in more detail later in the book.

My Wife's Nursing Career

Melinda was the first person in her family to attend college, and I encouraged her to simultaneously pursue her nursing degree at the local Lexington Community College. She was destined for nursing, especially for the elderly. What a saint she was! She even took her nursing boards fully pregnant, just two days before delivering our first child, Mindy. She sailed through her schooling, except for the first semester of chemistry with a non-English-speaking teacher assistant, who she could not understand. With the help of a fluent chemistry professor later on, she easily passed that course.

We managed to survive and even enjoy ourselves during these lean years with both of us in school. Early on, she worked many evening shifts at the University of Kentucky Medical Center as a CNA (Certified Nursing Assistant). Our paths crossed only briefly during the day. Thin-crust pizzas, hot dogs, chips, and Hostess "pink snowballs" became our cherished staples. I walked about a mile daily to the med school or hospital, no matter the weather, and she used our small Chevy car to drive to school and work. I could still shop at the grocery store anonymously then. Don't laugh!

Economics of Medical Education: More Delayed Gratification

I started my working career as a teenager by mowing lawns and performing other yardwork for my neighbors in the summer. My first "real job" was a 7-day gig taking care of and cutting flowers and roses (my avocation still to this day) for a local greenhouse nursery in Louisville. My best buddy, the humorous, brilliant Greg (and future architect), and I were a true team—very efficiently performing all our requisite tasks despite the 105°F degree nursery inside. We were sweating 2 gallons a day. But we only lasted seven days as we were too efficient, and we talked and joked too much, making us poor role models for the other workers there, who were mostly ex-cons and sadly unskilled folks. The boss just could not have the perception—someone could enjoy their job here and still converse!

Next up, in my youth, I worked two summers as a framing carpenter and then four more summers pouring concrete (level ground was much more to my liking). I learned that there were no cursing or vulgar words on a job site that were not amenable to yelling at an inanimate object or a fellow apprentice. NO big deal. This would serve me well later in my eventual occupation when encountering rare, hostile folks in life or in the office. Hard physical labor was fun for me, especially in the sweltering summer heat. I enjoyed using my hands. Nothing like smoothing out a long driveway or a large basement floor of freshly poured concrete every summer day. By then, upon learning I was going to medical school, co-workers started affectionately (Ha!) calling me "Doc" after a while, among other pejorative terms not meant for public consumption.

In contrast, all of one's friends and acquaintances were now gainfully employed and not borrowing large sums of money for the following economic sinkholes, in today's adjusted economic terms. Four years of college (about $100,000 to $200,000), four years of medical school (about $250,000 to $500,000), and being paid minimum wages during residency (often breaking even or losing money during these 3 to 5 years)—and then interest rate fees start accumulating at the end of medical school. On top of this massive debt burden, one must factor in the cost of buying a house beyond a matchbox or purchasing a "buy-in" to a medical practice or perhaps expensively starting one's own practice with all its new equipment and hiring office personnel. Alternatively, one could smartly "sell out" and become an "indentured servant," joining big-city corporate or hospital medicine. The educational debt being accumulated is staggering. However, a physician is always employable, practically anywhere in the developed world. Like I said, delayed gratification and poverty for about a decade is almost inevitable. It had better be true love with your spouse, eh?

Adding to other financial risks in the practice of medicine, note that nearly 50% of all primary care physicians, and 100% of most surgical specialties, will eventually face the nightmarish world of medicolegal extortion and lawsuits in their careers. And they say, "We only sue the 'bad doctors.'" Rubbish. Utter fiction.

University of Kentucky Medical School: 4 Years

Boy, was I "green" and a bit unprepared for the rigors of continuous studying required in med school. However, I wasn't as green as the four women who passed out upon their very first medical school encounter after observing the cadavers and formaldehyde smell in the gross anatomy lab. It was reminiscent of the novel *Coma* by Robin Cook. "Medical black humor" was essential for many of us guys like me to wade through all the intensity, gravity, and often bleakness of med school. Like many of my male cohorts, full-court basketball, several times a week, continued to be a mainstay for my mental health. But my real refuge and "shelter from the storm" (Bob Dylan) was my beautiful, calm, charming wife of one month upon entering med school. Kindness and empathy exuded from her aura. And she was beautiful, a *doppelganger* for Rita Hayworth, I am told. She surely did not marry me for my money—I was on food stamps and deep in debt with bank loans. I guess she saw potential there. "Love is blind, but love at least knows what is man, and what is mere beast," the American poet Robert Graves would pontificate. Still rough around the edges, as many would tritely say, I treaded full speed into medical school.

I usually studied late into the night for the first three years, but I never drank coffee. I found that a can of Coke every four hours was sufficient to sustain my wakefulness through those very long nights on call or while preparing for tests and studying the obscure medical subject *du jour*. The first year was brutal for me, as it consisted mostly of bench science and many *esoterica*, facts to be memorized and regurgitated for complex tests. Although in honesty, many of these "esoteric" facts would later be invaluable to me as a pediatrician. For example, concepts of genetic dominance (autosomal dominant or recessive conditions in family counseling), the Krebs cycle of energy metabolism (I have cared for infants with methylmalonic acidemia and propionic acidemia), neuroanatomy (pineal gland tumors), and gross anatomy (common talofibular ligament sprains). You name it, and I have had to dredge for so many of these old memorization facts buried deep within my own cerebral cortex.

The first two years of basic sciences—histology, anatomy, physiology, embryology, etc.—were a necessary requirement that I trudged through. I maintained a B average and performed respectably on both the course tests and, after two years, on the first of three levels of National Boards. Sadly, I never read a novel, newspaper, or magazine for four years of medical school and most of three years of residency. My reading and writing skills went totally dormant during this time. Who had time for such luxuries?

I had obtained a rural health scholarship from the state of Kentucky to be repaid by practicing primary care in Kentucky. But I still had to apply for food stamps during the first year of medical school. However, when I saw how poor and needy the other applicants were at the government office, I abandoned this approach. I couldn't bring myself to accept that I was actually at that level of poverty in my mind. Instead, I just borrowed more money from the bank and took a low-paying (frowned upon) part-time job at the Fayette County Health Department.

For the health department, on one or two short afternoons a week, I was sent to a multitude of low-income households in the inner city for assessments of the client's daily needs and basic disabilities, such as the ability to walk or live independently. I encountered patients with severe COPD, amputations, schizophrenia, and brittle diabetics, among other maladies. Cockroaches often roamed at my feet. The Health Department nurses were glad to see me, a male helper, to do their assessments in the many rougher sections of town. In the evenings, I also periodically performed screening and entry exams for new county jail inmates (Doc, got any pain pills on you, eh?) and new patient severe psychiatric admissions to Eastern State Mental Hospital. These patients were eye-opening for such a sheltered boy–the extremes of severe mental illness.

Through this experience, I saw the essential and humane need for a safety net for health care and economics among the poor. Some days I performed sexually transmitted infection (STI) exams, prescribed medications, and even administered penicillin shots to specific patients when needed—all for minimum wage. But the joy of helping someone less fortunate was worth it. These were often lonely, abandoned, and desperate people. *Noblesse oblige*.

Third-Year Rotation: Obstetrics and Gynecology

My first rotation in the third year was OB/GYN. Dr. Mike Guyler, a third-year OB resident, on my first night on call, told me, "Block, go start that IV in room 308 on that woman in labor." I had no idea how to do it or even where to start. I didn't even receive the ostensible obligatory medical student preparation on testing and procedures: "See one, do one, teach one." Luckily, a sympathetic OB nurse knew I was being "shafted," or institutionally degraded, to figure it out myself. With her quick tutorial, I did accomplish it, but that poor mother probably wished for a better technician and a few less pokes from a clumsy, apologetic med student.

But in my defense, later on in pediatric residency, I would be known as "that" resident who could, hyperbolically, get blood via venipuncture from a turnip, and "start an IV on a corpse." (Just kidding.)

Delivering babies was amazing and a joy for me, but I did not like the acute surgical crises frequently popping up, or popping out! Their job was very stressful. And on call constantly to just hurry up and wait till that little guy decided to pop out, or sometimes force you to surgically cut him out. And gynecological cancer surgery was so awful for these nice, hapless ladies, and occasionally demoralizing and disfiguring beyond belief. God bless their souls.

Hey, anyone who does not give their daughters the HPV9 vaccine should consider spending a week in the gynecological cancer ward! You will

NEVER forego this vaccine for your girls. Never. This HPV9 vaccine is the most important vaccine that we can now give to our own girls and boys. (I will discuss it later.)

I was not going to divulge the following. But what the heck. During the second year, we developed and emulated a variation of the infamous Chuck Barris *Gong Show* for our lucky professors. Occasionally, if after a long-winded or boring lecture or some unliked controversy, two or three fellow male classmates would pull out the metal garbage can lid and hammer it loudly with a single noisy, clamorous clang, to signal the class's "displeasure" with the lecture. Gong! Irreverent, I know. And it was all intended in good jest, and the professors just laughed along with us; sometimes we were a tad rowdy, eh? But if one has ever read the controversial medical school novel by Samuel Shem—*The House of God*—about interns in a famous Boston hospital, you would forgive the need for some "medical black humor" in our otherwise humorless, stressful, and rigorous lives.

Third Year Challenges and Rewards

As a third-year student, I was considered a "scut monkey," expected to perform all the grunt work—retrieving and reporting labs, test results, and patient progress all day long, including very early mornings before hospital rounds. And I had to do this amiably and without complaint. Thank goodness for all the prior "training" bestowed upon me by my ball coaches and brothers, eh? One can learn to tolerate a lot of emotional stress and abuse. This earlier training would prove to be beneficial during my later three years of residency at Wake Forest under the tutelage of the master Socratic and stern taskmaster, pediatric chairman Dr. Simon.

On the last day of my third-year psychiatry rotation in the summer, I was urgently summoned to come home. M's water had broken. I excused myself from the neurotic woman I had been interviewing, and ran full speed for one mile to our tiny 3-room apartment. Not a problem, since I had remained in good shape with routine full-court basketball for exercise. I gently put M in the Chevy, and we sped off one mile down congested Nicholasville Road to Central Baptist Hospital for the birth of our first daughter, one of four girls. She gave birth to a healthy six-pound, nine-ounce baby, Mindy. We were proud and excited. She delivered all four children vaginally without an epidural, while only using the LaMaze method of breathing. But I did suffer several deep scratches on my back as her nails "dug in" during most of the labor pains and delivery itself. BTW, she passed her nursing boards easily.

Melinda loved babies, all babies, any babies. So did I, which is partly why I chose pediatrics. My own kind mother later arrived at the hospital to hold our hands and guide us through the first few hours and early postpartum days. Quite an expert, too, after seven deliveries of her own. Just one baby of hers was really ugly.

The Med School Experience

Test Taking

Most of my med school colleagues considered me a class jester and perhaps an "accomplished" average student, relative to their brilliance during my first two years of medical school. These courses were tedious and uninspiring to me. But in the later, more patient-clinical-focused courses, I was captivated. Each of my seven third-year clinical courses had a final written exam with complex questions. For some reason, out of the 105 brilliant medical students, my name or identifier number kept popping up with the highest-class test scores in four of the clinical rotations (pediatrics, surgery, psychiatry, and obstetrics). My ability to answer questions on rounds accurately, along with my tendency to be unabashedly outspoken, sometimes earned me the label of one of "those brash guys" by both nurses and some precepting resident doctors. To me, it was just a statement and a response to facts that I knew. They asked, and I answered. No bombast, just simple, confident responses. In my case, *danged if you do, danged if you don't.*

On my final examination for my 3rd year surgery rotation, we were also required to undergo an "oral exam." This was not a dentistry "oral" exam. But rather, an academic faculty member would grill us about some finer details of the surgery rotation's basic knowledge. Terrifying, I know. Yet, not exactly like the judges in a Miss America contest. I had the lucky draw of being tested by the world-famous, serious, superb chief of surgery, Ward Griffin, Jr. As he was quizzing me, he had the misfortune of inquiring: "What do you want to be when you grow up, Dr. Block?" thus probing my future medical specialty choice. Never one to pass up a golden opportunity for self-deprecation. I quizzically and deferentially responded with the only stupid thing that popped into my pea brain. "A Fireman?" While he was still smacking on his gum, he proceeded to proffer:" I see we have a 'smart-ass' here." Then he continued his challenging line of questioning about hernias, gall bladder surgery, and post op complications. I still passed the course. Despite achieving the highest score on the written test in the entire class, eh?

As a fellow med school classmate and Wake Forest resident, jovial Cecilia Thomas, MD (God rest her soul), pointed out to me acerbically during residency that I was "seldom wrong, but never in doubt." And, as icing on the cake, my part 2 and part 3 national medical board scores may have supported this axiom. I scored in the 95th-97th percentiles on each part of these national tests among all medical students across the country. This remarkable pattern continued well after my pediatric residency, where I scored in the 99th percentile on my first national pediatric board exam, two years after finishing residency. None of the over 6000 testing pediatricians in the nation had received a higher test score than I. "Just the facts, Ma'am," as the detective, Sargent Friday, on the TV cop show, *Dragnet*, would matter-of-factly state.

All that lengthy, strenuous studying had paid off. Just an old Kentucky hayseed boy had succeeded? Rube, or ruby in the rough? Thus, I was now formally a "board-certified" pediatrician with all its honors. Only 2/3 of all pediatrician test-takers actually pass this "board test." I was now able to include the title "board-certified" and the **FAAP** (Fellow of the American Academy of Pediatrics) logo after my name. I had earned it. In later decades, I also happened to be one of only 10 older pediatricians in the entire U.S., who, although "grandfathered" in, did not need to take board recertification exams every 7 years to maintain "certification"; we still took the 4-hour written test and passed. My later test scores were 94% and 95% correct, respectively, 10 years apart. I just felt obligated to do so for my patient's reassurances that I was keeping abreast with pediatric knowledge.

Pediatric Residency (3 Years)

On July 1st, 1979, I approached the front doors of North Carolina Baptist Hospital at Wake Forest University with eager anticipation—riding 1.5 miles from my new tiny suburban home in Winston Salem, NC, on my new 27-inch Schwinn bike with my new haircut and new helmet, as I would do for the following three years. I chained it up and walked in.

When I arrived on the pediatric floor, we went on early morning rounds door to door, with the entire hospital staff, to discuss patients and patient care. It was remarkable—the teaching and Socratic methodology. Like most days for the next three years, rounds were led by the master of pediatrics and chief of the program, Jimmy Simon, MD. Later that afternoon, Dr. Simon held his weekly private-patient clinical rounds. He always asked for two leading residents to perform the patient examination and accompany him during these special visits. At this point, it was me and the affable Dr. Rusty Cook, who was the chief resident of the pediatric program. We accompanied Dr. Simon downstairs to the examination room, where we performed the examination of the young patient. Dr. Simon, with his expertise in rheumatology, took further history.

The patient was at her initial visit for what seemed to be new-onset juvenile rheumatoid arthritis. Dr. Simon was explaining the disease mechanism and the treatment options with the best medications available. During the discussion, he kept referring to Ms. Rogan as "Ms. ROGAINE." Of course, Dr. Cook and I giggled a bit at that. Then the ultimate *coup de grâce* occurred when Dr. Simon told Ms. Rogan that her daughter had a specific form of arthritis, an uncommon autoimmune arthritic disorder of children. He explained her prognosis as being: "No two people are different." Dr. Cook and I were truly overwhelmed with suppressed giggling as we tried to process this phrase. (Perhaps, "No two people are the same"?) That day, I learned that perhaps the most brilliant pediatrician in the state was prone to *malapropisms*. This was one of many endearing phrases we would hear over the ensuing three years.

Yeah, we can do this. This infection could "spread like wildflowers!" as he often announced on teaching rounds.

Although my pediatric residency was quite challenging and sleep-deprived, the first year of internship was probably the second most stressful interval of my life. We were either awake all night with several sick children or sporadically awakened on call every hour during every third night "on call." This meant we lacked sleep for 24 to 36 hours straight on shifts with no rest in between. We would start hospital rounds in the early morning and, by the end of the next day at 6 or 7 p.m., finally go home and crash. Frequently, we were really stressed, awake all night saving sick children and babies, resuscitating newborns by intubation (inserting a breathing tube down the trachea), or taking care of children with cancers who needed IVs, blood draws, medications, or adjusting orders on very sick children. Sadly, when some children died on us, no sleep would happen that next night for many of us, caught up in ruminating over the tragedy of death in such a young child or teen.

The 1980 "Plague" of Pediatrics: Reye's Syndrome

During my first year of residency, I received a phone call from the Wake Forest ER downstairs, that we had another one to admit to the ICU for you! He is 11 years old, he is incoherent and lethargic, and he does not appear to have nuchal rigidity or other signs of meningitis. His white blood cell count and electrolytes were normal, but his glucose level was slightly low, and his liver function tests were twice normal. Until that day, he had been recovering uneventfully from a chickenpox infection the week before. We had an IV in him and were pushing some normal saline fluids since he appeared somewhat dehydrated. Serum ammonia was pending; we did not perform a spinal tap on him.

"Thus, week by week, the prisoners of plague put up what fight they could. Some, like Rambert, contrived to fancy they were still behaving as free men and had the power of choice." —**Albert Camus, The Plague**

The unlucky patients had no choice. The parents also had no preventive choice during this era—no chickenpox vaccine was available, and the influenza vaccine was rarely administered to children. And we physicians had no choice in their invasive intensive care.

Thus, I began another winter week at Wake Forest Medical Center hospital ward as the eager, bright intern covering the ICU as well as the routine hospital "ward", in the 1979 to 1980 season—way before the chickenpox vaccine was available. We were admitting to the ICU similar horrific cases almost 2 times a week during this interval.

Being on call every third night and awake most of the evening, sometimes for 36 hours straight, was brutal. This sleep deprivation required that the next night off become one of make-up slumber within hours of getting home. Our poor spouses.

But I was dang good at the job, as Susan Primmer, MD, a third-year resident, would remark decades later, *"Block was always the intern you could depend upon to handle all the patients when he was on call."* But at a price.

That intern year, I truly learned so much about life and death, about decisions to terminate care, about the intense monitoring needed for the sickest group of patients ever, about the IV fluid and electrolyte balancing act needed, about brain pressure monitoring, and about desperate, hurting parents.

Despite great supportive faculty, highly capable nurses, and a technologically advanced ICU, we were still unable to save the majority of those with this particular illness.

We physician trainees in the early 1980s recognized the diagnosis as soon as we laid eyes on the child, very similar to present-day nurses who admit COVID-19 adult patients. We were no match for this horrendous disease either. We tried every known medical measure to save the kids and the teens. But you quickly came to know it well: the altered mental status, the erratic outlandish fevers (up to 106°F) or sometimes the contrasting opposite condition of severe hypothermia due to hypothalamic brain dysregulation, and the abnormal labs, which would continue to worsen and worsen over hours. The patients all shortly developed severely abnormal liver function tests (total liver metabolic failure) with a strangely normal bilirubin (no jaundice until the dying last days) and accompanying erratically low serum glucose, and very unstable usually quite low serum sodium (typically due to the abnormal, inexplicable syndrome of inappropriate antidiuretic hormone (SIADH) from hypothalamic dysregulation and/or high brain fluid pressure). And then you knew, you just knew.

This was our pediatric "COVID-19 era." Often, only their guardian angel could save them when they became moribund or comatose. This was due to the marked elevation in intracranial ventricular fluid pressure, known as intracranial hypertension. With this brain swelling in an unforgiving, sealed, bony cranial vault, the neurosurgery resident doctor must be summoned in to insert through an artificial, new hole in the skull an intracranial pressure monitor to try to prevent the brain swelling from herniating it down through the bony foramen magnum at the base of the skull. When the brain pressure exceeded a certain dangerous level, desperate attempts with IV mannitol and dexamethasone and permanently removing pieces of skull could sometimes forestall this terminal event. Oftentimes, the cerebral tissue just oozed out of these emergency holes.

Even though the patients were often circulatory hypotensive and needed more fluids to boost the peripheral circulation and blood pressure, this measure could paradoxically raise the intracranial fluid pressure to dangerous levels. With the high likelihood of developing SIADH, they were all placed on IV fluid restriction to prevent the accompanying severe, hazardous hyponatremia. But we still had to maintain the blood pressure and peripheral circulation to the heart, kidneys, and, yes, even the brain. This could become an often-impossible balancing act. Thus, all of these organs were now also susceptible to failure as well.

Early on in their initial presentation, we obtained the pathognomonic (diagnostic) **serum ammonia from their blood,** which was rarely elevated for any other pediatric illness condition, except for severely vomiting newborns with metabolic disorders. This blood sample must be drawn into certain extra tubes, iced down, and immediately rushed to the lab, since it was such a fickle test. If it was elevated, you had confirmed what you truly suspected and dreaded.

Reye's Syndrome

The Wake Forest medical catchment area encompassed the entire western part of North Carolina. Before routine vaccines and the following measures, the rate of Reye's syndrome was about 1 to 2 per 100,000 population. It only affected those under 18 years old and was most commonly triggered by earlier infection with chickenpox or influenza A.

So once diagnosed, for the next 1 to 3 weeks, each of these pediatric patients required continuous monitoring in the ICU in hopes that this patient was one of the minority of patients able to fend off all these bodily insults to the brain and liver, especially.

Nonetheless, many of these survivors were permanently brain-damaged as well, furthering the parents' worst nightmare. History often repeats itself, as we have witnessed:

> *"Many continued hoping that the epidemic would soon die out and they and their families be spared. Thus, they felt under no obligation to make any change in their habits as yet."* —**Albert Camus, *The Plague***

Then...

The blessed *coup de grâce* happened; an epidemiological study of Reye's syndrome by the unfettered, astute CDC doctors was able to establish in 1981 that **salicylates or aspirin products** were the missing key trigger for Reye's syndrome. The good news: once the public and the health systems became aware of this association, aspirin use for fever in pediatric patients plummeted, as did the concomitant rates of Reye's syndrome.

The Reye's syndrome era was almost over. Almost.

Later, we would find out further that **anything with salicylate-like products**, including adult Pepto Bismol, wintergreen liniment, etc., could trigger it under the right circumstances. (see later story).

Residency Knowledge and Skills

Working in the newborn intensive care nursery for two to three months a year was highly stressful but extremely rewarding. Although we hated to see the suffering, we were saving babies, and it was intellectually and medically challenging. One had to know all the parameters of intravenous fluids, oxygen and carbon dioxide levels, and ventilator settings—what requirements were needed for oxygen, respiratory rate, and lung pressures. These factors led to an interesting dynamic, each interacting with the others. The team of respiratory therapists and nurses worked with us to try to get this algorithm correct for each unique, ever-changing newborn. We battled illnesses like premature lungs, respiratory distress syndrome, meconium aspiration, hypoxic encephalopathy, brain bleeds, pneumonia, and more. We frequently had to perform technically challenging, painful procedures such as the insertion of chest tubes, umbilical (belly button) artery catheters, IV catheters in tiny veins, and sometimes spinal taps—commonly on "micro-premie" babies, many weighing less than a pound or two. Numbing with lidocaine injections sometimes became one's best friend. But this was the heart of newborn intensive care medicine on a pediatric floor. Better bring your "A" game here, too. And the nurses were magnificent and knowledgeable, and essential for everyone's survival. Including my own!

During my three years of residency, like my colleagues, I acquired an astounding encyclopedia of specific pediatric medical knowledge, which integrated well with the unbelievable fund of knowledge from medical school, like physiology, histology, embryology, etc. After all, our small pediatric program test scores were ranked as the **number 3 program** in the entire U.S., second only to Harvard and Stanford. Chairman Dr. Simon would not have it any other way. He attended morning rounds almost 7 days a week, grilling us residents and med students on each case in the hospital. He was the original "Dr. House" TV showman. You could learn something new even on routine admission cases. I also achieved some interpersonal skills in dealing with parents and families. However, to truly perfect the latter, a few additional years of experience in private practice would be required.

Trust Your Physical Examination

During my second week as a first-year intern at Wake Forest University, a 13-year-old pleasant, quiet young lady came in with a history of recurrent vomiting and weight loss. She also had ongoing headaches. Occasionally, she stumbled and had a subtle, wide-based gait.

Several medical trainees and students, along with house staff physicians, conducted examinations that were all thought to be normal. The patient also underwent a normal evaluation by a second-year pediatric neurology fellow.

When I examined her, I—the intern—felt that her Romberg (balance) test and gait were equivocal. Something just didn't add up. Dr. Bob Baumann, a first-rate pediatric neurologist at the University of Kentucky, had taught every third-year medical student that with increased intracranial pressure, spontaneous venous pulsations originating from THE OPTIC NERVE AREA at the back of the eye disappear first, followed by blurred optic disc margins, and then more intense retinal changes like flame hemorrhages— all indicating increasing intracranial pressure.

Pediatric neurologist Dr. Baumann emphasized that physicians must perform fundus/retina exams for any severe, persistent, or atypical headaches. **You will save a life**, as I've come to realize on multiple occasions in my career. This complex exam with an ophthalmoscope requires much patience, persistence, and time.

When I performed her fundoscopic exam, I saw that her optic nerve disc margins were sharp, but she had **no spontaneous venous pulsations— the earliest sign**.

My team initially dismissed the findings I presented. "What does an intern know, after all? You are just a rube from Kentucky." The pediatric neurology fellow outright denied my concern, claiming she had never seen a case where mysterious venous pulsations disappeared in a similar patient. Still, I kept insisting something wasn't right. Later, they returned after rounds to take another look—curious now.

Now, everyone was paying attention.

Thank you, Dr. Baumann.

As opposed to the previously normal CT scan of the head, the lower CT scan of the cervical spine was obtained, and it revealed an **ependymoma**

tumor located beneath the upper cervical part of the medulla oblongata. The tumor compression explained the vomiting, headaches, and balance problems due to increased intracranial pressure. But her head CT scan was normal, which had confused all of us.

The neurosurgeon successfully removed the tumor. Post-surgery, she underwent radiation therapy combined with chemotherapy. She left the hospital after a week and had a full recovery over a year.

Home Life During Residency

In my third year of pediatric residency, Melinda and I had our second child, Misty. She was a full-term, healthy, and active baby. In the middle of the night, her delivery required me to drop off our little girl, Mindy, at my best friend and fellow pediatric resident, as well as former Protestant preacher, Dr. Lee Finklea's house. He was married to Melinda's best friend, Kathy Finklea. From their house, I rushed to the hospital with Melinda, and we (loosely defined "we") successfully delivered a happy little 8lb4oz Misty. She had pooped 5 ounces of meconium first.

We were now outgrowing our small house in Winston-Salem, NC. Due to lack of space, and then because of her colic and nocturnal crying, to obtain some quiet, and so as not to wake her older sister, we had little Misty sleep in the bassinet on our floor. We patted her to sleep, sometimes for hours. The door was often open during these first few months until we could finally have her be a sleep partner in her older sister's bedroom. Desperate times now that the nest was filling up. It was now time to exit the nest— time for interviews for private practices in Kentucky.

CHAPTER 2

Starting My Practice: The Big Fish in a Little Pond

Doc Holiday (movie title about a country doctor)

On a dreary, drizzly December morning in Central Kentucky, I jumped out of my VW Passat and scrambled for the shelter of our local strip mall's Radio Shack to purchase some batteries. An SUV roared up behind me, blaring its horn, sending my sympathetic nervous system—and my sphincters—into overdrive. Jim, the driver, an acquaintance from the office and a local entrepreneur, rolled down his window and exasperatedly blurted out, "Doc, we've been up to the emergency room. It's so crowded they said it would be a 3- or 4-hour wait. Little Amos has been screaming and crying for the last 6 hours. I didn't think we could wait that long. I tried Doc Jones, who is on call for your group, but after 5 minutes I got no response. You gotta help me."

As the drizzle soaked my thinning hair and chilled my scalp, I contemplated my alternatives in front of the Shack. I could run for shelter and ignore him. I could politely say I'm not on call—try the on-call doc again. Or I could say the ER docs are perfectly fine, and a little "watchful waiting" never hurt anyone, especially a child. So, they say!!! Or I could do the "right thing" and arrange to help him.

I chose the last option. Over the years, I've learned that my self-induced pediatric angst becomes overwhelming whenever I don't follow the "Golden Rule of Pediatrics": Treat all families as you would want to be treated yourself. Whenever I have not followed this pithy aphorism, many a waking hour and night has been needlessly disrupted with anxiety and guilt over what I *should* have done.

So, I asked him if he'd mind meeting me at my home—where I had some medical instruments and, more importantly, some Bob Dylan-esque "shelter from the storm." The Shack, although carrying an extensive inventory, did not (to my knowledge) carry otoscopes and stethoscopes. Unfortunately, all my medical equipment was still at the office—not at my house, as is my usual habit. So, we made a second stop further down the road at my office, where I quickly discovered this youngster's malady: a bulging acute otitis media. I delivered some antibiotic and ibuprofen samples from the cabinet to tide them over until they could get a prescription the next day. (Yes, I firmly believe *bona fide* acute otitis media should be treated.)

"How much do I owe you, Doc?"

"Oh, don't worry about it. Someday, I may need your help."

Although most people respect a physician's private time, desperate times sometimes call for desperate measures, especially from frantic parents. As a physician practicing in a small town, who frequently sees families and patients in passing every day, we often try to remove ourselves from the uncomfortable process of billing and collections. Propriety, cordiality, nice-guy manners—call it what you will—it remains a task considered too mundane and crass to perform personally by many doctors. However, as he walked out the door, he spontaneously offered to pay me in free video rentals from his store for a few months—perhaps *Patch Adams* or *Doc Holiday*. Consider it continuing medical education, I suppose.

I still had the problem with dead batteries, which were not amenable to medical intervention or resuscitation, nor free delivery from the Shack.

Curbside Consult: Literally

I often struggle to get my essential exercise with my hectic office and family schedule. On a cloudy, cool autumn night, I was strolling along the sidewalk with my wife and our friendly leashed mutt when a Taurus passed, then suddenly screeched to a dead halt just 20 yards ahead of us—half on the curb and half on the busy road. My friend, the painter, screamed: "You gotta help us, Doc! We were just headed to your house to see if Junior here is breathing OK! He got choked on a barbecued rib a few minutes ago and has been choking and crying that he can't breathe ever since!"

"Pull over into the side street ahead," I yelled.

With my ACL-deficient knee and frantic, leashed, gregarious dog, I hobbled over to the car to find a calm 8-year-old boy. First, my never-met-a-stranger canine quickly hopped into the back seat. Once I jerked her back on her leash and prevented the additional deluge of dog drool, the little boy said his chest was hurting beneath the sternum and that it "really hurt so bad" to swallow.

Yes, he could still speak quite eloquently. He could still swallow and drink fine—but he really couldn't breathe (allegedly).

"You mean it hurts when you breathe in?"

"Yeah, and the pain is so bad."

I poked my head into the back seat and found a well-perfused, calm youngster in no distress, whose breath sounds from his mouth were smooth and steady. His neck and chest wall exam were normal to palpation. (What, did you expect a complete examination during a *true curbside consult*?)

Words of calm reassurance were offered for the family's assimilation: *probably scratched his esophagus from the hard meat; breathing and speaking normally means no major airway obstruction; no cough means no aspiration; give lots of fluids; for the scratch, try some Mylanta—several teaspoons, several doses tonight and tomorrow; let me know if anything worsens.*

"Boy, Doc, you just saved us an expensive trip to the emergency room— and a long wait. I tried to tell that boy to slow down and chew his food."

My wife just shook her head, and my dog just wagged her tail. The stroll had to continue. Doctor Heimlich would have been proud.

A Rock and a Hard Place

The night of my daughter's big rivalry game arrived after a full schedule of sick children in the office. Influenza was taking its toll in our community. As the lead cheerleader for the boys' varsity basketball team, her parents' attendance was expected—particularly by the daughter. I had already missed half of her games that season, as our office rarely shuts down before 7 p.m. in flu season. My promise: *Tonight, I will attend your game. Daddy will be there.*

I arrived home in time to grab a 20-minute sit-down dinner and prepare for the short trip. The phone rang. My wife looked at me, you know, the death stare look. My skin crawled. *I am not on call, that's right.*

My wife answered—it was for me. Our friends, the Holyfields.

This upper-crust but down-to-earth family lived nearby. We occasionally dined together and shared social outings and family war stories. I had been the primary physician for their five children for a decade. I had even correctly diagnosed enigmatic temporal lobe seizures in the father by history, which had gone undiagnosed for years, allowing him to finally get the right treatment.

Tonight, their 8-year-old boy had sustained a laceration of the scalp after falling on a rock. The phone conversation was terse. I was already late and almost out the door.

"Doesn't sound too bad. Would you mind taking him to the emergency room tonight? I'm really in a hurry."

"Sure."

"I'm sorry."

Click.

The Big Chill has never really thawed.

I suppose it was partly my fault, as I never really explained why I was in a rush or why I couldn't find the time to partake in the vital "cranial sewing class." I rationalized: any parent would surely understand that sometimes even the doctor has other family commitments. Otherwise, I would have missed that important, sacrosanct father-daughter outing.

Months later, I realized I had become the recipient of a social brush-off, and their children were no longer coming to see me at my office.

But did I need to justify my needs to a friend, somewhat in need? After all, a simple laceration wasn't major surgery. *Rue that day.*

Such a nice, enjoyable family, too—and such a tangled web we weave. That cut really hurt.

Home: Bardstown, KY. How Did I Get Here?

I had always promised Melinda that we would return to Kentucky if I could choose the pediatric residency program of my choice and my location. Both of our parents lived in the Louisville area. I had interviewed at multiple locations throughout the state of Kentucky, most of which were rural, and this appealed to me more than urban-center practices. Notably, when I interviewed in Bardstown, KY, a bearded, loquacious young pediatrician named James Hedrick was using two locum tenens to fill in for his second pediatric partner spot. His former partner, the erudite Dr. Chris Harrison, together for five years earlier, had left this practice to pursue pediatric infectious diseases at an academic center. Oh yeah, Dr. Hedrick had obtained a degree in "nuclear physics" from the University of Illinois at Urbana-Champaign. OMG. That intellect was way out of my league, I knew.

When I arrived at his house for an interview, for about an hour, we talked about the future of me joining his practice. He then excused himself to pick up some groceries and run errands, since he had been handling on-call duties alone for most of the past week. While I was visiting, his father, who had Alzheimer's disease and was in the late stages of dementia, was sitting quietly in a recliner. He asked me to watch his father for him. Uh-oh! His father started leaning over in his chair, nearly falling out about a hundred times. I had to adjust him into an upright position repeatedly so he wouldn't fall over out of the chair. (A harbinger of my future destiny with my wife.) Finally, Dr. Hedrick returned a few hours later, and we moved his father into a more secure spot on the couch using a pillow fortress.

Later that evening, we met at one of the finer local restaurants. Over a steak dinner (and he paid!), we discussed the parameters I was interested in if and when I joined his practice. These included seeing patients for an average of 15 minutes per visit and expanding the age range of the practice from 13 to 21, possibly 23 years old. I was particularly interested in adolescent medicine and felt that we could provide an invaluable service to the community by doing so. (My prophecy was correct.) We reached an agreement that I would join his practice as a full partner with equal pay, right from the start. This was unheard of, as most practices required a buy-in agreement. However, I later found out I was making more money as a pediatric resident than he was as a full-fledged practicing pediatrician. Still, I felt this would be an opportunity to make my mark in the world of pediatrics in a small community.

Both of us being "astute" businesspeople, we signed a contract on one of the signature restaurant's paper napkins. Add a handshake, and you have an agreement. Really!

And that was the beginning of my tenure as a general pediatrician in Bardstown, KY, which has lasted for over 43 years. I've also lived in the same 120-year-old farmhouse for 43 years. Granted, there have been numerous improvements and additions to this small farmhouse on three acres since we first moved in over 40 years ago. And then, two more beautiful female children were added to the nest over the ensuing six years—four beautiful daughters in total. Thank goodness their looks favored their lovely mother.

The newspaper *USA Today* selected Bardstown as the most beautiful small American town due to its unique rural Kentucky charm. This is also the world's bourbon whiskey capital, where distilleries such as Jim Beam, Maker's Mark, Barton, Bulleit, and Heaven Hill manufacture bourbon. They serve and sell this connoisseur liquor to the worldwide community. Agriculture still functions as the leading economic force in this county's community of 44,000 people, who often maintain a bond with one another. Bardstown provides the peaceful atmosphere of a small rural town with rolling hills. It sits between Louisville to the north and Lexington to the east at distances of 40 miles and 65 miles, respectively. The Local Gethsemani Monastery was the inspiration site and home for the famous Catholic philosopher, Thomas Merton, who wrote extensively, inspiring numerous philosophers and spiritual seekers across the world. And then there would be the renowned impact of the office of Physicians to Children and Adolescents.

The Big Fish in a Little Pond: The Rural Pediatrician

Being a community pediatrician is the best job in the world for the *right* person—like me. You must truly enjoy hanging around, talking with, and yes, even carefully examining babies, children, and teenagers. You must have patience and a high tolerance for "gross stuff" like vomit, spit-up, poopy diapers, sweaty teens, skin conditions, and boils, being called ugly or stupid by teenagers, and dealing with totally uncooperative crying children who *occasionally* calm down with your patient reassurances. You'll have countless babies and toddlers screaming in your ears—inches away—while you examine them or coughing and spitting on you during a mouth exam. And the list goes on. And I cannot count the number of times a baby infant has "whizzed" on my pants. That makes it a "smelly pants" day for me. And if you do not have an after-hours phone answering service, a pediatrician can receive over 50 phone calls on each weekend day or holiday that you must respond to. Literally tethered to the phone all day.

At times, working with the youngest patients (and many teenage boys) feels much like veterinary medicine—they often cannot or will not tell you what is wrong, what hurts, or what feels abnormal to them. You must develop a sixth sense—a pediatrician's intuition—to recognize who is truly sick or what is the true agenda for the visit. This skill can make the difference between helping a child, potentially saving their life, or missing critical information. In over 40 years in practice, I estimate I have saved the lives of over 500 children—more than half due to that intuitive "tingle up the spine," that nagging worry, and those many sleepless nights. About 5% were saved due to my having a guardian angel, I surmise. As my middle brother Bruce (the family's official Shakespearean Falstaff, ribald and irreverent) often said to me: "Better to be lucky than good some days." He often gambled successfully at the horse racetrack of Churchill Downs.

To be really skilled at this job, one must develop keen powers of observation, an empathic rapport, and a mastery of reading between the lines in conversations with patients and parents. One must hone patience and sensitivity to the "Oh, by the way, doctor..." moments—often shared just as you're leaving the room, with your hand on the doorknob. These latter times are frequently the *real* reason they came in.

"Oh, by the way, he's been losing weight lately." *(New-onset diabetes mellitus.)* "By the way, she doesn't come out of her room much anymore." *(Cutting, depression, suicidal ideation.)*

"Hey, Doc, Mom said you need to look at his foot," per Dad. *(Turns out to be a raging, hospital-worthy MRSA cellulitis.)*

As a country doctor, you don't have a specialist or consultant immediately available. You must become a jack of all medical trades and develop basic mastery in many branches of medicine: cardiology, dermatology, orthopedics, psychiatry, endocrinology, and more. For instance:

Psychiatry/Mental Health: Counselling a grief-stricken little boy or teenager after the death of a parent (think car wrecks and COVID-19).

Caring for a victim of physical or sexual abuse. Screening for under-the-sleeve arm cutting, depression, or anxiety. Picking up on the demeanor and subtle clues of hidden self-harm. Uncovering the deeper reasons for drug usage, school underachievement, or failure.

Orthopedics: Evaluating bruises, sprains, tendonitis, stress fractures, major fractures, overuse syndromes, joint effusions, even bone cancers or juvenile arthritis.

Endocrinology: Monitoring growth curves and growth rates, routinely identifying thyroid enlargement or failure or even cancer, managing menstrual irregularities, and even recognizing hidden teen pregnancies. For instance:

During my third year of practice, I was called by the nurse to the ER for my 15-year-old patient, who was having some vaginal bleeding. *We think she is having a miscarriage.* When I arrived, I told the nurse, "That is not a miscarriage!" But rather, a full-term newborn baby was "crowning". I needed some lidocaine for a pudendal nerve block (the old days) and to get her up to the delivery room STAT. And to call over the family practice doctor.

Too late. I had to deliver the descending 8lb, full-term baby, cut the cord, deliver the placenta, and tend to the newborn as well, who was healthy and vigorous. No one else knew that she was pregnant—she was a much taller, stockier girl who always wore baggy sweatshirts, thus hiding her pregnancy.

Next, I called the girl's mother. "I got good news and I got bad news, Mom: first, your grandbaby is healthy, and second, you are a new grandmother. That is the good news and the bad news. She was totally shocked. She will keep this quiet, for now. Come visit her in the hospital."

Gastroenterology: From stress to chronic abdominal pain to celiac disease, constipation, gastric reflux, food intolerances, IBD, IBS, to gastric tumors, and more.

You are their first line—their primary interface with the medical world. It's your responsibility to assess severity, determine the most likely diagnosis, and decide when to order additional imaging (X-ray, MRI, CT), blood work, or other tests. You must also decide when a referral is needed—and balance that with the knowledge that over-referring can be just as frustrating, time-consuming, and inefficient as missing a necessary referral.

On top of it all, you're constantly managing long-term "adult" problems that aren't traditionally considered pediatric: hypertension, pregnancy prevention, thyroid disorders, severe mental health conditions, high cholesterol, PCOS, metabolic disorders, type 2 diabetes—the list goes on. And for most of these, *you* will be the sole clinician managing them for years.

Background: Rural U.S. and Rural Kentucky

About one-third of children in the U.S. live in rural areas—and roughly half of these are enrolled in Medicaid, the government-funded health insurance program for low-income families and their children. This is a critical health safety net for so many families who otherwise would not survive the health system. Yet less than 10% of pediatricians practice in rural communities. To further complicate the picture, over 90% of pediatricians entering the field in the 21st century are women, many working part-time. That is a good thing. But, as a result, male pediatricians are recently considered the "unicorns" of the profession. Lucky if you can find a young one in your area now.

A problem can be that teenage boys similarly often feel uncomfortable discussing private, genital, or sexual health issues with a female provider. Many also refuse to see a counselor or psychiatrist, fearing the stigma—*I'm not crazy.* So, who becomes the default mental health expert? Their pediatrician. Like me. Or my partners. With the pediatrician, there is no divulging, no apparent threat that people can call you crazy, since everyone in the waiting room visits their pediatrician for a sundry of reasons.

Nearly all rural pediatricians accept Medicaid, unlike some of our suburban or metropolitan counterparts. But Medicaid's meager reimbursement rates already strain the economic survival of rural practices. Any disruption in payment structure, such as delayed payments, reduced rates, or disenrollment of eligible families, could lead to the collapse or severe restriction of our services. We are that price-sensitive in rural America.

If government cutbacks further disenroll children, teens, and young mothers from Medicaid, it won't just result in missed well checks or skipped appointments. It will mean missed opportunities for life-saving, morbidity-reducing vaccines, and medical interventions, leading to increased ER visits, higher long-term costs, and unnecessary suffering and death.

Note politicians: **The law of unintended consequences** from short-term cost-saving will wreak havoc on public health—and, ironically, government budgets. Health care cannot be short-sighted! In rural areas, poverty and lack of higher education are more prevalent than in metro settings. High-paying jobs are scarcer, and Medicaid dependency is naturally higher. So, when coverage is cut, families rely even more on the goodwill and compassion of country doctors. But this economic "failsafe" has limits. You can only stretch a rubber band so far before it snaps. And if it does, the loss of rural pediatric and family practice care will also further devastate small-town hospitals—the backbone of health for many communities. There are only so many of us "rubies" out here. Many essential rural hospitals will begin closing with Medicaid cuts.

Some Keys to Success in Pediatrics

Various principles may help ensure a successful pediatric practice:

- Always listen to the mother. The mother intuitively understands her child's situation and issues better than anyone and should be respected, in most circumstances. There are obviously rare exceptions—such as those with Munchausen by proxy (child sabotage), drug addiction, and severe mental health disorders.

- Show kindness and friendliness to children and teenagers. Goofiness and self-deprecating humor may work to gain trust.
- The patient should usually receive a complete, thorough physical examination for most illnesses and well visits. Such diligence will often improve diagnostic detection/accuracy.
- Sometimes a tiny yet essential detail may be the key. As my friend Lee Finklea, MD, once taught me in residency, "Even the blind hog finds a nut once in a while."
- Always be calm and considerate. This provides a sense of security to adolescents and their families during the visit
- ****And during an office emergency, we joke that you need to take your own pulse first. Staying calm improves your performance.
- Forcing Occam's razor theory as a single diagnosis will often mislead you in pediatric patients. The majority of the complex medical cases present with several diagnoses. Most adolescent girls will have at least four or five medical diagnoses. Theirs is an extremely complicated stage of life.
- Hire a good, friendly staff. They serve as one of your main communication channels with the community.
- An early diagnosis, proper treatment, and referral for severe pediatric diseases/infections and cancers will improve the odds of a favorable outcome.

A Visit from the Undertaker: A Day in the Life

It's 6:20 p.m. After a long workday, I've invited my fourth-year medical student to dinner at my home—a tradition I've maintained for decades with pediatric trainees. It gives them a taste of rural life and a glimpse into the heart of a medical family in our community.

I show him around my 3-acre property, shaded by mature white pines, ash, and birch trees. Over 30 hydrangeas and more than 30 hybrid tea and grandiflora roses bloom beside hostas scattered across the grounds. This very property has been featured on the Bardstown Garden Club's home tour three times in the past 20 years—a reflection of my favorite pastime, aside from raising four spirited daughters.

Just as we're sitting down to enjoy my wife's classic country cooking, there's a knock at the back kitchen door. It's the local undertaker from New Haven—with his unhappy 3-year-old son.

"Sorry to interrupt dinner, Doc," he says, barging in. "But Johnny's been crying with ear pain for the past couple of hours. Thought maybe you could take a quick look. Sorry, Mrs. Block—how are you, ma'am?"

I respond warmly, though with restrained amusement. "Of course, I'd be happy to help." My daughters keep eating as if this is completely normal—because for them, it is. The medical student, however, is slack-jawed in disbelief.

I grab my medical bag and otoscope, and I check Johnny's ear—infected. I write a prescription for amoxicillin, reassure Johnny that he'll feel better soon, and ask the undertaker to give my regards to his wife. The whole thing plays out like a familiar short play I've performed a hundred times before.

"How much do I owe you, Doc?"

"Nothing," I reply. "Maybe you can repay me somehow, someday."

Gee, I hope not, I mutter to myself. Bartering services with an undertaker is not exactly a comforting proposition.

Gymnastics of a 'Drive-By': Rural Style

Another time, I had just wrapped up a long clinic day and was taking my blonde, athletic 5 y.o. daughter to gymnastics. She hopped out of the car with excitement. I was turning the car around in the gravel parking lot when I heard someone calling.

"Dr. Block! Dr. Block! Just a minute—could you look at my daughter?"

The mother was holding her 4-year-old, who had just started crying with arm pain during a gymnastics routine. Now, she wouldn't move the arm at all.

Well, I thought, **drive-by** *care, not* **drive-thru** *care.*

I asked the mom to stretch her daughter's arm through my open car window. I palpated her forearm, upper arm, clavicle, and wrist—no fracture. But she was cradling her elbow in flexion tightly. I told the mom I suspected a **nursemaid's elbow**—a common elbow dislocation from an unintentional, harmless, too-firm pull on the hand.

"I'm going to twist her forearm in a particular way. It will hurt briefly, but it should fix the problem immediately," I explained.

I had the mom place her fingers under the elbow for support and to feel for the following: I grasped the girl's wrist, twisted gently—*pop.* A very subtle sound and sensation. Within seconds, the child was moving her arm freely—completely pain-free.

"Amazing—that's it?" the mom said. "How much do I owe you?"

"In the parking lot?" I smiled. "Your daughter's smile is payment enough."

And just like that, I returned to my ordinary, out-of-office life—until the next drive-by.

No S...t! A Snow Day Story

It was a heavy snowfall—maybe 12 inches—one of those true isolating winter days in rural Kentucky. *No one* should have been out on the roads, much less at the stores. Or so I reassured myself.

I hadn't set foot in Kroger grocery in over a decade of practicing pediatrics in Bardstown. Why? Because every trip turned into an impromptu clinic in aisle six. And others.

Dr. Block! Dr. Block, could you...?

Or worse—into a 15-minute discussion about ADD medications for Little Johnny that never seem to work, right between frozen peas and cereal.

But on this snowy noon, I decided to gamble. Snowdrifts don't bother me much behind the wheel, and the roads were deserted. I grabbed my cute, blonde-haired daughter—just the two of us—and we set off for Kroger. I used to enjoy grocery shopping back in Winston-Salem, when no one knew who I was. My wife enjoyed it too—mainly because I was the one doing the grocery run.

We filled our cart, checked off the list, and were just 50 feet from the empty checkout lane when I heard the dreaded call.

"Dr. Block! Dr. Block!"

Uh oh.

"Little Johnny hasn't pooped in three days," the dad announced loudly—helpfully broadcasting it to the only other two shoppers in the store. "Now he's crying with a bellyache. What should I do?"

I resisted the urge to respond with sarcasm. Instead, I walked back with him toward the pharmacy, pointed out the saline enemas and the laxatives I usually recommend. Little Johnny stared at me, confused—probably trying to place who I was in an out-of-office context. I smiled and introduced him to my 6-year-old daughter, Lindsay, now shyly hugging my side. She looked up at me like this was completely normal.

It kind of is.

My wife now reminded me—without fail—to wear a baseball cap, tip the brim down, and *never stop walking* in a local store. Otherwise, it's 20 to 40 extra minutes of curbside consults disguised as casual conversations. The joys of being the big fish in a small pond—the pediatrician version of a lawyer at a party. Everyone has a case they want to run by you. What's it cost them, right?

Football's <u>Friday Night Lights!</u>

It was a Friday night in autumn, cool and crisp, and dark by the time I arrived home after work—a busy, tiring office day. I was greeted warmly by my wonderful wife with a hug (which always makes me melt. Damn, I miss her still). As I sat down for a tasty supper of grilled chicken, she reminded me: "It's Friday night, dear. 7 p.m. They need you."

I had committed to being the football team doctor over a decade ago. At home games or even at away games. Hot summer nights or frigid fall nights. It was *Friday Night Lights*, just like in the TV series of the 1990s. Similar to their fictitious high-powered high school football in Texas, where it is almost a religious experience, likewise, Bardstown football was always rated highly in the Kentucky state rankings for small schools. They had some fantastic, dedicated coaches and amazing, speedy athletes. AND great cheerleaders—often with the Block girls representing this contingency.

This night was atypical. The speedy fullback went down on the ground after a head-to-head collision with the opposition's big linebacker. I rushed onto the field (my old torn ACL knee injury meant it was more like a brisk hobble for me). Our fullback seemed woozy and could not answer simple questions about the score or date. He was clearly disoriented. The "usual" concussion protocol of the 2000s decade was to put him back on the field as soon as he was able to walk again.

However, I intuitively knew better as a pediatrician. I sidelined nearly all of them who had any fogginess, amnesia, or unconsciousness. For years, this often brought the wrath of the parents or the spectators. I had to stand my ground despite the criticism and occasional epithets hurled at me. *Put him back in*, they yelled. *You don't know squat...* Mine was quite an unpopular decision, until the last decade, when we began to understand the gravity of a concussion in youngsters and the implications for CTE, or chronic traumatic encephalopathy, from repeated concussions, especially with susceptible pediatric patients. My job as an unpaid team physician in high school sports was to put the athletes' welfare first. Over time, I was finally vindicated.

Within 5 minutes of this concussion and while he was sitting on the bench, I was next summoned onto the field again. Our star linebacker was laid out on the ground, moaning with arm pain. I checked the forearm, elbow, wrist, and clavicle—all normal. However, he could not move his shoulder at all. He had tried to arm-tackle their hefty fullback, and now his shoulder seemed to be painfully dislocated. Under the shoulder pads, it seemed to be protruding anteriorly out of the shoulder socket. An anterior shoulder dislocation? Only two joint dislocations can be fixed on the sidelines. This was one of them. So, I had him lie down on his stomach on the bench with his arm and shoulder hanging over the edge. With tremendous downward pressure on the arm, I was able to pop the joint into normal anatomical alignment and thus improve his pain 100-fold. I swaddle-wrapped his arm fully with an ACE bandage to immobilize the arm for now. Applied an ice pack. He was now in need of an orthopedic doctor, months of physical therapy, and rehabilitation.

This night continued to be one of endless numbers of players going down on the field. I must have been summoned for both teams about 12 times—mostly for sprains, leg cramps, and bad muscle and bone contusions, which temporarily forced the players to go down on the field. After the game, I went back to the locker room to check on my guys' condition, and all but these initial two were recovering nicely.

When I returned home, my wife asked, "How was your evening?" I just shrugged. We do not have enough time.

Plus, I had missed another episode of *Blue Bloods*, my favorite TV show, to compound the rough night.

"Dr. Block, When I saw my son laying on the sidelines I wanted to run down from the stands. I would have been hysterical but seeing you there gave me peace of mind. Thank you so much for being there for our son. I know I speak not only for myself, but for all the parents. We appreciate your dedication, time & caring for our sons. Thanks, and God bless you." —**Don & Rita P.**

Medical Survival in Rural America

In rural practice, the pediatrician is often the first—and sometimes the only—line of defense, both in the clinic and in the newborn nursery for youngsters. That means we have to be available, recognize, stabilize, and act quickly when things go sideways and dangerously. And we did procedures—in the past—*a lot* of them in the office as well. But now we perform about 1/100 of the number of daily in-office procedures (blood cultures, lumbar punctures, IV/IM antibiotics) as in the 1980s and 1990s. Thanks to the routine use of HIB, pneumococcal, flu, and rotavirus vaccines in babies.

But in our nursery, sick babies still may need chest tubes for spontaneous pneumothorax, intubation and ventilation for respiratory failure or meconium aspiration, or umbilical artery catheters for fluid resuscitation and blood gases. Even more commonly, it's a radial arterial stick or IV line for fluids and antibiotics. It's hands-on medicine—real-time, no delay.

For over 40 years, we've been "on call" every day for every potentially complicated birth at our local rural hospital. Obstetricians depend on us heavily. Saving that baby often means sparing them that later trial lawyer's subpoena, some dreaded day in the future, for a damaged baby beyond the doctor's control. That is just how the malpractice system works.

The seconds after delivery can be intense, even harrowing. Success relies on our superb training, instinct, and having a good nursing team by our side. Decisions are made in seconds, then reassessed multiple times over hours, as the baby's condition can quickly deteriorate. When needed, it's a welcome sight to see the neonatal transport team arrive, with tools and treatments—like surfactant—that only they can provide.

Earlier decades in my career, if a critically ill child needed transport to a tertiary hospital—say, with meningitis or sepsis—I had to ride in the ambulance with them for the full 45-minute journey. Our small hospital didn't have pediatric ICU coverage, and ambulance crews weren't trained for severely ill pediatric patients.

So, I'd pack my own emergency kit: laryngoscope, different-sized endotracheal tubes, a vial of lorazepam for sedation, mannitol in case of brain herniation, extra IV gear, an ambu bag, etc. Thus, that day's office schedule—or my night's sleep—went straight out the window. When awakened at night, I could never go back to sleep after the massive adrenaline rush.

However, this brings me to another major medical issue: obstetricians. Our fine surgical colleagues, whom we and the community rely on, unfortunately, only last 5 to 10 years in a rural community like ours. We have had 8 different obstetricians leave in the last 40 years. Retaining and recruiting will be getting worse with recent Medicaid budgetary cutbacks, which means even less access and lower pay for them. Their rate of burnout is fierce from the stress of being on call every 2 to 3 nights, limited vacations or time off, and constant emergencies for placental abruptions/previas, fetal distress, etc. These continuous episodes of adrenaline excess take a toll as one ages. Then there is the 100% certainty that they will get crushed with one or more deflating medicolegal liability cases in their career—perfect outcomes are always expected. These cases require years of defending against the destruction of their reputation by the unrelenting trial attorneys. Their brutal PTSD and rumination, already from the bad outcome, are now under the microscope.

Our hospital's birthing center continues to face tremendous economic pressure to close already. Pregnant mothers will likely need to drive up to an hour to see an obstetrician if it closes. Car births, ER births, baby deaths, and bad outcomes will increase.

Lifestyle Trade-Offs

Rural Opportunities

Life in rural practice comes with a unique blend of freedoms and challenges. In many areas, people still leave their doors unlocked—a testament to trust and close-knit communities. Everybody knows you—you are the town's pediatrician. Even the unsavory criminal and drug-dealing element in town respected me—I took care of their children with unbiased and high-level care. I was accepting of their children's needs first and foremost. They, too, were welcomed in our office with the expected civil behavior.

But this simplicity comes with a price: time with your own children and wife is often sacrificed, especially when you're on call or handling emergencies, often daily. While there may be fewer available elite extracurriculars like ballet or orchestra, rural children may grow up with a deep connection to the outdoors—basic sports, fishing, hunting, exploring the woods, and learning firsthand about farming, animal care, and weather patterns.

Your spouse quickly learns that you are "married" to your medical specialty as well.

Professionally, rural physicians enjoy a high degree of independence. You're often not tied to a large corporate medical entity, which means you have full control over your practice—from setting your schedule and patient volume to office hours to hiring and firing staff. But with that autonomy comes full responsibility for everything, including workplace drama and all the business aspects and equipment that need to be managed in a busy practice.

Community gossip and local social dynamics play a more noticeable role in daily life and can affect patient relationships or office atmosphere. On the flip side, acts of office-based philanthropy, like giving a bit of cash ($100) to a struggling patient, family, or homeless person, or providing free formula for a newborn, are more frequently used and deeply appreciated. But you are like a priest—all issues and "confessions" in the office are relegated to the grave with you. Confidentiality is sacrosanct. Thus, your circle of friends must understand that you cannot have loose lips about anybody you know or don't know. Anybody! Because you never know if there is a connection. Thus, it makes one appear quite aloof in conversations, especially with non-medical people.

There's also a persistent stereotype that country doctors are less sophisticated. Poppycock. In reality, rural clinicians often need broader medical and psychiatric knowledge and must be more hands-on with most pediatric procedures. We also make it a point to avoid the "office mill" model of medicine—the rushed, high-volume practice style. And with the internet as a knowledge-leveling tool, access to evidence-based medicine and sophisticated medical references is no longer a limiting factor for rural doctors.

City Opportunities

City life offers a contrasting set of advantages. There's easier access to arts and culture, from professional sports to concerts, galleries, and theater. For your spouse, urban areas often mean more career opportunities, making it easier to build a dual-income household.

Most physicians in urban and suburban settings are employed by larger hospital systems or insurance networks. This reduces the administrative burden. You don't have to worry about payroll or HR issues, but it also means giving up autonomy. Work hours, division of labor, and income distribution are often determined by the system, and there's typically less incentive to see more patients.

On the plus side, cities offer quicker access to specialists and hospitals, streamlining patient care. And perhaps best of all, you can walk into a grocery store without being recognized. Being anonymous at Kroger? That's a luxury rural docs can rarely enjoy.

Challenging Medical Conventional Wisdom: The Start

Two Issues with the Diagnosis and Treatment of Rocky Mountain Spotted Fever

1) Diagnostic Tests

Early in my rural Kentucky practice, I encountered a case of presumptive tick-borne Rocky Mountain spotted fever. The medical textbooks of that time stated that the diagnosis was primarily based on serum blood titers for Proteus OX19 and other similar, esoteric bacterial antibodies unrelated to Rocky Mountain spotted fever (RMSF). This was purported in the second edition of one of the most prestigious infectious disease textbooks. I called the editors and suggested, as deferentially as I could, that these tests were outdated and not very sensitive for the diagnosis. I explained that clinicians would probably miss the diagnosis of RMSF in far too many cases—a real problem for such a deadly disease. Our pediatric group in North Carolina had vast experience with this ominous and lethal pathogen, and at my urging, the next edition would soon correct the misinformation.

It all started at Wake Forest Medical Center, where I trained for 3 years as a pediatric resident. We would seemingly see at least one case of Rocky Mountain spotted fever per week during the summertime. The typical child presented with a notable fever, usually a history of a tick bite (over 90% of the time), and a spotty-looking, peculiarly bumpy rash. This rash would start on the hands and feet and spread centrally, a pattern known as centripetal spread. Critically, the rash was often petechial, meaning it had small purple spots, and sometimes purpuric, appearing as bruising. Along with the rash, children would often experience severe headaches and appear moderately to extremely ill.

Through my own and some of my trainees' observations, I noticed three laboratory values that were almost pathognomonic (diagnostic) in children presenting with Rocky Mountain spotted fever. These were: 1) a low white blood cell count with a high band count (immature neutrophils), 2) a low platelet count, and 3) a low serum sodium level. If a child had two or three of these findings, there appeared to be about 95% certainty that they had been infected with the Rickettsia bacteria causing either Rocky Mountain spotted fever or the other similar tick-borne illness, Ehrlichiosis. If they had only one lab abnormality (maybe drawn too early), they still probably should be treated empirically with appropriate antibiotics, or at least have the labs rechecked daily until certain. RMSF was too deadly to be left untreated. So, some overtreatment was highly acceptable for clinicians. But if caught early enough with these ancillary findings, oral doxycycline could be used on an outpatient basis, if there was guaranteed follow-up within 24 hours and trustworthy parents. (I will explain the doxycycline story below.) Only a few other terrible illnesses presented with a few of these lab findings, rarely. In pediatrics, one in particular is meningococcemia—another imminently life-threatening bacterial condition that requires immediate antibiotic treatment with intravenous antibiotics and IV fluids.

Although I acknowledged that I was just a simple country doctor (and that I had not been imbibing the local world-famous bourbon), I called the textbook editors and suggested they consider revising their recommendations. These three lab tests could more than likely provide diagnostic clarity within 60 minutes, allowing treatment to begin immediately. In the emergency department, we also found that liver function tests were sometimes elevated in these cases, but this finding was more typical of Ehrlichiosis, another similar, deadly rickettsial bacterial disease. By using these three lab parameters in the presence of fever and a suspicious rash and tick history, we could more rapidly and confidently diagnose the disease and start antibiotic therapy promptly, saving lives. Interestingly, its tick cousin, Ehrlichiosis, has, in the last decade, become more common in our area.

RMSF (and Ehrlichiosis) has a high geographic endemicity for southeastern states, especially North and South Carolina and Oklahoma/Arkansas, but it certainly can occasionally be found in most states. The organism enters human skin via a tick bite, with the tick having been feeding off an infected dog or cat. The illness usually appears within 2 to 14 days of the tick bite. It is widely reported that the tick must be attached for more than 24 hours to cause disease, but I have witnessed otherwise rarely.

Uncannily, this diagnostic laboratory approach was soon published in a pictorial textbook of pediatric infectious diseases. Written about ten years after our observations, this textbook detailed the same diagnostic criteria we had established. Drs. Mandell and Wilfert, pediatric infectious disease experts, advocated the use of these same three parameters for the rapid presumptive diagnosis of RMSF in their 1999 pictorial textbook on *Pediatric Infectious Diseases*. Confirmatory diagnosis may be through the use of PCR or the latex agglutination test (which takes 2 or 3 days for results) or an IFA blood titer, by comparing a sample taken at presentation with a follow-up blood sample taken two weeks later, showing a rise in antibody titers. None of these other tests is much help for the febrile acutely ill child!!! PCR testing is used more commonly in diagnosis now. It still may take a few days for results.

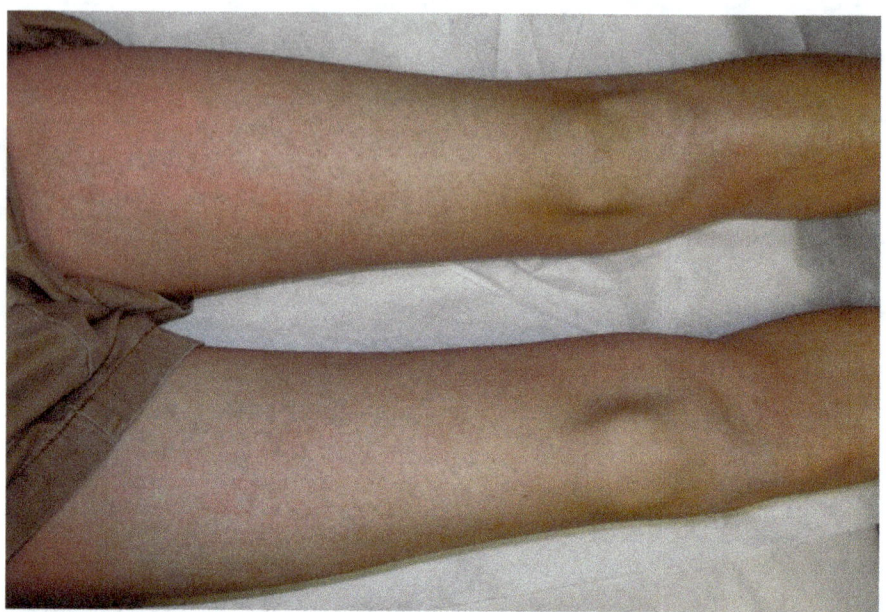

Figure 1(a). A 17-year-old boy with Rocky Mountain spotted fever (leg view).
Source: Dr. Block

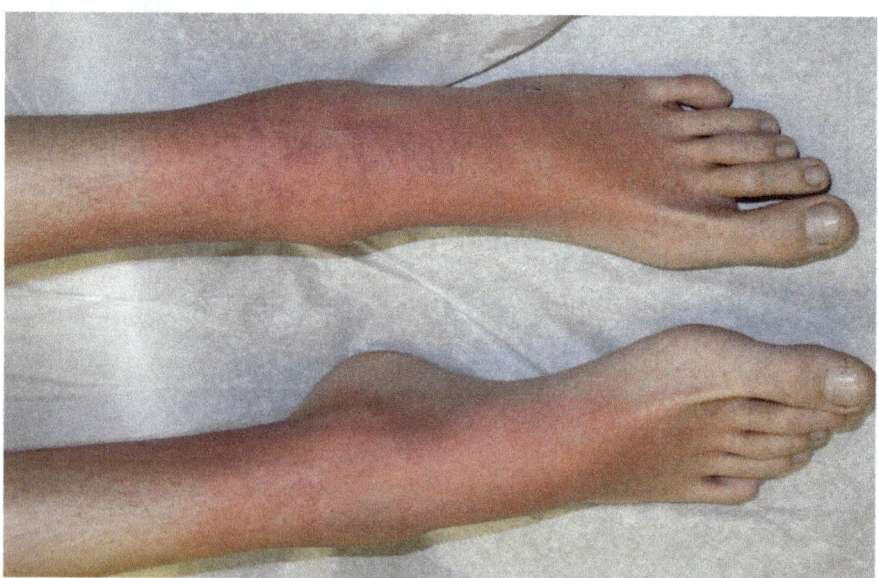

Figure 1(b). A 17-year-old boy with Rocky Mountain spotted fever (feet view).
Source: Dr. Block

In another example involving one particularly memorable phone call a few decades ago, a 27-year-old man who had been admitted to the local hospital with fever and a somewhat petechial and bumpy rash (Figures 1a and 1b are examples of this RMSF rash). A colleague, who was the attending internal medicine doctor, called me for advice about him because she had witnessed my expertise in acute infectious disease diagnoses in some patients we had shared. She told me that this patient had received over 5 days of IV ampicillin and gentamicin, then more recently switched to Rocephin, yet he remained feverish and his medical condition was deteriorating badly. During this phone call, I asked her to check for the following three laboratory tests: Was there a low white blood cell count with a high band count, low platelet count, and low serum sodium? When she confirmed he had all three, I told her with certainty, "You have a case of Rocky Mountain spotted fever, and if you don't switch antibiotics soon, your patient is likely to die." She immediately switched him to IV doxycycline. Within 24 hours, he was improving and appeared to have gone from his deathbed to being ready to eagerly return to work. That is how rapidly doxycycline works in many of these cases of RMSF (and Ehrlichiosis).

2) Revolutionizing Treatment: Doxycycline for Young Children?

Before the 1980s, the standard therapy for Rocky Mountain spotted fever in **children younger than eight years old** relied on chloramphenicol. Tetracyclines were thought to stain their developing teeth. The high treatment efficacy of tetracyclines for RMSF in patients older than 8 years was well established as the standard of care, in whom it did not cause teeth discoloration. Notably, chloramphenicol, the former antibiotic standard of care in children, was reported to cause deadly aplastic anemia in 1 in 25,000 courses, and also posed significant risks for erythroblastopenia in red blood cells and neutropenia in white blood cells through its bone marrow toxic effects at any age.

As a pediatric resident in 1980, I decided to examine three original articles from the early 1950s that focused on tetracycline use among pediatric patients.

Oxytetracycline, a close cousin to regular oral tetracycline, was the treatment drug commonly used in previous decades. But oxytetracycline, like tetracycline, shows higher water solubility properties, so it easily enters developing teeth because these tissues primarily consist of water-soluble elements. By contrast, the antibiotic doxycycline remains largely soluble in fat; therefore, it poorly penetrates dental structures. I thought that doxycycline would be a potential replacement for chloramphenicol subsequently.

The early available literature showed that tetracycline teeth staining happens mainly in posterior molars, and typically develops only after consuming three or more repeated tetracycline antibiotic courses. I began to wonder why we would need to avoid an effective "fat-soluble" antibiotic, particularly when used as a single course. It showed reasonable tolerance. But arguably, data about a single short course was very limited about it causing any major teeth staining in younger children. Thus, most of us were avoiding the use of doxycycline for children younger than eight years old at that time due to the fear of tooth staining as well. But let's put this in proper perspective. Parents were provided with two equally effective treatment options for RMSF in children: 1) chloramphenicol, which provided a choice with small but very serious risks of bone marrow toxicity (e.g., aplastic anemia), including a risky bone marrow transplant; or 2) doxycycline, which could <u>potentially</u> cause minimal teeth staining after a single seven to ten-day short course. Which did they opt for?

In the ER, all my parents of children younger than 8 years old consistently opted for doxycycline as their treatment choice. This really challenged the conventional wisdom of RMSF treatment at our university and elsewhere in the U.S. at the time. Eventually, the approach I had started at Wake Forest had expanded to Duke and UNC Chapel Hill until it became acceptable as a standard of care option during that decade onwards.

Furthermore, Dr. Lochary, a pediatric dentist from North Carolina, routinely examined the teeth of children under the age of 8 for dental staining after they had taken a course of doxycycline. Dr. Lochary then reported two different large observational studies, which confirmed that doxycycline usage as a single treatment course did not cause significant tooth staining. Occasionally, he observed that doxycycline treatment produced only limited tooth staining that mainly affected posterior molar teeth. These additional research results confirmed my new approach to use doxycycline as the primary treatment option for Rocky Mountain spotted fever and some other rare infections in young pediatric patients under the age of 8. Even a standard pediatric infectious disease textbook by Drs. Mandell and Wilfert had adopted this approach in 1999, and a bit later, so would the American Academy of Pediatrics' "gospel"—the *AAP Red Book* on infectious diseases.

Serious Skin Signs to Watch for If Your Child Has Had a Tick Bite

If your child has been bitten by a tick:

1. Promptly remove the tick with firm and steady traction—preferably using tweezers if possible.

   If the tick has never been attached to the skin, or attached for less than 24 hours, your child is *usually at no risk* from this particular tick-related incident.

2. Clean the area with soapy water.

3. Assess whether the tick was a deer tick (tiny), a dog tick (larger, average size), or a fully fed and bloated tick.

4. Most serious tick-related infections show signs within 2 to 14 days of the tick attachment.

5. Deer tick attachments:

   These bites carry a slight risk for Lyme disease, depending on the region of the country in which you live. At the tick bite area, you should watch for any red, ring-like rash (Photo I) that is expanding around the bite. Any rash at the tick-bite location requires prompt evaluation by your doctor.

6. Dog tick attachments :

   You should watch for three possible problems:

   • Staphylococcal or methicillin-resistant *Staphylococcus aureus* (MRSA) infections, which often start with a reddened tender area of skin, or a small boil, or a red streak going toward the chest. Sometimes near the tick bite you will find a small, tender kernel or lymph node, which often requires medical evaluation (Photos IIA and B).

   • Rocky Mountain spotted fever (and ehrlichiosis) nearly always begin with many of the following signs: fever, aches, headaches; and usually (but not always) a rash initially on the hands/arms or feet/legs. The rash may be red, spotty, and raised; or with small, flat purplish dots that do not blanch when you press on them (Photos IIIA and B); or with larger, bruise-like splotches (Photo IV); or any combination of these.

   • Tularemia (very rare) mostly shows signs of a swollen tender, red lymph gland (Photo V) near the tick bite, and is sometimes associated with a small ulcer within a few inches of the tick bite as well.

If your child develops any of the above findings in relationship to a recent tick bite, please contact your doctor promptly.

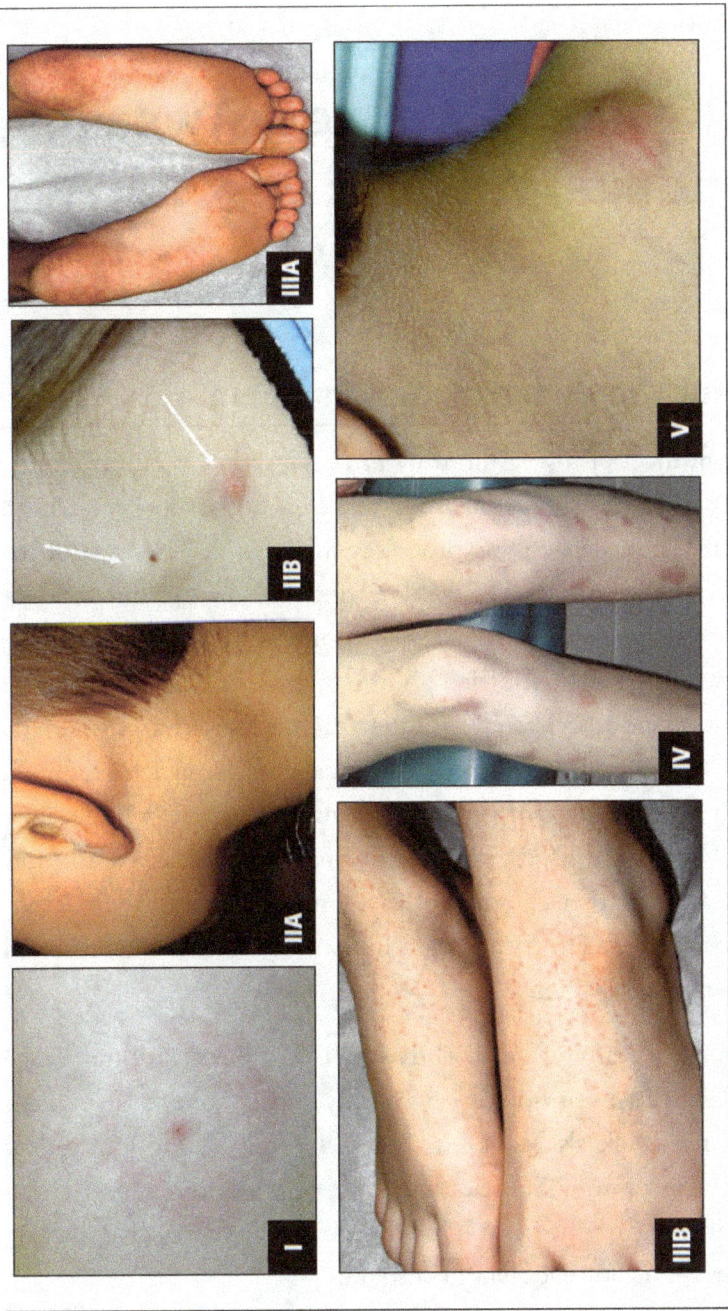

Figure 2. Tick bite complications
Source: Block SL, Spots and Lumps: Treacherous Tick-Borne Problems, *Pediatric Annals*, 43 (7), 2014

CHAPTER 3

Pediatric Annals Articles—Tweaking Conventional Wisdom: Part 1

Purpose for the Pediatric Annals Column

My purpose for most of my 37 monthly *Pediatric Annals* columns in the 2012-2014 years was to discuss the following: common issues pertinent to general pediatricians; the thinking process involved with ferreting out the "zebras" from the bovine herd when hearing hooves in your field of practice; to publish many of my own office's numerous informative photos (over 1000 available personal office photos of patient illnesses) on both strange and mundane cases I had seen; and to examine and challenge several conventional wisdoms, I guess. However, each of these articles required approximately five full days of my time per month to research, develop, write, carefully edit, and re-edit with the journal's peer-reviewed critique. This allowed me to gather up some of my compiled interesting, relevant photos and cases. Like all my other scientific publications, I never received any payment either. Silly boy.

I was sitting poolside after a vaccine advisory board meeting about a new vaccine for pediatrics. I was sipping on my only drink of one of Kentucky's finest bourbons—Maker's Mark—in South Florida. A most respected academic colleague of mine, Stan Shulman, MD, the world-renowned head of pediatric infectious disease at Northwestern University in Chicago, plopped down on the lounge chair next to me.

As long-time buddies, we began discussing topics ranging from his affinity for Detroit Tigers baseball to the latest in Kawasaki disease—one of his many areas of expertise. Suddenly, he changed focus and asked me if he should become the chief editor of the monthly CME journal, *Pediatric Annals*. I told him that it was a prestigious, well-read monthly journal for pediatricians and that he should definitely consider the editor job.

Then he turned the tables on me. He said, "Stan, I will do it only if you agree to come join me on the editorial board and write me a monthly column about general pediatric topics." I said, "Stan, ugh, that would be adding to my already very busy plate of pediatric clinical trial articles and managing my prolific pediatric outpatient research group." He said to me again, "Stan, I will only take the role if you join me." I mused: *The general pediatricians of the world would treasure your brilliant doctor's insights and leadership for a favorite magazine.* We both sipped our bourbon drinks and pondered our future friendship and future topics for the journal.

As Jimmy Buffett sings: "It's OK to be crazy, just don't let it drive you nuts," which medical writing will do to you. Let the lunacy begin. "Fruitcakes," anyone?

After 3 years, for my last column in Pediatric Annals, Dr. Shulman remarked in that 2014 issue of Pediatric Annals ... "as noted by Stan L. Block, MD, FAAP, this is his last 'Healthy Baby' column—at least for a while. Stan, the self-styled small town "country doctor," has done a fabulous job of writing a column each month on a topic relevant to general pediatrics. We are greatly indebted to his outstanding efforts and his eagerness to share his wisdom from his long service in the trenches. Thank you, Stan! Job well done!" **—Pediatric Annals Editor-in-Chief Stanford T. Shulman, MD, is the Virginia H. Rogers Professor of Pediatric Infectious Diseases at Northwestern University and Chief of the Division of Infectious Disease at the Ann & Robert H. Lurie Children's Hospital of Chicago.**

Petechiae and Purpura: The Ominous and the Not-So-Obvious? [Heavy science; intended for clinicians]

(Adapted from Block SL, Petechiae and Purpura: The Ominous and the Not-So-Obvious?, *Pediatric Annals*, August 2014)

Case 1

An 11-year-old male who was being treated with amoxicillin for typical streptococcal pharyngitis develops a morbilliform measles-like dermatitis 4 days into therapy. He still has a sore throat and remains febrile at 101°F; his cervical lymph nodes and abdomen are normal; his leukocyte count is normal.

His rapid test for mononucleosis is positive today. Thus, you assume this is just the purported "typical" mononucleosis rash triggered by amoxicillin and not a drug hypersensitivity reaction or other complication. The rash is non-pruritic and not urticarial. Four days after you switched his antibiotics to oral cephalexin, he has now developed a petechial and lumpy purpuric rash over his entire body, much more so below the waist (Figure 3). He is non-toxic, talkative, and feels fine. He is afebrile with normal vital signs and an otherwise normal physical examination.

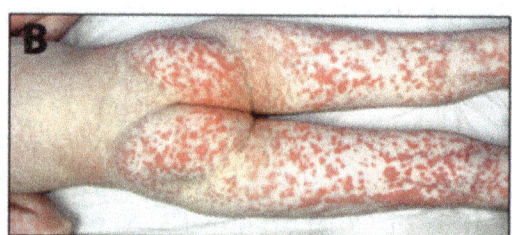

Figure 3. An 11-year-old White male who developed this scary morbilliform measles-like rash 4 days into treatment with amoxicillin for streptococcal pharyngitis. His fever is still 101°F, his lymph nodes and abdomen are normal, and his leukocyte count is normal. Further testing? When the patient showed a positive monospot test, his doctor switched him off amoxicillin and substituted oral cephalexin. Four days later, the patient developed this full-body "lumpy" purpuric rash. He is now afebrile and has minimal other symptoms. Allergic reaction? Refer? Hospitalize? Treatment? The morbilliform purpuric rash in the 11-year-old male would markedly dissipate 24 hours after being treated with which drug? (Answer can be found in the text.)
Source: Dr. Block

Diagnosis

Although he has classic palpable purpura, the distribution of the rash is too extensive to be typical of HSP or immunoglobulin A (IgA) vasculitis (Figure 3). Or is it? After all, you have been taught that the rash rarely goes superior to the waistline or on the arms. (Look closely.) But one of the other keys to this diagnosis is the usual lack of any systemic illness signs or fever.

You obtain a CBC, UA, and CMP (serum chemistries) to ensure you are not witnessing a dangerous case of early meningococcemia or hemolytic uremic syndrome, ITP, or lupus. All laboratory tests are normal, thus you default to the HSP diagnosis.

How common is HSP? You audited your charts for the diagnosis of either anaphylactic purpura/HSP over the past 5 years. In your busy, seven-pediatrician private practice of children and adolescents, you found 27 cases within the 60-month interval—about one episode every 2 months may occur in your rural office. Only three patients were adolescents. You personally saw 15 of them. Crazy, huh? Lucky perplexed me.

You are well aware that IgA vasculitis can primarily affect (early on or later) four other organ systems besides the skin, such as: 1) glomerulonephritis (kidney inflammation), 2) severe abdominal pain (rarely along with intussusception), 3) arthritis, and 4) orchitis/oophoritis (testes/ovaries). Although these sequelae have been reported in 50% to 75% of children (who were mostly hospitalized referrals), they are actually uncommon (< 5%) in your experience with outpatients in the general pediatrics office. You are quite attuned to possible secondary nephritis, which may have particularly severe long-term sequelae. However, in fact, you have only seen this occur in two patients during 30 years of general pediatric practice. Both these patients are doing well, but both still require antihypertensive medication. And, you learned this week in the office that one young girl had just finished receiving immunosuppressants for over three years.

Only a few of your patients have also experienced severe abdominal pain to the point of requiring surgical evaluation and hospitalization. In one of these patients who was febrile, despite 48 hours of an initial diagnosis of HSP and the later development of a typical HSP rash, the blood culture obtained in the emergency department revealed that she actually had a meningococcal serogroup B infection. **So be very, very careful with the diagnosis of HSP in the febrile child.** Continued physical and laboratory monitoring is very vital.

Monitoring in HSP

Careful follow-up over the first few weeks is still essential, despite the low incidence of nephritis. In the otherwise uncomplicated afebrile case after HSP diagnosis is made, you may typically recommend: 1) two additional visits within the first week, and then two more weekly visits; and 2) to return at any time if the family notices the child has developed puffy eyes, bad headaches, tea-colored urine, decreased urine output, abdominal/genital/joint pain or swelling; 3) at each visit, a CBC, UA, and serum chemistries as well as obtaining weight, vital signs (blood pressure especially), and a physical examination.

Treatment of HSP

This is a fairly controversial area, but the literature suggests a possible role for steroid therapy, particularly in hospitalized or sicker patients. I think that two recent studies conducted by Weiss et al. have shown that steroids may cause a modest reduction in renal disease and significant reductions in surgery (odds ratio: 0.39), endoscopy (odds ratio: 0.27), and abdominal imaging (odds ratio: 0.5).

When the child with HSP did not have severe abdominal pain, I have personally only used oral steroids in an outpatient setting one time—in this case. And the results appeared to be dramatic within 24 hours of initiation of oral steroids. My rationale was based on the severity of his vasculitic rash in this case and the fact that steroids have also shown a modest benefit in some cases of severe mononucleosis. The earlier steroids are started in more severe cases of HSP, the greater the benefit will be, in my opinion. Obviously, I did not want to wait for a severity requiring hospitalization.

Mononucleosis Rash Due to Amoxicillin: Mythology?

I believe this may be one of the most unsubstantiated mythical "factoids" in pediatric medicine, and any entrenched mythology is hard to extinguish. For years in our office, we have been treating streptococcal pharyngitis with amoxicillin as the first-line agent. We observe probably 50 to 100 cases of mononucleosis annually, of which at least 5% are co-infected with streptococcal pharyngitis, and several will also develop acute otitis media or sinusitis, which we have almost uniformly treated initially with amoxicillin, as well. We have rarely ever observed a rash in this group of children. A recent report regarding Israeli children seems to confirm our anecdotal findings. Among children with mononucleosis, the incidence of rash was not any different for children who had received amoxicillin versus those who had not (29.5% versus 23%).

Diagnosis: Petechiae/purpura secondary to HSP; possibly related to mononucleosis or I doubt Group A strep.

Case 2

The following child (age 13, who was otherwise healthy and afebrile) shows the uncharacteristic distribution of the palpable purpuric and petechial rash in HSP. The rash was distributed all the way up the back up to the arms. The rash may be associated with pruritus and excoriations. In each case, the CBC and platelet counts were normal.

This patient with streptococcal pharyngitis showed a worrisome distribution of petechiae (i.e., on the feet and palms, extending up to the knee). Because RMSF classically presents with a rash starting on the hands and feet, which spreads centripetally, you must be particularly attuned to this diagnosis and carefully assess for a history of any tick bites and fever. This is summertime, after all. You think that a CBC, serum chemistries, and UA are a prudent starting point in the evaluation.

But this patient does not appear ill. Thus, if you were to carefully assess his oropharynx, you would have a distinct likelihood of uncovering some red, round, yellow-centered blisters in the posterior pharynx or on the lips. Remember that the peak season for very commonly encountered enteroviral infections is also summer, and enteroviral infections can also cause petechiae, which they did in this case.

Diagnosis: enteroviral infection

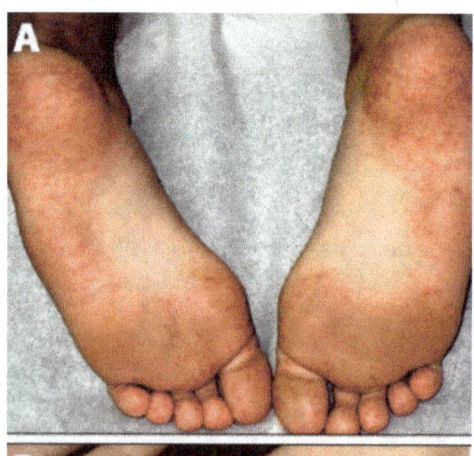
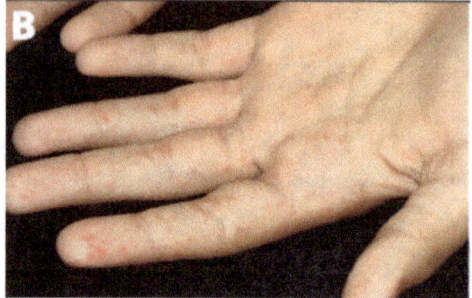

Figures 4 (a) and (b). Worrisome petechiae rash on the soles (2) and palms (3) of a 13-year-old male who has a sore throat and fever (102.5°F). It is summer, and he has been camping, but his mother recalls no recent tick bites. Further testing? Or a more thorough physical examination?
Source: Dr. Block

Case 3

The eight-year-old boy presents with a fever of 102°F, some joint aches, vomiting, and severe headaches. Your exam is unremarkable except for some tiny petechiae on his hands and feet that you see (Figure 4A and 4B). He appears mildly ill. His neck is supple (bendable).

In your office, you obtain a CBC, UA, and serum chemistries, which only show a low leukocyte count. Because your automated office hematology machine does not perform a leukocyte differential, you send the bloodwork to the hospital. Although you were not initially certain of the severity of his illness, when the WBC band results (28%) arrive a few hours later, you call the patient back into the office. You have observed enough.

You decide to admit him to the hospital for blood culture and parenteral ceftriaxone antibiotics. His mental status and neck suppleness remain unchanged over the next several hours, so you do not think a lumbar puncture is worthwhile. He does not have meningitis, so you do not think that he initially needs either vancomycin or steroids as well. Within 24 hours, most of his fever and illness symptoms have dissipated, except for the joint aches. His blood culture is now growing a gram-negative cocci. Your index of suspicion was correct: He was affected by both the ominous and not-so-obvious early meningococcemia.

Diagnosis: Early meningococcemia.

CONCLUSION

Petechiae and purpura are among the most alarming findings a pediatrician will occasionally observe in the office. The severity of the cause of illness can range from a simple temper tantrum or vomiting to common viral infections, to the deadliest of infections (meningococcemia) and diseases (hemolytic uremic syndrome). Although no cases of the following were presented here, I have seen several cases of idiopathic thrombocytopenic purpura, aplastic anemia, and leukemia present in a similar manner to these cases.

To avoid many of the pitfalls in diagnosis, practitioners will need to be thorough in history taking, assessing fever and immunization status, and careful physical examination. Also, you will usually need to resort to a few simple laboratory tests and likely request a manual differential on the CBC, paying meticulous attention to the details in all these reports. Index of suspicion and clinical gestalt are key as well. Be especially wary of any child who has fever with his petechiae/purpura. These petechiae and purpura will test your mettle!

Managing Cervical Lymphadenitis—A Total Pain in the Neck! [Interesting but heavy science; intended for clinicians]

(Adapted from Block SL, Managing Cervical Lymphadenitis—A Total Pain in the Neck, *Pediatric Annals*, October 2014)

Abstract

Patients presenting with cervical lymphadenitis are a complex and common occurrence in a general pediatric practice. Although *Staphylococcus aureus* (often methicillin-resistant S. aureus [MRSA]) and *Streptococcus pyogenes* (strep throat) predominate as causative pathogens, the next most common pathogens—*Bartonella*, atypical mycobacteria, and mononucleosis—must also be considered early on. The best way to diagnose and manage these cases initially is to proceed methodically, with a detailed history and physical examination, initial rapid tests for streptococci and mononucleosis, serial office visits, and complete blood counts. In non-viral cases, an empiric oral antibiotic trial is usually prescribed as early as possible to cover for MRSA or *Bartonella*. Very tender or reddened lymph nodes larger than 5 cm that are unresponsive and/or worsening may likely require inpatient parenteral antibiotics, biopsy and sometimes surgical removal. The practitioner must also realize that submandibular and supraclavicular node locations are highly suggestive of atypical mycobacterium and cancer, respectively.

Text: In your private general pediatric practice, almost daily, you are on a "nodes-to-know-basis" with the multitude of cases of cervical lymphadenitis you assess and manage. Worried (about cancers), stymied (about the huge differential diagnosis), and perplexed (by the complexity of etiologies), you still plodded onwards with your assessment.

Over the years, you have found, however, that proceeding methodically along certain levels of complexity in pursuit of an accurate diagnosis often leads to your improved successful management of this common enigmatic problem. Etiologic diagnosis often requires astute history taking and physical examination skills, along with selective and appropriate laboratory testing in stages. Often, this must be combined with reasonable empiric antibiotic therapy for specific targets to determine whether the clinical response corroborates your suspicions.

Nonetheless, you will be dealing with some clear exceptions to this approach. While you are pursuing the diagnosis, here are some general rules and some exceptions to remember during the evaluation that are helpful, but by no means pathognomonic.

History

Obtaining a history of each of the following may be helpful: level of fever, sore throat, oropharyngeal blisters, nearby impetigo lesions, and tuberculosis exposure.

TABLE 1

Laboratory Evaluation of Cervical Lymphadenitis

Level 1. Rapid antigen detection test (ADT) for strep; complete blood count and monospot (by simple easy finger stick); without a significant pharyngitis, be wary that a positive ADT may actually be strep carrier state.

Level 2. If high leukocyte count (>15,000 white blood cells/mm³) or increased erythrocyte sedimentation rate and negative strep ADT, strongly consider oral therapy for methicillin-resistant Staphylococcus aureus (MRSA), particularly prescribing oral clindamycin or trimethoprim-sulfamethoxazole and amoxicillin; earlier treatment is better. If no response, highly febrile, or marked worsening, consider hospitalization for intravenous therapy of MRSA and surgical consultation.

Level 3. If normal leukocyte count/ESR or history suggestive, consider:
- Serum testing for Bartonella henselae, Francisella tularensis, and Epstein-Barr virus (EBV) titers.
- Intradermal tuberculosis (TB) skin test (uncommonly positive in patients from private practice with atypical mycobacterium).
- A trial of targeted empiric antibiotic therapy almost as a diagnostic test:
Oral azithromycin (10-12 mg/kg/day for 5 days) should be considered with any history of recent local cat (or even dog) scratches; a trial of oral clindamycin if any recent regional tick bites to cover for MRSA first.

Level 4A. If fluctuant or markedly enlarging, consider ultrasound to determine abscess vs solid node. Consider fine-needle aspiration or "incision and drainage" as a starting point, along with empiric intravenous clindamycin or even vancomycin or linezolide.

Level 4B. Consider surgical extirpation if ill, unresponsive, or markedly enlarging (>5 cm), or if atypical TB is most likely, especially for submandibular nodes. Your experience suggests that nodes that are initially >5 cm will most likely need surgical extirpation. Most nontender supraclavicular nodes >2 cm will require biopsy.

Be very cautious if there is a history of a tick bite, with a nearby skin ulceration-tularemia is considered a Centers for Disease Control and Prevention level 3 biohazard for the surgical team and laboratory personnel. They should be warned appropriately.

Table 1. Laboratory Evaluation for Cervical Lymphadenitis

Furthermore, you should inquire about exposure to the following rarer zoonoses (animal vectors: Just remember cats, farms, rabbits, ticks):

- Above the shoulders, a scratch by a cat (or rarely dog) within the last approximately 2 months (*Bartonella henselae*—cat scratch disease)
- Aquarium or farm animal or (this is a real thing now, unbelievably) **unpasteurized milk** exposure (atypical mycobacterium (TB), Brucellosis, Listeria)
- Nearby tick bite, with or without an ulceration (*S. aureus* or, rarely, tularemia)
- Rabbit exposure via hunting or skinning (tularemia)

Physical Findings

The cervical gland(s) should be carefully assessed for size, pain, redness, discoloration, induration, fluctuation, mobility, and probably for any additional satellite nodes in the cervical, axillary, and inguinal areas (including for the **stealthy lymphoma or leukemia)**.

The following ancillary findings on physical examination may often point you in certain diagnostic directions:

- High fever: *S. aureus* and *S. pyogenes* top the list
- Exudative pharyngitis: *S. pyogenes* and mononucleosis
- Scarlatini or morbilliform rash: *S. pyogenes* and mononucleosis
- Hepato- or splenomegaly: mononucleosis and lymphoid cancers
- Scalp and facial sores/lesions, such as insect or tick bites
- Dental or periodontal disease or salivary duct inflammation (sialadenitis)
- Puffy upper eyelids in the morning: present in half of the cases of mono
- Scalp kerion: Epidermophyton (ringworm)

Etiology of Cervical Lymphadenitis

S. aureus and *S. pyogenes* are by far the most common pathogens identified, accounting for 65% to 89% of the pathogens. The next most commonly identified group of pathogens is EB virus (mono), Bartonella, and atypical mycobacteria. But, also note that both *S. pyogenes* and EB virus uncommonly present with unilateral lymphadenitis (except in your private practice, of course, as you will see).

A more esoteric and quite rare etiologic group includes Brucella, leptospirosis, tuberculosis, Kawasaki disease, thyroid nodules, branchial cleft cysts, cystic hygromas, and finally, the most dreaded of all—lymphomas and leukemia types.

CASES

Solitary Lymphoid-Like Neck Masses (Figure 5)

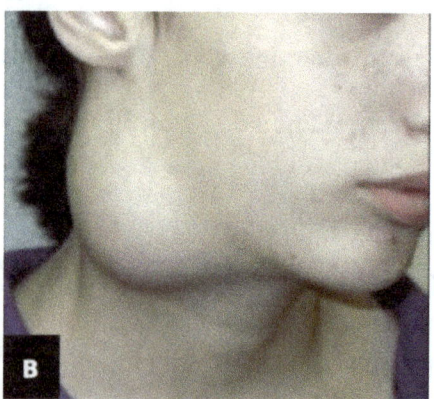

Figure 5. A previously healthy 11-year-old female presents with a markedly swollen, mildly tender anterior cervical node. She has had some malaise, fatigue, and "low-grade fevers." She has no cats, tick bites, or tuberculosis exposure. After 2 weeks of multiple oral antibiotics, including azithromycin (10 mg/kg/day) and clindamycin, her node has continued to enlarge notably. She has been seen by two different surgeons this week; neither wants to pursue a surgical evaluation. What further tests and diagnoses are you considering now that she is back in your office? In an "Oh, by the way" moment, as you review her history again, you just learned that her dog had scratched her on her right shoulder a month ago.
Source: Dr. Block

During week 3, the surgeon was finally ready to operate. During the surgical removal of the massive node, she was discovered to have a **branchial cleft cyst** with a congenital tract tunneling into her esophagus. However, to cover for the positive *Bartonella* titers (cat scratch), another course of azithromycin was prescribed. She did well postoperatively, with a good cosmetic outcome. And once again, your patients do not read the textbooks: branchial cleft cyst in an 11-year-old? And an abrupt onset? Who knew??? This condition is typically slow-growing and becomes very obvious by age 2 years. Not in my practice.

Figure 6. This 3-year-old female with a retro-auricular smaller lymphadenitis and no external otitis really baffled you. Her 10 days of persistent constitutional symptoms of malaise, fevers, and anorexia all seemed totally out of proportion to a typical staphylococcal lymphadenitis. Her ESR was elevated at 45 mm/hour, but her leukocyte count was normal. But you had warned the mother about the other possible etiology of this lymphadenitis, so that when your partner saw the patient in your absence, she had reassured the mother that the new small ulcer in her scalp was merely a herpetic reaction. Dr. Block tends to be an alarmist? OOPS!

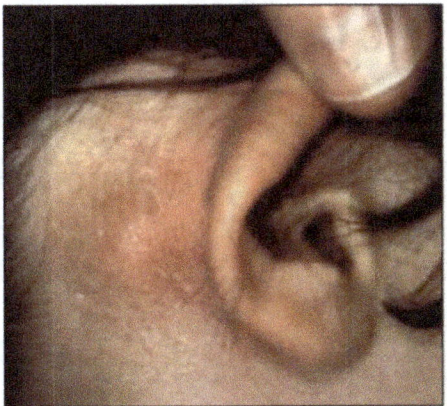

Figure 6. This previously healthy 3-year-old female has had this posterior auricular node for 10 days. This is the node's appearance after four different oral antibiotics. The lesion is now fluctuant, and she has just recently developed a small ulcer in her scalp, near a previous tick bite. How should you proceed? Should you aspirate it?
Source: Dr. Block

Seeing the skin ulcers in the next 48 hours clinched your earlier suspicions. You very carefully (and perhaps cavalierly) needle aspirated about 5 mL of pus from the node and submitted the specimen for culture. Along with a large note for the lab to process it as **a CDC level 3 biohazard!**

Yes, you had your first of 4 cases of *Francisella tularensis* that year! Think tick bite, fluctuant node, and nearby skin ulcer—and you have **ulceroglandular tularemia.** You discussed with the parents the antibiotic choices for outpatient treatment: twice-daily intramuscular gentamicin for 10 days that would require baseline plus two more hearing tests, and a series of about three serum chemistries and gentamicin levels by venipuncture as well. Gentamicin = Potential for ototoxicity and renal toxicity.

Or, since Dr. Block has firmly tweaked the conventional wisdom on doxycycline in youngsters, you could prescribe twice-daily oral doxycycline liquid with a slightly lower cure rate than gentamicin. There is a chance of adverse effects of gastrointestinal distress (mostly when given without concomitant food), along with a slight risk of mild posterior molar dental staining when using such a short course of this lipophilic antibiotic in children under 6 years old. Thanks to my prodding, the *American Academy of Pediatrics Red Book* Report Committee had already long-considered a single course of doxycycline to be safe to use in children with suspected rickettsial infections, a different infection.

Subsequently, you elected to use oral doxycycline to treat the node at this point, and she had a rapid, successful response. Perhaps needle aspiration of the abscess, which likely helped significantly, would have been preferred in the pediatric surgeon's office, too?

Only about 60 pediatric cases of tularemia are reported annually in the entire U.S. I have identified five pediatric cases in rural Kentucky in forty years. Who knew? Why me?

Figure 7: The purplish-red node seen in this image is highly suspicious for our esoteric pathogen again—tularemia. The history of a nearby tick bite and lack of any response to multiple antibiotics, including doxycycline, is suggestive. But the patient also lacked any constitutional symptoms of fever or malaise as far as you could tell. Additionally, his CBC and ESR results were normal. However, his tularemia IgG titers were positive at 512:1, proving the diagnosis of the dangerous tularemia.

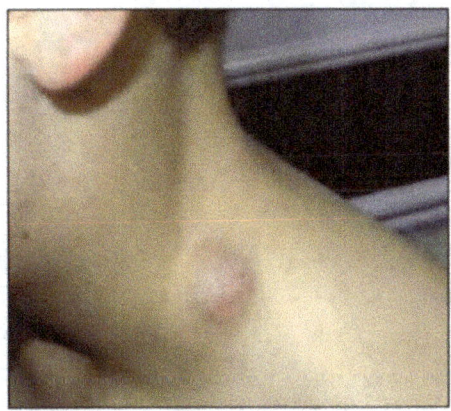

Figure 7. A previously healthy 7-year-old male presented with a swollen, tender, and moderately reddened node in the supraclavicular area. He has a history of a dog tick bite in his scalp. This is the node's appearance after 3 weeks of multiple oral antibiotics, including azithromycin, clindamycin, and even doxycycline. The node is now quite fluctuant. What are you thinking, and how should you proceed? Note the location.
Source: Dr. Block

Should you aspirate the node? Perhaps too risky for you. Hospitalize? The child is not acting ill. So, you do the next best approach—send him to the pediatric surgeon for total node extirpation with cultures. His culture never grew a pathogen—probably due to doxycycline suppression. But he responded well to the node removal and a switch to IM gentamicin antibiotic, with all its monitoring for kidney and hearing toxicity.

Figure 8. Perhaps you would like to perform all your diagnostic lymph node tests on this patient in Figure 8 right out of the gate. Do not bother! This is a very large, fixated, nontender or minimally tender supraclavicular **mass or lymph node of somewhat abrupt onset**.

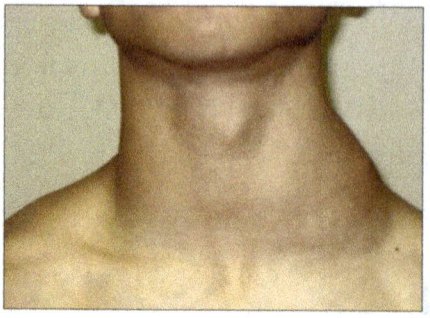

Figure 8. This previously healthy, afebrile 15-year-old African-American male has abruptly developed a slightly tender, very large node in his left lower neck. How should you proceed? Note the location. Supraclavicular.
Source: Dr. Block

Just send the patient to the hematology-oncology group directly, as you did here. Not much good would usually arise out of a huge supraclavicular node. The patient needed immediate further evaluation and treatment for his non-Hodgkin lymphoma. Henry is still alive and in remission to this day.

You may not know it when you see it.

The previously healthy 4 y.o. boy presented to the office with a history of tonsillitis, fevers, and swollen neck glands.

He was seen by one of the partners over a 3-week period with a presumptive diagnosis of strep throat initially, despite the negative rapid strep test, and despite the initiation of what should have been effective antibiotics for strep. Yet his sore throat, low-grade fevers, and swollen neck nodes persisted. He was then tested for mononucleosis, which was negative. But in defense of the decision, up to 50% of children under the age of 6 years old will have a false negative test for mono, despite having an actual mono infection. He was given more ibuprofen and a short course of oral steroids, which can occasionally help the symptoms of severe mono in children.

After three weeks, his mother, whom I knew well from taking care of several of her older children for years, sought my opinion.

When I examined him, he was afebrile; he had 3 cm anterior cervical nodes bilaterally, which were nontender, and a few shotty, small nodes a bit lower in the neck. His throat was no longer red, but his tonsils were still mildly enlarged. His chest was clear, and OH No! His abdomen had a moderately enlarged spleen, with a slightly enlarged liver.

But the critical finding was several large, 3 cm non-tender lymph nodes in the inguinal (groin) and axilla (armpit) areas. This was the missing link not found yet on his previous physical examinations, because they are not routinely checked in mundane respiratory illnesses. I then understood the gravity of his illness. I explained to the mother that I wanted him to see the "blood doctors" for a total evaluation of his blood system.

Then that fateful question popped up: *What could it be, Dr. Block?*

I stood by my standard answer: "The list is as long as my arm, and we will not know until further testing is performed."

Unfortunately, the biopsies confirmed my number one suspicion. They showed a non-Hodgkin lymphoma version. He underwent several rounds of chemotherapy and radiation, but despite episodes of remission intermittently, after about a year, he succumbed to his cancer. A tragic loss—devastating to this super nice family, or to any family.

The death of a child is always unfathomable. And I estimate that in over 90% of those parents who were previously married, the marriage will fall apart, as most cannot withstand the horrific grief and irrational guilt that accompany the heartbreaking death of a child.

Some days, I do not want to be right with my diagnosis.

When the grandmother visited the office a few years later with one of the other healthy siblings, she asked me: "Did you know his diagnosis, Dr. Block, when you saw him in the office that day?"

I just responded: "What do you think, Karen?" (But, I also know that occasionally the more "obvious" bad diagnosis upon further testing may prove to be devastatingly or unnecessarily wrong. Thus, the hedging.)

She just nodded her head to me.

Some days I just don't want to be right.

You will probably never know it when you see it!

Words of advice: In the child with "nonsuppurative" (no abscess) cervical lymphadenitis, **routinely examine the child's other node regions** (i.e., inguinal, axillary) and the liver and spleen on each serial visit. You may again, just like you did a few years ago, uncover a child who has leukemia or lymphoma despite his presumptive diagnosis of mononucleosis, etc. A life may possibly depend on it.

When encountering a really sick child, why do I say, "The differential diagnosis list is as long as my arm"? Some may protest that it is not fair to the patient's family.

For example, with lots of flu circulating, the day was a busy one in the office during the winter of 1998, so much so that the front desk was overbooking patients on the schedule of all the doctors. I would really have to hustle and perform at peak efficiency.

When I walked into the room of this sick-looking two-year-old girl whom I had just met, I knew that I had encountered a child with a severe infection or worse. By merely visually examining her skin, I saw that she was pale and covered in non-traumatic petechiae (tiny dark blood spots that did not blanch upon pressure) and sporadic bruises over the skin of most of her body. She had some fevers up to 102°F over the last four days as well. Most of her other physical examination was normal, except for the spleen, which was enlarged about 5 cm, and the liver, enlarged about 2 cm above normal. She had some small, non-tender cervical lymph nodes as well.

I explained to the mother that her daughter had a likely severe infection or severe blood disorder in my experience. I obtained the obligatory CBC, which showed a very low platelet count (65000), low white blood count (2400), and low hemoglobin or red blood count (8.1). This confirmed some of my following speculations as my brain was going through the list: the very long shots like Rocky Mountain spotted fever and meningococcemia; the most likely diagnosis of blood/cancer disorders, particularly leukemia and lymphoma; and unlikely here, an autoimmune disorder like hemolytic uremic syndrome (HUS). I was next calculating— that all of these disorders, if diagnosed early, should have a very high survival rate, even with the most likely diagnosis of leukemia, which I am "confident" he has. But to discuss most of these conditions without any certainty would take over an hour, and would be terrifying for any parent, especially at the mention of the treacherous word "cancer." The diagnosis would depend, of course, on many more confirmatory tests that needed to be performed at the children's hospital.

"But Dr. Block, what could he have?"

As I am eager to give her some somewhat comforting news, I tell her, "**The list of possibilities is as long as my arm**. Yet, I think that the odds are very high that most of these possible diagnoses are treatable."

As is expected, "Could it be cancer?" she then asks. I defer and deflect, and explain that we will not know anything until further tests are done (a very prescient statement in this case).

So I had her promptly drive her down to the excellent emergency department in Louisville. She was stable overall with normal blood pressure, pulse, respirations, and oxygen levels. (Sadly, we can no longer talk with the attending subspecialty physician for a direct admission and an explanation of our findings. This "ER-first" approach is rarely hazardous for patient care, as I have discovered over the years and as you will read later.)

From my home that night, I called down to the hospital at 11 p.m., optimistically seeking an update on her condition from the nurses. The mother explained, "She is on a ventilator, her organs are failing, and she is dying. They do not expect her to live much longer, because they say she has MODS (multi-organ dysfunction syndrome), which was too far advanced for any treatment. And I do not even know for sure what MODS means."

"OMG. (Showing my ignorance) I have not even heard of the term either." I am flabbergasted and deflated.

"They say her immune system is attacking all of her blood organs."

I apologize profusely and tell her that she is in the best of hands for her care where she is, and that I will pray for a turnaround. But I had no idea yet what we were dealing with.

I called the ICU nurses' station and received an explanation from the on-call doctor. Her labs were all diagnostic of MODS or HLH (**hemophagocytic lymphohistiocytosis**), an extremely rare, severe genetic blood disorder, which supposedly occurs mostly in infants. Recently, it has been reported to be common in adults, too. However, they both involve an uncontrollable activation of the immune system with multi-organ failure. In the earlier workup on her admission, the extremely savvy hematologist had checked her ferritin level. So, along with her low blood fibrinogen, her ferritin was diagnostically elevated for MODS at several thousand (normally about 20 to 40), particularly in light of all the other abnormal physical and blood findings. It can be triggered by all sorts of conditions. But almost no outpatient pediatrician will ever see a child with this illness in their lifetime. My entire office, with over a total of 200 years of experience, had only seen one case before.

Needless to say, I did not sleep that night. I called down to the ICU several times to get updates over the next two days. She expired after 48 hours in the ICU. Her funeral service was so sad. Sometimes life is so fragile.

Rethinking Pediatric Conjunctivitis: "Pink Eye" Is Rarely Viral Under Age 5

For years, pediatric conjunctivitis—commonly called "pink eye"—was thought to be mostly viral, especially by academicians and textbook authors. However, I led a study on conjunctivitis where our office cultured eye discharge from 250 children under the age of five in our practice. We found that the overwhelming majority had bacterial infections detected. The primary pathogens were *Haemophilus influenzae* (non-typeable), *Streptococcus pneumoniae*, and, rarely, *Moraxella catarrhalis*. In addition, this was also among the first reports indicating that many eye infections caused by pneumococcal bacteria were now penicillin-resistant and refractory to typical topical antibiotic drops.

Most young children under the age of three with bacterial conjunctivitis did not actually even present with a "pink" eye. Instead, they had clear conjunctivae, along with green, pus-filled discharge at some point. However, by the time they arrived at the doctor's office, often their parents had wiped away the discharge, making the clinician's physical diagnosis more difficult. Our study showed that if a child had green discharge—either observed in the office or reported by the parent—there was an extremely high likelihood of bacterial infection. Rather than waiting to see if symptoms resolved, it became standard practice to topically treat most bacterial conjunctivitis in children to reduce both the duration of eye discharge and the contagiousness to daycare, school, and family members.

Additionally, we found in an earlier study (1986) that 25% of these young children with acute conjunctivitis under three years old also developed acute otitis media. Our research demonstrated that over half of the cases of bacterial conjunctivitis involved beta-lactamase-producing *Haemophilus influenzae*. When a concomitant ear infection was present, first-line amoxicillin would often prove to be ineffective for this concomitant ear infection because the bacteria in the eye were the same as in the middle ear. Its beta-lactamase enzyme would inactivate plain amoxicillin. Instead, second-line antibiotics, such as amoxicillin-clavulanate or cefdinir, should be used in cases of **"conjunctivitis-otitis" syndrome**. This helped shift the standard antibiotic approach to treating conjunctivitis associated with ear infections in young children.

By contrast, older children with conjunctivitis presented differently, often with red, irritated eyes rather than pus-filled discharge. However, our research found that even in these cases, bacterial infections were common, particularly *Streptococcus pneumoniae* and Group A strep. Again, treating bacterial conjunctivitis was not just about symptom relief; it also helped prevent the spread of infection in classrooms and daycares.

A rare, distinct form of a weeklong, severely reddened and painful conjunctivitis in older children was, on the other hand, usually caused by adenovirus.

There are epidemics of adenoviral conjunctivitis, but while it is often talked about as a widespread issue, in reality, it is not as common as many believe. The key symptoms include fiery red eyes, excessive watery discharge, and significant eye pain. When these characteristics are present, bacterial conjunctivitis becomes far less likely. This form of viral conjunctivitis is extremely contagious, and children with it need to be isolated from their classmates and daycare peers to prevent the spread of infection. No treatment is available.

Newborn Conjunctivitis: Is it Different, Really?

(Adapted from Block SL, Etiologic and Therapeutic Pitfalls of Newborn Conjunctivitis, *Pediatric Annals 41(8)*, August 2012)

The following article helped to clarify the approach to infant acute conjunctivitis as being caused by bacteria typically found in ear infections, just like those in older children. It also clarified: 1) the very limited role of chlamydia in conjunctivitis etiology; and 2) to avoid the use of erythromycin ointment after several days of life.

With some trepidation, a bleary-eyed, pallid-looking young mother brings her 7-day-old infant boy into my office. Baby care is all so new to her that she reports relying heavily upon her grandmother for advice. The child developed purulent drainage from the right eye yesterday. The grandmother, who was afflicted by some eye discharge 3 days earlier, remarked that the baby should be "checked out" by a doctor. A 2-year-old sibling at home has been well. Incidentally, the baby was born at 38 weeks gestation by emergency caesarean section after placental rupture during a motor vehicle accident. Fortunately, no other serious injuries were sustained by the mother or newborn.

Upon examination, the newborn appears to be well-fed, growing, and robust. The right eye has an obvious green, purulent discharge exuding from it. Upon a careful and technically very difficult examination of the tympanic membranes (TM), they appear flat and dark grey. The usual TM landmarks observed in older children are virtually never discernible at this age. Similar to many pediatricians, the 4th-year medical student on his outpatient rotation in my office apparently was unable to adequately visualize the appearance of the TMs. He was using those poorly designed disposable speculums that he was given at the hospital. The remainder of the newborn's examination was normal.

"Pink Eye"

"Pink eye" is a misnomer for young children because very few children younger than 36 months have a pink or red bulbar conjunctiva when it becomes infected. Typically, it remains white or merely somewhat injected-looking. The salient manifestation of childhood "pink eye," or bacterial conjunctivitis, is heavy green or yellow discharge on the eyelids or in the conjunctival sac (Figure 9).

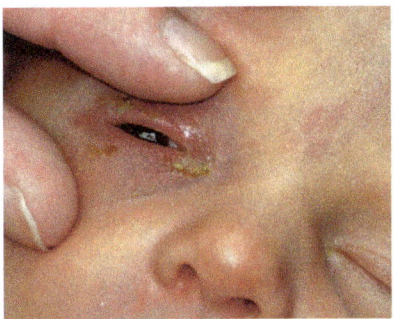

Figure 9. A 7-day-old infant with abrupt onset of unilateral acute purulent conjunctivitis. **Source:** Dr. Block

Because of his very young age, the infant's conjunctival sac was cultured for aerobic bacteria. Polymixin-trimethoprim ophthalmic solution was prescribed four times daily for 7 days. When the patient returned to the office after 48 hours of treatment, his eye had cleared completely. Three days later, his eye culture grew beta-lactamase–negative *Haemophilus aphrophilus*, possibly a genital tract isolate, or a mistakenly identified nontypeable *Haemophilus influenzae* strain, in light of the grandmother's infection, which was likely infectious conjunctivitis. In most children, *H. influenzae* (not HIB) accounts for 50% to 70% of bacterial conjunctivitis pathogens.

Predominant Pathogens of Neonatal Conjunctivitis

Many pediatricians consider *Chlamydia trachomatis* to be the true pathogen of newborn acute purulent conjunctivitis in the United States. But does the literature after the advent of universal neonatal topical antibiotic prophylaxis truly support this notion? Emphatically: No. Time to tweak the conventional wisdom.

At birth, prophylactic topical erythromycin ointment is administered into the conjunctiva of all newborns. During an erythromycin shortage, silver nitrate, tetracycline, or azithromycin ointment can be substituted.

These ophthalmic antibiotics are intended only to prevent the very rare and wickedly purulent gonococcal conjunctivitis. According to the 2012 *AAP Red Book*, conjunctival prophylaxis at birth will not eradicate *C. trachomatis* conjunctivitis. I assume this is due to its limited penetration of deeper conjunctival tissue, and, critically, the ointment will also fail to eradicate the associated nasopharyngeal infection.

Furthermore, most studies have reported a very low rate of chlamydial infection in neonatal conjunctivitis, usually in the range of 0 to 2%.

Note also that the rate of infection with *C. trachomatis* is even lower in mothers older than 25 years.

About 65% to 80% of purulent conjunctivitis infections in children older than 2 months grow a single typical bacterial ear type of pathogen that is predominantly beta-lactamase–producing, nontypeable *H. influenzae*, and less frequently *Streptococcus pneumoniae*. Likewise, I have reported earlier that 60% of eye cultures in a subset of infants younger than 2 months old similarly grew these same typical ear types of pathogens (Figure 10).

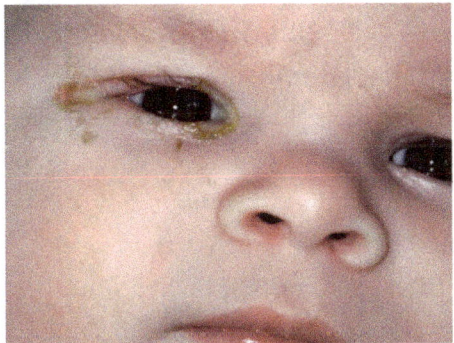

Figure 10. An 8-week-old infant with persistent purulent conjunctivitis despite topical therapy with polymixin-trimethoprim, ocufloxin, and moxifloxacin over a 2-week interval. His culture grew penicillin-resistant pneumococcus, requiring additional oral therapy with oral clindamycin for 10 days to eradicate the infection. Note the eyeball conjunctiva is not red or pink.
Source: Dr. Block

Although many clinicians claim that *Staph* bacteria are conjunctival pathogens, most microbiological studies have found *Staph* at the same frequency in asymptomatic children as in those with conjunctivitis. Thus, not an eye pathogen.

Neisseria gonorrhoeae, an extremely rare cause of newborn conjunctivitis, presents with continuous severe and profuse purulent discharge within days after birth. On the other hand, manifestations of chlamydial conjunctivitis are more similar to a typical purulent conjunctivitis caused by the ear types of pathogens, but symptoms usually develop within 5 to 14 days of life. It is still very rarely identified.

Viruses are alleged to be a very common cause of "pink eye." However, most recent North American studies that evaluated young children (<5 years old) with true purulent conjunctival discharge by history or by clinical assessment have reported a bacterial ear type of pathogen in 65% to 80% of cultures.

Erythromycin Ointment

In my opinion, topical erythromycin should not be prescribed to newborns (or any age child) anymore. I believe this for the following reasons: 1) the rate of chlamydial conjunctivitis is probably less than 1% to 2%; 2) the drug of choice for chlamydial conjunctivitis is oral azithromycin; and 3) topical erythromycin does not eradicate *Chlamydia* in either conjunctiva or nasopharynx, nor in pneumonitis, which occurs concomitantly in 5% to 20% of children with chlamydial conjunctivitis. Although data on newborn infections are limited for both antibiotics, I prefer to use oral azithromycin (10 mg/kg daily for 5 days) instead of poorly tolerated oral erythromycin (50 mg/kg/day divided four times daily).

Oral azithromycin is much better tolerated, has much better adherence because it is dosed once daily instead of 4 times daily, and it requires only 3 to 5 days total therapy versus 14 days of therapy. It also probably has much less risk of inducing **secondary pyloric stenosis** in infants younger than 6 weeks. Note that coverage of topical erythromycin for the two most common conjunctival pathogens, *H. influenzae* and drug-resistant pneumococcus, is minimal.

By contrast, if penicillin-resistant pneumococcus or Staph aureus is recovered, then prescribe oral clindamycin or intramuscular ceftriaxone (for 2 or 3 days), or oral clindamycin or trimethoprim/sulfamethoxazole, respectively.

CONCLUSION

Please note the following concepts about neonatal conjunctivitis: the conjunctiva is rarely pink; rather, it will have purulent discharge by history or by examination. *C. trachomatis* is a very rare causative pathogen in this age group.

The following article provided further impetus to the expert early management of infantile hemangiomas with oral propranolol, which was just being investigated in the literature at the time of its publication.

Treating Infantile Hemangiomatosis: A Case Study

(Adapted from Block SL, Treating Infantile Hemangiomatosis: A Case Study, *Pediatric Annals 42(6),* May 2013)

Infantile hemangiomas, which occur in about 4% to 5% of all children, create a difficult management dilemma in routine pediatric practices and continue to stir debate and controversy. Practitioners are aware that all elevated hemangiomas and most flat hemangiomas typically grow throughout the first year of life, and that most elevated ones spontaneously involute over the next 5 to 10 years. The flat, less conspicuous hemangiomas often do not. Nonetheless, why should a clinician be concerned about these benign lesions?

I think it may become incumbent upon the pediatric community to alter its approach to most hemangiomas. At birth, 65% of hemangioma precursors were present. A recent photographic report showed that the most rapid growth of hemangiomas occurred between ages 5.5 weeks and 7.5 weeks. This age factor may be critical when deciding upon using a more prophylactic type of treatment, such as propranolol, because most children with hemangiomas are not referred to a dermatologist until age 5 months. These authors have even suggested biweekly monitoring for any high-risk hemangiomas after the first month of age.

Although the lesions are always benign and usually self-limited, some of them may be located in areas that become life-threatening or function-threatening, some may ulcerate and bleed, and some may lead to significant psychosocial distress or may cause permanent residual skin changes that are cosmetically undesirable. Importantly, clinicians cannot reliably predict which hemangiomas in the first few months will create any of these problems. In addition, one must be very diligent about the further evaluation of children with possible PHACE syndrome, or multiple hemangiomatosis, as additional expert consultation will be needed.

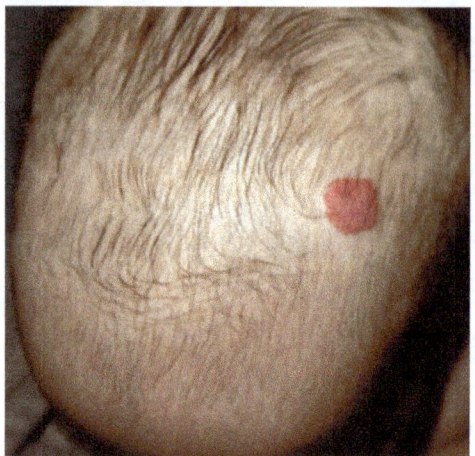

Figure 11. Photographs of a single scalp hemangioma
Source: Dr. Block

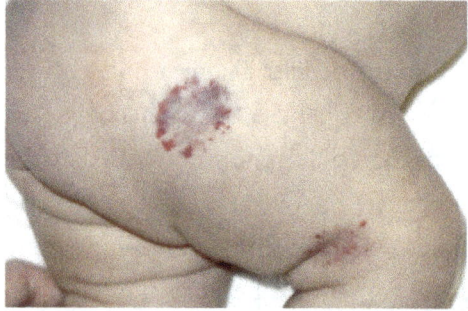

Figure 12. Photographs of 2 leg segmental hemangiomas with mild regression when treated with propranolol.
Source: Dr. Block

With propranolol treatment, the hemangioma sequentially fades to much less bright red and eventually becomes totally flattened and has no more satellite metastasis after 2.5 months of treatment. This fading is a more acceptable cosmetic result. But parents may want to consider further laser therapy for cosmetic reasons, as these hemangiomas have a tendency not to dissipate further over time, unlike the hemangioma in Figure 11.

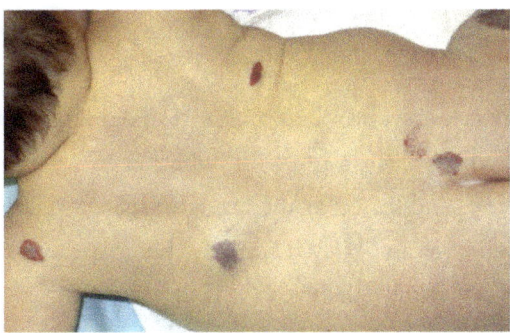

Figure 13. Photographs of 5 focal hemangiomas of the back. Each of the hemangiomas sequentially fades to much less bright red, eventually totally flattens, and develops no more satellite metastases after 5 months of treatment. This dramatic fading is a much more acceptable cosmetic result. Further laser therapy for cosmetic reasons for these proximal three particular focal hemangiomas will probably not be necessary, as they are likely to totally disappear, and the well-faded segmental ones on the sacral area are smaller, barely perceptible, and will remain covered by clothing.
Source: Dr. Block

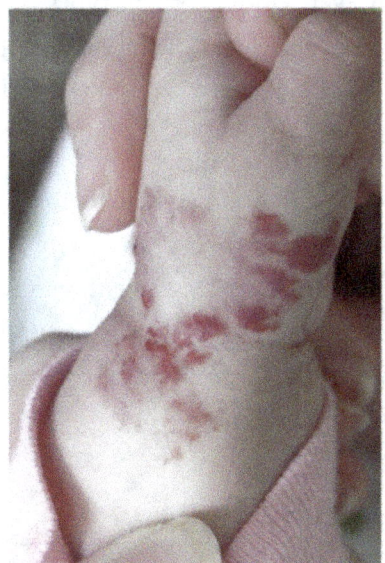

Figure 14. Photographs of a larger solitary segmental hemangioma of the hand show that the hemangioma sequentially faded to much less bright red and became totally flattened with no more satellite metastases after 2.5 months of treatment. This fading is a marginally acceptable cosmetic result. The parents will likely consider further laser therapy for cosmetic reasons, as the location of this segmental hemangioma is more conspicuous and will be unlikely to dissipate further over time.
Source: Dr. Block

For the practitioner, it is the numerous smaller hemangiomas, the less conspicuous ones, or the more cosmetically subtle but noticeable hemangiomas that can create difficult psychosocial or emotional dilemmas for parents and practitioners when deciding upon whether to treat. Hindsight is always much better, and once again, as with other more cosmetic conditions such as plagiocephaly, early timing of therapy may be much more critical than previously widely believed. It is also much more difficult to be prescient about the severity or complexity of these types of hemangiomas.

Although treatment timing and therapeutic choices have been completely revolutionized in the past 4 years with the use of propranolol, they still remain controversial. Before 2008, corticosteroids and laser therapy had been the mainstay of treatment for life-threatening, function-threatening, complicated, or difficult lesions. However, most other types of hemangiomas have been "treated" with benign neglect, knowing that most would eventually spontaneously involute and dissipate by 6 to 10 years of age, leaving only minor or no residual signs.

But is this last assumption true? Nearly 75% of nodular hemangiomas reportedly create discernible residual skin changes. The growth rate of hemangiomas is unpredictable and quite variable, and 12% are significantly complex. Adding to the clinician's consternation, a new prescription pharmacologic agent has been approved by the U.S. Food and Drug Administration for the treatment of infant hemangiomas.

Use of Propranolol in Outpatient Settings

Overall, propranolol appears to be a very safe drug to use in infants. Monitoring for pulse and blood pressure is advised only at baseline, 1 and 2 hours after the first dose, or with any significant increase in dose (>0.5 mg/kg/day). Routine electrocardiogram or Holter monitoring is not indicated for otherwise healthy infants. Subsequently, how does one decide when and whether to "pull the trigger" and when to start therapy for many of these more benign, non-threatening lesions? When does the risk-to-benefit ratio become worthwhile?

What to Expect with Propranolol Therapy

The recent article by Hermans et al.[1] showed that nearly all of the 174 patients responded strikingly to propranolol therapy with a fading of abnormal color, immediate cessation of growth (a critical component of the early timing argument), softening, and rapid induction of regression. Medication was effective even though the mean age of patients was older (4.8 months old), and all of the lesions were potentially threatening or complicated.

The same white female infant (my granddaughter) is shown in each of my images.

Tweaking conventional wisdom: this article's approach to the following complex problem was recently adopted as the standard of care by the Ohio State University Department of Otolaryngology. The retro-auricular cellulitis is now included as a distinct diagnosis in several of the newer pediatric infectious disease textbooks.

Mastoiditis Mimicry: Retro-auricular Cellulitis Related to Otitis Externa [Heavy science; intended for clinicians]

(Adapted from Block SL, Mastoiditis Mimicry: Retro-auricular Cellulitis Related to Otitis Externa, Pediatric Annals *43*(9), September 2014)

---

[1] Hermans, D. J., Bauland, C. G., Zweegers, J., van Beynum, I. M., & van der Vleuten, C. J. (2013). Propranolol in a case series of 174 patients with complicated infantile haemangioma: indications, safety and future directions. *The British journal of dermatology*, *168*(4), 837–843. https://doi.org/10.1111/bjd.12189

Case 1

A previously healthy, afebrile 7-year-old male was seen in your office last week with moderate otalgia and an "apparent AOM" (the physician could not see the patient's tympanic membrane [TM] due to the combination of swelling and whitish discharge). After all, ear pain and ear discharge equal AOM, or do they?

Due to concerns that he might have a "secondary" otitis externa or "swimmer's ear" from otorrhea, not only was he prescribed twice-daily amoxicillin for apparent AOM, but he was also prescribed topical combination steroid-antibiotic drops four times daily. But do these drops actually get past the canal or anywhere near the canal skin?

Today, when you see him, his right ear is now protuberant with redness of the skin behind the ear and loss of the ear sulcus (Figure 15).

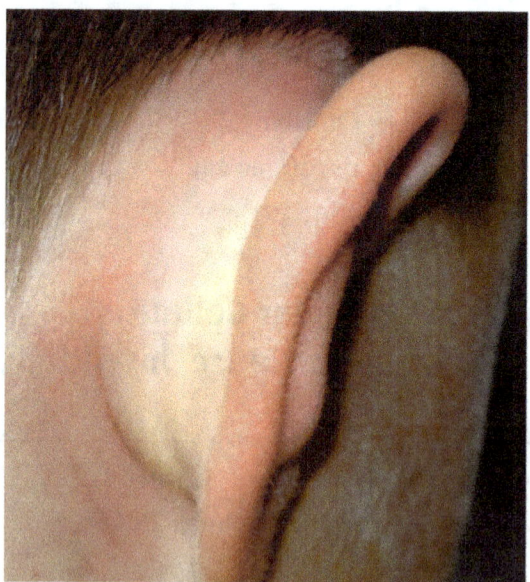

Figure 15. A 7-year-old male with a 1-week history of severe ear pain, particularly the tragus, and mild otorrhea during the summer that has acutely worsened in the past 2 hours. Therapy with oral amoxicillin twice daily was started 4 days ago, along with topical ofloxacin otic drops twice daily. How should you proceed?
Source: Dr. Block

You are completely surprised at the degree of pain with any motion of the pinna; the boy screams and cries real tears every time you attempt to insert your otoscope speculum into his ear canal, and he begs you to stop. You are perplexed; as a novice practitioner, you have never seen this type of reaction before. Surely this is mastoiditis. So, you blithely order a complete blood count (CBC), plain films of the mastoid (despite their low yield), and in the diagnostic *coup de grâce*—a computed tomography (CT) scan of the mastoids. You are also aware of all the recent "brouhaha" about head CT scans' association with a slightly increased risk of cancer.

All of the tests are normal, including the blood leukocyte count. So, what is going on here? You now assume that this must be a case of *S. aureus* cellulitis associated with otitis externa. You wish to provide antibiotic coverage for methicillin-resistant *S. aureus* (MRSA), which has been so prevalent this summer, so you prescribe thrice-daily oral clindamycin, along with some oral narcotics for the severe pain. He returns to your office in 48 hours, with no change in pain and redness. The ear is only slightly more protuberant.

You consider hospitalizing him for parenteral antibiotics and pain relief. You explain this to the mother and child, who both promptly ask you, "Is there not anything else we can try first, doctor?" You tell them that we can always try a large dose of parenteral IM ceftriaxone at 50 mg/kg for a few days. You assume that this will stop his AOM and otorrhea, but you doubt it would do much good to ameliorate MRSA cellulitis. Thus, you also add oral trimethoprim-sulfamethoxazole to cover for the possibility of clindamycin-resistant MRSA, as recently reported for some strains. But what about coverage for the most common pathogen of otitis externa? The next day, he has still made no progress and still complains of intense pain. You consult your pediatric infectious disease expert and decide whether to hospitalize him for parenteral antibiotics.

Case 2

The same week, a previously healthy 4-year-old female presented to your pediatrician partner 5 days earlier with a swollen ear canal and a very reddened TM, which he thought he could see despite the canal swelling. She was prescribed amoxicillin clavulanate for AOM.

When you see her today, she is afebrile and nontoxic, with an otherwise normal physical examination. However, as you attempt to examine her left TM, she cries vociferously when you put pressure on her pinna. You pull her hair back and see redness behind the earlobe and the loss of ear crease. From this perspective, you can now see that the earlobe is protuberant (Figure 16).

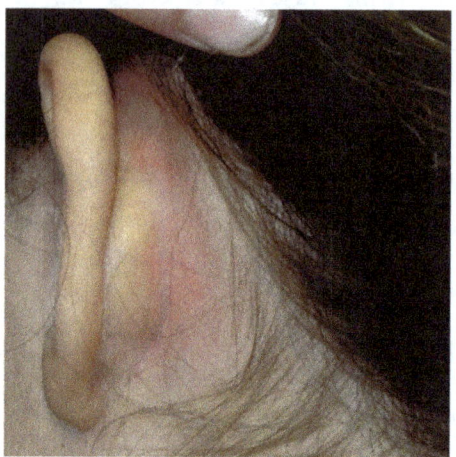

Figure 16. A 4-year-old female presents with severe worsening ear pain despite amoxicillin clavulanate for a presumed acute otitis media, when her physician observed a swollen ear canal with purulent discharge last week. When you touched her pinna or tragus in order to examine her ear, she yelled out in pain. Pulling back the hair, you find this red area. How should you proceed?
Source: Dr. Block

Are You Seeing a Mini-Epidemic of Mastoiditis?

You grab your smallest ear speculum (original equipment's tapered 2.5 mm size) and try to talk her through the painful TM examination. Yet, all that you can see now is a swollen canal with thick white debris. Her blood leukocyte count is 13,500 cells/cm^3.

A plain radiograph of the mastoids shows some cloudiness in the mastoid air cells. But you also remember from your AOM lecture in residency that more than 50% of cases of routine AOM may have some mastoid cloudiness. And, you also recall your infectious disease text, which states that when it comes to plain radiograph films, only coalescent mastoiditis is considered diagnostic for acute mastoiditis. Should you perform a CT scan of her mastoid, which is a more definitive test? But even cloudiness on the CT scan may be considered normal.

Since she is afebrile and nontoxic, should you instead just proceed with additional oral antibiotic coverage for MRSA cellulitis localized to the skin? Or is there another choice? What about the primary pathogen of otitis externa?

Discussion

In each of the two cases presented here, the child had developed retro-auricular cellulitis. But Cases 1 and 2 had retro-auricular cellulitis with loss of ear sulcus, a markedly protruding ear lobe, and potential for a hidden AOM infection, as visualization of the TM was unobtainable or questionable. In the past, many practitioners and emergency departments seeing these children have diagnosed them with mastoiditis, triggering a full evaluation. Mastoid radiographs, CT scans, hospitalization, and otolaryngology consultation would have been ordered. Parenteral treatment for otopathogens and possibly MRSA would have been ordered, too. Rarely, the unconventional selection of antipseudomonal antibiotics would have been ordered. But each of these six patients was managed as an outpatient, and no radiographic imaging was obtained. How did that happen?

Each of these two cases demonstrates the practical difficulties in determining the origin of retro-auricular cellulitis or pre-auricular cellulitis:

A. Potential mastoiditis (very rare today) secondary to AOM, which is most commonly related to gram-positive organisms such as *Streptococcus pneumoniae* or *Streptococcus pyogenes*, or

B. Skin structure infection like cellulitis (uncommon in this anatomic area) due most commonly to methicillin-susceptible *S. aureus* or MRSA, or

C. Cellulitis infection strictly secondary to otitis externa, which is mostly related to *Pseudomonas*?

Thus, how does one differentiate the three potential causes of retro-auricular cellulitis?

The Diagnosis of Retro-auricular Cellulitis

In general, fever and any appearance of toxicity are most likely related to mastoiditis. Elevation of the leukocyte count, or other inflammatory markers, is too nonspecific, but may direct you more toward mastoiditis. To simplify, the key is in a meticulous and detailed clinical examination, looking for each of the physical findings shown in the table below.

TABLE 2

Retro-auricular Cellulitis Secondary to Otitis Externa versus Mastoiditis Secondary to AOM versus Staphylococcus aureus Superficial Skin Infection

Characteristics	Retro-Auricular Cellulitis	Acute Mastoiditis	Superficial Skin Infection
Redness of skin behind the pinna	Always, unless it is preauricular cellulitis	Almost always	Usually, unless it is preauricular
Protuberant ear	Typically if retroauricular	Almost always	Rarely, unless related to insect bite or sting
Loss of posterior ear sulcus landmark	Always, unless it is preauricular	Always	Possibly
TM with AOM	Occasionally	Always	No
Otitis externa: swollen canal with canal discharge	Always	Occasionally from spontaneously ruptured TM or draining tubes	No
Severe pain of ear canal	Always	Very rarely	No
Severe pain over tragus and pinna	Always	No	No
Pain on skin behind pinna	No	Always	Yes
Plain radiograph of mastoid	Normal typically	Usually cloudy or rarely coalesced air cells	Normal
Positive CT scan with cloudy mastoid air cells, etc.	Normal typically	Almost always	Normal
Fever	Very rarely	Usually	Very rarely

AOM = acute otitis media; CT = computed tomography; TM = tympanic membrane.

Table 2. Retro-auricular Cellulitis Secondary to Otitis Externa versus Mastoiditis Secondary to AOM versus *Staphylococcus aureus* Superficial Skin Infection

When marked pain both over the tragus and in the ear canal is associated with ear canal swelling and some non-cerumen debris, it is nearly pathognomonic for otitis externa. Furthermore, the skin over the retro auricular cellulitis associated with otitis externa is uncommonly very tender, in total contradistinction to either mastoiditis or staphylococcal cellulitis. But one needs to be aware that the skin involvement with otitis externa-related pre-auricular cellulitis is usually quite tender.

Treatment of Retro-auricular Cellulitis Related to Otitis Externa

Thus, when a definitive diagnosis of otitis externa (including a very painful tragus) is combined with either a pre-auricular cellulitis or a retro auricular (minimally painful) cellulitis, then the antibiotic should target *Pseudomonas*.

In previous decades, this generally meant resorting to parenteral ceftazidime or other parenteral anti-pseudomonal antibiotics. Currently, we can readily treat this infection as an outpatient with oral ciprofloxacin in any child older than 12 months. The earlier concerns about the general safety and joint issues of ciprofloxacin in children younger than 18 years of age have been dispelled. Ciprofloxacin has been approved by the U.S. Food and Drug Administration to treat any complicated or refractory urinary tract infection in any child older than 12 months.

However, there are a few important caveats to consider when using ciprofloxacin:

- **Occasionally**, otitis externa may mask an underlying acute otitis media (AOM), for which ciprofloxacin provides inadequate coverage against common otopathogens.
- If the cellulitis is caused by **Staphylococcus aureus**, ciprofloxacin is ineffective.
- There is a **rising trend of Pseudomonas resistance** to ciprofloxacin in the United States, which could limit its effectiveness.

Thus, when you encounter a child with retro auricular cellulitis associated with definitive otitis externa, you should consider proceeding as shown in the table below.

Optimizing Outpatient Management of Retro-auricular Cellulitis

- Consider plain radiographs and/or computed tomography scan of mastoids when uncertain or inexperienced practitioner, or if febrile child.
- Assess carefully for severity of pain in external canal, pinna, and tragus to confirm the diagnosis.
- "Aural toileting: "Gently clean out debris in the ear canal with a small, dry, Calgiswab-like device. This can be quite painful but important debridement.
- Insert cotton wick; instill the first dose of topical antibiotic drops to moisten it. A few drops of lidocaine may be helpful.
- Prescribe ciprofloxacin otic (or ophthalmic, which is cheaper) drops every 2 hours for the first day, then four times daily.
- Prescribe oral ciprofloxacin twice daily for 7 to 10 days.
- Consider oral narcotics for a few doses.
- Follow up daily for 1 to 2 days; remove wick; replace if not much better.
- (very rare) Consider hospitalization for parenteral ceftazidime or meropenem if not much better; or may need addition of staphylococcal coverage for possible methicillin-resistant Staphylococcus aureus cellulitis.

Table 3. Optimizing Outpatient Management of Retro-auricular Cellulitis

Clinical Course

Case 1

After your phone consultation with your pediatric infectious disease physician, you decide to try one more oral outpatient antibiotic—twice-daily oral ciprofloxacin. You combine this with good aural toileting during the visit. You insert a cotton otowick, then you prescribe oral ciprofloxacin topical drops every 2 hours for the first 2 days, along with some oral narcotics for the first 24 hours. On follow-up 24 hours later, he has improved, and at follow-up 48 hours later, he has almost regained his full daily functioning.

Case 2

Similar to Case 1, you begin twice-daily oral ciprofloxacin in each patient with a remarkable turnaround in symptoms within 24 hours. As recommended by the textbook of Feigin et al., I think that the initial gentle debridement of the canal and the insertion of an otowick are also keys to the rapid positive response in each of these patients. The clinical response was again amazingly rapid, with full resolution of the canal pain and swelling along with the cellulitis within 48 hours.

CONCLUSION

As reported in 1994 by Hopkin, retro-auricular cellulitis associated with otitis externa is now the great mimicker of mastoiditis. It may be the most common cause of this specific cellulitis/auricular protrusion—particularly when it is associated with otitis externa. In the era of the highly efficacious HIB and PCV vaccination programs, mastoiditis has almost seemingly disappeared from the office in most general pediatric practices. The diagnosis of otitis externa is relatively straightforward (severe pain over the tragus and in the ear canal, with swelling and discharge in the ear canal). When otitis externa is associated with retro-auricular cellulitis, you will probably need to target your antibiotic toward the bacteria, *Pseudomonas* (i.e., use oral ciprofloxacin). This should be combined with good cotton swab wiping and insertion of an otowick.

Once you become comfortable with this diagnostic constellation, you will likely be able to avoid the significant time, sedation procedures, expense, days of ineffective antibiotics, and radiation created by the CT radiographic exposures to evaluate for possible mastoiditis in your young patients. Patient response at careful, early, daily follow-up visits is critical to ensure that you are not dealing with untreated MRSA, underlying AOM, or very early mastoiditis.

CHAPTER 4

Pediatric Conundrums

The "Boy" Who Cried "Wolf"

It may be important to remember Aesop's fables when dealing with some patients.

(Adapted from Block SL in *Infectious Diseases in Children*, January 2008.)

As physicians, we still must take care of those who get "stoned," one way or another.

Our office policy has always been to take care of the sick patient first, then later ask questions about insurance, payment, custody, follow-up, etc.

As I entered the examination room, Mary, aged 18, from Louisville, KY, was writhing in apparent abdominal pain, swearing at me to stop her pain. She used some choice scurrilous words to describe her abrupt affliction within the last four hours. Thank goodness no nurses in my office were present in the examination room with me. They take great umbrage at anyone who curses in the office.

Not me. I have been through a ruptured lumbar disc three times in my life, worked with construction crews most school summers, and played street basketball with motley crews all my life. I have heard it all. Still, I hesitated to supply Mary with pain medication. Why? You may ask.

One must realize that Mary has been a patient of mine since birth. She has had remarkably recalcitrant attention-deficit/hyperactivity disorder, which was real. Yet she never seemed to respond to stimulants because she was selling her pills on the street, sometimes abusing them herself, and had established a drug habit over the last four years. This wound her in jail twice and in rehabilitation once so far, despite the fact that she was raised by the nicest mother a girl could ever have. Her father abandoned her while she was in middle school. She also treated her mother unhappily, swearing at her and belittling her, even while in the office in my presence over the last several years. I finally advised her to take up the notion of tough love, encourage her to live with a relative, and finally, to cut off financial support.

When I asked her where she had eaten the day before, to consider the possibility of food poisoning, she begged off. I did not relent with the questioning, and her evasiveness gave way to her exasperation, with cries of "give me some pain medicine."

Trouble is, Mary did not know what she ate yesterday because she was so stoned on seven or eight hits of drugs throughout the day—a detail she finally divulged.

A ploy?

As I always do in most cases like this, a few years ago, I had basically cut Mary off from her stimulants and any other abusable prescription drugs, although that never stopped her from coming in and requesting them. She repeatedly complained that she needed her stimulants to help her ADHD and to keep her out of jail. She would often say, "Atomoxetine never works, Doctor Block." Bear in mind that atomoxetine has no abuse potential and has no street value. Or sometimes she complained that she had "really bad headaches," and insisted on Vicodin, since she would say, "Ibuprofen works like water for pain."

So you can understand my reluctance to treat this young lady's pain with narcotics. Was this another ploy?

Yet something was nagging at my cerebrum.

Look at the patient.

Mary had no recent history of fever, nausea, vomiting, diarrhea, or respiratory illness. She had basically been healthy physically all of his life. My examination of her and her abdomen revealed that she really seemed to have significant left mid-abdominal pain. No guarding, no rebound tenderness. Nothing surgically amenable could possibly be there, I thought. On the other hand, the young lady craved her drugs. But her persistent barrage of epithets and apparent writhing told me to look at the patient first.

Much to my office nurse's chagrin, I asked her to make arrangements so that I could get her to the hospital for further evaluation. She really had no way of getting there because her license was revoked, her mother was estranged, and her boyfriend was unavailable. I could clearly see it was going to take a while to get her over to the nearby hospital. I would need to call her mother and beg her to bail her out with transportation. This would be a hard-pressed favor, I knew.

She was well-groomed, articulate, and appeared to me to be in major apparent distress. Her complete blood count was normal, she could not urinate, and she was slightly febrile. I had nothing else to rely on, except my gut intuition, that even miscreant or malingering folks get real diseases sometimes.

Thank goodness for mother's instinct, because her mother came through, much to her disdain, and transported her to the hospital.

Once she was in the hospital, I placed orders for repeat CBC, abdominal X-ray, and computed tomography scan of her abdomen, along with an order for a single dose of morphine and intravenous fluids.

Somehow, this ruffled the feathers of the nursing staff. First, I received a call from the charge nurse who asked, "What do you think you are doing? She admits to drug use and has been using and dealing with drugs for years. Everyone in the community knows that."

Then I received a telephone call 10 minutes later from the hospital social worker, who told me they found a rehabilitation center for her in

Lexington. I calmly reassured both parties that I really needed to evaluate her for the bad abdominal pain. I thought the pain was significant. I appreciated their concerns about giving a drug addict a dose of narcotics.

How Doctors Think

Jerome Groupman, MD, recently published a book titled *How Doctors Think*, in which he states that physicians tend to use shortcuts and heuristic approaches to streamline the daily flow of patient encounters.

Groupman also advises doctors to be careful when using these approaches and to always consider listening carefully to the patient or parents as we assimilate our deductions as to the diagnosis. He details in his book numerous examples where physicians will jump to conclusions based on prior history, past medical records, or where we tend to judge a book by its cover, before even perusing the pages, by ignoring pertinent findings that contradict our diagnosis. He also emphasizes the importance of occasionally using "gut instinct," or a *gestalt*, and to avoid the oversimplification of a patient's problem, especially when the data presented does not fit the diagnosis we may be pursuing.

In the book, Groupman alleges that **the quickest way to a bad medical outcome is to apply Occam's principle to anything other than the simplest of cases.** To refresh your memory, Occam's razor is the theorem that the simplest, most direct diagnosis will always be the correct diagnosis.

Crying Wolf!

Groupman further elaborates that "flesh and blood decision making" often relies on "pattern recognition," which is often visual, and reflects an "immediacy of perception." Such was the case here. This patient was a known drug addict, complaining of abdominal pain and seeking narcotics. Was I to be one of the physicians he describes, who often put patients in a narrow category and ignore information that contradicts a fixed notion or presumptive diagnosis?

In this case, possible real abdominal pain. Could Mary be the boy who cried "wolf" too many times, and who has now placed herself in the precarious position of lacking any credibility?

I guess it came down to two things:

1. Did I trust my own physical examination?
    The answer is yes. After 28 years, I have very good skills. But I occasionally get fooled, of course.
2. Did I believe in redemption, forgiveness, and human frailty?

Oftentimes at my dinner table, my four daughters, as they grew up, would heatedly cast aspersions upon my judgment when they found out I was the physician for their school's local drug dealer, promiscuous teen, pregnant 14-year-old teenager, etc. "Why can't you make them stop?" they would ask. My daughters were raised in a quite moralistic background and were taught to avoid people like this in their personal lives. Now, whether they listened or not, that seemed to be the case learned for them.

Subsequently, I would have to defend my actions to them. "Somebody has to take care of them, dear. They are people, too. They get sick or need help just like any of us, good or bad. That is what I am trained to do as a pediatrician."

Remember, in our practice, with a sick child, we do not question whether they can pay or not, whether they are going to be ethical or not, or whether they are going to take their medicine or not. People make mistakes and nobody is perfect. If I do not help them, who will? As long as they are willing to work with me or trust me and my clinical judgment, they will have a medical home here.

Call me Pollyanna, but these young folks may still have a good future. Redemption is possible. Over the last 3 decades, I have seen many of these folks rise like a phoenix above the ashes of their self-destructive behavior.

Truly "stoned"!

Within a few hours of Mary's hospitalization, I had my answer to her affliction. The wolf cry was real.

Her urinalysis contained scads of erythrocytes (blood). She had a single 5 mm stone lodged midway in the ureter as seen on the CT scan. I continued another single dose of morphine (of course, she said the dose was too low!) along with forced hydration and diuresis. Within two days, her pain had subsided. She was headed toward the halfway house in nearby Paducah at discharge.

Checking on her two days later by phone, she never showed up. I think she headed for Florida to get away from the drug-using friends. One can only hope.

The Rant: The Office Zoo, Shooting From the Hip

Also, Tips for Changing the Worst Habits of Your Menagerie of Patients

(Adapted from Block SL, *Infectious Diseases In Children*, March 2005)

Some days during an office visit, or when I write my column about some people, I feel like the new television show's heroine, "Ugly Betty."

This television sitcom features a somewhat average adolescent girl who is serendipitously the glue both morally and officially in a high-powered, chaotic fashion office. She is always sticking her nose in other people's business and often makes a humorous mess of the situation. Through television magic, she often seems to pull it together within the hour and save the day. But sometimes she fails, as well; I empathize. Her role is sort of like the Steve Carell of *The Office* scene.

I have had some experiences analogous to "Ugly Betty" recently. For instance, I was concluding an office visit with one of my shorter young teenage patients, who became mortified when I told her that she was unlikely to grow any further after menstruating for two years. I cajoled her, trying to cheer her up by saying, "Look, dear, you can be petite, cute, and smart like you are now, or you could have been big, dumb, and ugly like me."

Her rapid-fire response: "You're not so dumb, Dr. Block. After all, you ARE a doctor."

I retorted, "But what about the 'big and ugly' part?"

She responded, "No hope there."

I looked over at her mother and said, "Brutally honest, isn't she?" and we both chuckled.

It is my role in life to be the whipping boy and verbal punching bag for teenagers, both in the office and in my own household of four daughters—perhaps, karma's payback for all my prior transgressions. Hey, if it defuses their situation, and they are able to smile again and realize that it could always be worse (thanks a lot!), I am thrilled with the teasing aspersions. Thus, the Ugly Stanley title must stick.

My office actually runs very smoothly most days, and I can imagine no other career that I would enjoy more or that would provide such fulfillment. However, there are moments!

The purpose of this opinion piece is for me to vent—to explain those occasional peccadilloes in my office or my life that drive me to the ranting of a King Lear. (He only had 3 daughters.)

Perhaps you may agree with my pet peeves. Remember that the rants are not to belittle my young patients, as they are probably perfect. Rather, most of these transgressions originate from parental or societal cluelessness or indifference.

Teen "Raptors" of Rapture

I am always highly alarmed when parents allow a daughter to start "dating" a male 2 years older or more than she is <u>during high school</u>. Having raised four young daughters and cared for countless teens in my practice, I am a seasoned warrior. If one of our goals when treating adolescents is to postpone sexual involvement—at least until after high school graduation—then parents and young teens should be forewarned about the perils of this age discrepancy.

In many states, a 14-year-old or 15-year-old female becoming sexually involved with a 17- or 18-year-old male is legally considered sexual abuse or statutory rape. And yet, in the National Longitudinal Survey of Youth, at age 15, the first sexual partner of experienced females was "typically" three years older—clearly a worrisome statistic. Sadly, the reason for first intercourse for these females was stated as "to please the partner" (20%), "my partner forced me" (15%), and "did not wish to engage in it" (25%). Importantly, 70% of female adolescents sexually involved by age 16 reported later that they wished they had waited longer—clearly, at this age, an impulsive and often dangerous situation. Thus, early intercourse for young females in high school often results from a sexual predator situation.

My personal observation in my mostly white rural population is that when the female-to-male age discrepancy is more than 2 years, sexual activity assuredly will occur within six months of the relationship's start. And we should counsel them accordingly. These young girls are also at much higher risk for sexually transmitted diseases, cigarette and drug use, and, of course, teen pregnancy. I also observe a very high frequency of total male dominance/control and serious male jealousy issues in these relationships, and the stifling of the girl's healthy emotional and social growth in high school. Most of these girls are placed under a social martial law under the thumb of the boyfriend, and become stressed-out and miserable while in this relationship.

Suggestions: Have parents swoop down "raptor-like" and confront the daughter's dating life. It's either parental tough love early, or daughter tough luck later (babies, partner abuse, drugs). As the poet Robert Graves noted: "**Love may be blind but Love at least/Knows what is man and**

what is mere beast." These young girls are blinded by the "prestige" and "social security" of the older raptor. They too often become impulsively involved and relinquish control of their social lives and sexuality. Otherwise, parents may become premature grandparents or start paying for their daughter's psychotherapy.

Personal pearl: Each of my daughters was warned that during high school, dating any male 12 months older was not allowed under my gentle version of martial law. Too many other younger male fish in the sea for them to become oppressed bait and to spawn all types of other regretful high-risk behaviors and consequences in high school.

Gummy Bears and Office Grazing

The epidemic of dental caries in practice is staggering. Too many children walk around all day at home or in the office with a bottle, sippy cup, or bag full of Cheerios or gummy bears. Not only is this disrespectful to the office/home cleanliness, as they spill their liquids and solids on our floors, but it also truly destroys their tooth enamel, rots teeth to the "gummies," and predisposes them to obesity.

Suggestions: Have a sign in each room stating "No food or drink in the exam rooms." Counsel all parents of toddlers about the need for children to eat or drink only at the kitchen table and to have nothing by mouth in bed or after parents brush the child's teeth at night (except water). Dispose of the bottle forever after 12 months of age.

Pack of Wild Jackals

Discipline and the total lack thereof. Ever watch the children on *Super Nanny*? This had to be the best show on television for parents. Well, children of that elk, er ilk, seem to permeate the office on some days. Unruly, petulant, and demanding, this overindulged child has no respect for you, your property, or the (usually ineffectual) mother. These are the same "sweethearts" who are insomniacs and whose parents insist they must sleep in their bed to assuage both parties. Talk about an eventual sure-fire visit to divorce court!

Suggestions: parental discussions, AAP booklets, and books about discipline; forecasts such as, "You think the tears are bad now when you tell your child NO—wait 'til you try saying NO at age 14 or 15 when their future is on the line." And emulate the "Nanny" in action.

Phone-us Interruptus Birdies

What is the aural fixation that mesmerizes parents and teens into believing that any warbling that emanates from their Apple phone is more important than anything you have to say? Surprisingly, they can obtain reception anywhere in the recesses of our office. And of course, hearing other little birdies chirp about the latest gossip is much more entertaining than and always takes precedence over an antibiotic discourse or a synopsis of herpangina. They can always just call us back and ask questions to the phone nurse later. The doctor should have time to peripherally listen to the latest lovers' spat or when to pick up the little chickies.

Suggestion: Post a sign in each room that says, "Turn off all cell phones when the doctor is in the room." Alternatively, consider installing a wireless phone jammer in your office—I wish!

Go-fer Two-fer

I really need the antacid when this ugly go-pher-beast pops its head during the visit. "Oh, by the way, Doc, could you just look at lil Johnny's brother's rash, ears, lungs, belly, [fill in the blank]." This is the perpetual "innocuous" two-for-one phenomenon that parents love to spring on us good-natured, non-confrontational pediatricians.

Suggestion: No longer do we just "go-fer" it. Put a sign in each room: "We are obligated to ask the nurse to obtain the chart, vital signs, history, and charge slip for the two-fer or add-on child. We are medically and legally bound to do so. We will be 'happy' to see the child if time allows and in the next available time slot. Thanks for helping us with our busy schedule." Even our nonpaying Medicaid patients usually respect this. I like to accommodate them if I can.

Herd Immunity: Nonvaccinators

Most parents who believe in nonvaccination also truly believe that vaccines are important for everyone else's child to receive, to prevent their own child from getting ill with vaccine-preventable diseases. Some feel they are just too smart to allow the doctor or government to force (trick) them into taking any risk for a vaccine adverse reaction in their child. As Blanche DuBois stated in *A Streetcar Named Desire,* "**I have always depended on the kindness of strangers.**" The same can be said for some non-vaccinators. The only problem is that these children are a (preventable) potential infectious disease biohazard (think measles, pertussis) in your office and waiting room for all those unvaccinated newborns and infants. Thank goodness we asked the children of our chiropractor to seek care elsewhere a few months before his two children acquired a bad case of pertussis. This could have devastated some of our infants.

Suggestion: Reinforce the following additional vaccine concepts: the necessity of herd immunity, "**The Golden Rule: Do unto others as you would have them do unto you,**" and the strict office policy of prevention and avoidance of unnecessary aerosol biohazards.

Boots of Pig Farmers

Porcine olfactory wonders that linger for hours from those boots are best left outdoors. Ah, the perils of rural pediatrics.

Pork Barrel Politics

Speaking of pig stuff at the trough, our state legislature, like many other state legislatures around the United States, has recently legalized the performance of high school sports physicals by chiropractors. The medical lobbyists were asleep when this occurred. And this legislation was purchased fairly cheaply. Who cares about medical science, the powers of auscultation, seven years of medical training, screening for real diseases, and ensuring physical fitness for contact sports? Check for proteinuria, anemia, an absent testicle, vision defects, aortic stenosis, or tetanus vaccination? Why, these are not important when most backs (and I am not talking fullbacks or tailbacks) are misaligned and need diagnostic radiography and manipulation. Next, let's allow the spine guys on the sideline to evaluate players who get injured: spine adjustments for that anterior cruciate ligament tear.

Suggestion: Maybe send them to medical school first if they want to participate like doctors in the big game.

Teaching New Tricks to Old Dogs

I can't express how overjoyed a parent can become when listening to the 6 p.m. evening news daily (tongue in cheek). With the opportunity to learn not only about the latest war, tragedy, economic crisis, or healthcare crisis, we must also daily endure a barrage of dinnertime commercials to cure one of the hazards of aging. The big pharmaceuticals should be ashamed! Talk about destroying quality family dialogue with your high school or middle school daughter (a few in my household). Do you look forward to a nightly dinner discussion with your 16-year-old daughter about the critical importance of "Daddy, what is ED?" "I dunno, go ask your mother?"

Suggestion: Wake up, FCC! This advertising abomination belongs long after bedtime hours. This is tenfold worse than the Janet Jackson exposure. How about a stiff fine for their really bad taste and their license to licentiousness!

Of course, these are just my opinions; "I could be wrong"—to paraphrase Dennis Miller in *I Rant Therefore I Am*.

Tricks of the Trade for Managing Adolescents

(A report adapted from the *Infectious Diseases in Children* national meeting, February 2007. New York City)

> *You have to be a medical jack-of-all-trades to manage adolescents in your practice. That's according to Stan Block, MD, a clinical professor at the University of Louisville and the University of Kentucky, who spoke about the nuts and bolts of caring for adolescents at the 19th Annual Infectious Diseases in Children Symposium.*

"Teens crave adult opinion; they want your feedback. They desperately need us to tell them if they're doing well or not," said Block, who has been practicing in Kentucky for more than 40 years. When dealing with the adolescent patient, your knowledge must span the gamut from behavioral problems to sexual issues.

Optimal Adolescent Care

The demand for adolescent physicians is high in 2007. Only a smaller % of pediatricians are going into rural pediatric/adolescent medicine today compared with 14% in the past, according to Block, who considers this type of practice a great experience. "Finally, you have a patient who can talk with you, can interact with you. It's really fun," he said.

But when is the right time to suggest the teenager stop coming to their pediatrician? For some adolescent practices, it is 16 years of age, some 18 years, and some up to 23 years. "If they still want to come to you, don't chase them off," Block explained. "I feel honored they still want to visit with me."

The office itself plays a big role. When dealing with adolescents, the office should have separate waiting areas, paper gowns, curtains for privacy, non-baby tables, and stirrups. The visits may also be longer, so allow an extra 2 to 20 minutes per visit. The staff must be friendly, positive, and nonjudgmental, Block said.

A Pediatrician's Approach to Adolescents

Attention is key, but only through a nonjudgmental and non-condescending eye.

"You've got to coach them. I tell them, 'You need to do this,'" said Block, who said teens and adolescents really do listen. "You have to know that some teen girls are drama queens, but really most are sincere," said Block, who is a father of four daughters.

Update patient history on a regular basis. Block said one way to get the most from questions is to ask how things are affecting the teen. Examples include: How do you feel/mood? Are you happy lately? How are your grades? What activities are you doing after school? How are things going with your family?

Using open-ended questions can open up the discussion much more. Some additional tips to get the most out of each adolescent visit:

- Take a firm approach.
- Do not preach, but rather advise.
- Maintain good eye contact.
- Greet the adolescents warmly, for example, with a handshake and a smile.
- Use humor, if that is your style, but don't use it to belittle them.
- Try self-deprecation.
- Ask them about their day.
- Give compliments, especially for what they do right, such as grades or extracurriculars.
- Be somebody they can trust.

Handling the Parents

Confidentiality is very important for teens and adolescents, and also for parents. "I say, what you have to say to me is confidential unless you are going to hurt yourself," he said. There are many things kids in this age group won't say around their parents or adults in general, so gaining their trust is vital.

After age 14, parents may not need to be in the examination room for many problems, according to Block. But I like them to stay for the initial history and exam. If they want to be in the room, accommodate them, and then, perhaps after, ask them to leave to have the opportunity to speak with the teen alone. Remember, they will often just stand outside the door, trying to listen in. Be very aware of this for confidentiality reasons.

For gynecological, breast, and genital examinations, always have a nurse in the room. Also, it may be beneficial to have the opposite-sex physician available for the chance to give valuable wisdom from another point of view.

Back to School: The Underachiever and the Slow Learner

Your young patients have begun their annual trek back to school. Some gladly, some reluctantly. Some children and teenagers with educational problems may be brought into your office specifically for that particular evaluation. Others with educational problems will often be uncovered in your office by routinely obtaining a history, specifically asking, "How are your grades in school?" I suggest avoiding the too-generic inquiry, "How is school going?" as this will often lead to a monosyllabic answer such as "fine," even when the grades are Ds or Fs. Beauty is in the eye of the beholder, it seems. Another valuable question for the mother of an elementary-age child who is struggling: *At what age do you think that your child functions, relative to his peers?*

Whenever a student answers that he received more than one D or F letter grade, or a lot of "needs improvement," this should send up major red flags for you to obtain a more detailed educational and social history. You should also obtain any available recent report cards, achievement tests, and the rarely already performed psycho-educational tests. A recent vision and auditory evaluation is prudent as well. Thus, educational problems are an area where the resourceful pediatrician can be very helpful to the child's overall academic and emotional health.

ADHD follow-up leads to a discovery

This autumn, a 6-year-old boy is in your office for his biannual follow-up for a diagnosis of attention-deficit/hyperactivity disorder given by your office last year. You re-examine his initial ADHD checklists from early first grade, where he was noted by his parents and teachers to have significant issues with focusing and completing tasks, along with problems of disorganization and distractibility. At that time, his mother had no concerns about his level of work. Stimulant medication was prescribed, which improved his completion of schoolwork, and it also seemed to improve the amount of time spent on tasks and behavior. But during the year, he was still observed as struggling with his schoolwork.

At his 1-year medication follow-up near the end of first grade, the teacher commented on his ADHD checklists: *Puts anything down on assignments. Does not take time to try to figure things out. Does not ask for help.* When asked about his grades, the mother admitted that the teachers mostly evaluated his work as unsatisfactory or needs improvement. She also said he seems to be unable to keep up with his peers academically.

Being a perceptive and proactive pediatrician, you subsequently requested more formal psycho-educational testing due to his poor academic progress. You know that nearly 23% of students may be categorized as slow learners or with a borderline cognitive disability, according to Voight and colleagues. Although much inattention and distractibility were observed during his psychological testing, his intelligence testing revealed that he was functioning in the lower academic range, receiving an overall or full-scale IQ score of 75.

But what the heck does this mean to anybody but the psychologist? This is where you, as a pediatrician, are a key player in translating the techno-babble to parents.

Thus, this child was likely affected not only with a mild version of inattentive ADD, but also he could be categorized as a slow learner. This latter problem is among the most perplexing for the child, the parents, and the school. No formal educational avenues, programs, or remedial courses are readily available for the slow learner.

Definition of "slow learners"

The slow learner is generally considered a student who achieves a full-scale score between 70 and 85 (or 89) on formal IQ testing. This range of IQ is thus considered a borderline intellectual disability (cognitive impairment) or low-average intellectual capability. These IQ scores are not low enough (less than 70) to place them in the mild cognitive impairment group (old term = mild mental retardation). Nor is there usually enough discrepancy between their IQ and academic ability to place them in the learning disabled group as well. Surprisingly, this group of children may represent about 23% of the entire student population, compared with a rate of 5% to 10% for remediable learning disabilities in the population. Yet, you likely may not have observed such a high rate of slow learners in your private general pediatric practice.

The worrisome aspect of being a slow learner is the fact that they usually will not qualify for any special services, special education, or even a helpful individualized educational plan (IEP).

In the typical classroom setting, most teachers tailor their academic coursework to the average learner, who typically has an IQ of 90 to 110. These children, who are slow learners, are likely to struggle here. Thus, it is incumbent upon you as the pediatrician to help the family interpret what these lower IQ scores mean for the child's projected academic achievement.

Note that IQ scores have also been shown to be predictably stable over time. However, in some areas of academics, the child may show major scatter and spikes in different subjects. Meaning, for instance, that he may perform much better or much worse in verbal than in math or performance-type skills.

Critical Interpretation of Full-Scale IQ Scores

To further simplify it: an IQ of 75 means that an 8-year-old child will function intellectually overall at 75% of the average 8-year-old's intellectual functioning, i.e., at an average of a 6-year-old level. As he ages, he will commensurately function intellectually as a 12-year-old at age 16 years. This correlation continues to the assumed intelligence peak of an 18-year-old. Furthermore, it is important to remind parents that oftentimes the mental age will correlate well with the social maturity age as well. This lack of age-appropriate maturity, too, can lead to major problems in the classroom, with a lot of acting out, acting up, and acting unfocused.

Like most experts, I also think it is important to attempt to diagnose the slow learner before second grade.

The first reason early diagnosis is best is that it really helps parents to acknowledge the slower learning pace and to take the pressure off the child for not maintaining high academic achievement. In addition, one school tactic can be used. A controversial stopgap remedy may buy the child some vital extra time to gain some early additional academic and social competence and an early positive school experience. You may have the parents strongly consider holding back or retaining the child in kindergarten or first grade. However, any later grade retention is considered counterproductive by most experts.

At this younger age, I have rarely seen self-esteem issues with very early grade retention. And yet, the parents must be reminded that the child with an IQ of 70 or 75 will never fully catch up to his same-age peers. Thus, the discrepancy in academics with the early addition of one year chronologically (e.g., cognitively a 7 versus an 8-year-old) will eventually become more difficult to overcome and more noticeable (cognitively a 13-year-old versus a 16-year-old).

Corroborating this approach during the early academic career, Zoega and colleagues recently published data showing that students with later birthdays, i.e., the younger one-third of the classroom, tended to have more long-term academic struggles (language arts and mathematics) at age 9 years. The study also found that these children were 50% more likely to be placed on medication for ADHD. This usually results from their inability to perform their grade-level work and their social immaturity in the classroom.

Adolescent ADHD and the Ramifications of School Failure

You are seeing this very pleasant and articulate, previously healthy 15-year-old female from Loretto, KY, for the first time in 2 years for a sore throat. As part of your routine generic review of systems at this age, you briefly inquire not only about her menses, home life, boyfriends, and mood, but also about her schoolwork. You specifically ask about her grades to expedite your process in this limited amount of time. You receive some hesitancy from her and a monosyllabic reply of "OK." You ask her: "What specifically were your grades?" And she just looks at her mother and says, "You tell him."

You discover that she had two failing grades last year as a freshman, and that she has been struggling since high school began. But, she did very well in middle school with an A/B average. Her mother says that now she is always irritable and angers easily. She mopes around a lot and tries to avoid the family by going into her room alone most evenings. Your patient admits that she cries many days of the week.

However, you are actually quite impressed with her lofty goals for the future (as a physical therapist) and by her insightfulness, diction, and articulateness.

And her spaciness. How can this bright girl be barely surviving high school academically?

You now conjure up your quick and salient differential diagnoses for academic failure in high school that include:

- Inattentive ADD
- Drug abuse, particularly marijuana
- Slow learner
- Severe mood disorder or anxiety
- Home life chaos
- Adolescent adjustment reaction (severe rebellion)

You arrange for a follow-up visit the following week for further evaluation and discussion of the academics and mood issues. By then, you will have received her recent report cards, ACT/SAT standardized test scores, and achievement tests, along with some current ADHD checklists from a few teachers (an onerous task in itself during high school). Today, along with your streptococcal testing, you will also have obtained a current urine drug screen in your office (negative).

As you peruse her achievement scores, you are perplexed that most of her achievement scores were in the upper quartile for her grade, her ACT scores were 26 as a freshman, and her freshman grades were mostly Cs and Ds, with an A in chemistry. Her teachers' ADHD checklists were markedly positive for inattention, daydreaming, and even some defiance and sadness in the classroom.

After further discussion with the teenager, you surmise that she is afflicted with a moderately severe case of **inattentive ADHD**, along with some mild reactive depression and adolescent adjustment reaction issues.

In your experience, inattentive ADHD is the most common cause for school failure or underachievement in high school among female students who have otherwise average or above-average intelligence. Their academic potential may be commonly readily gleaned just by evaluating annual school achievement test scores, and somewhat by your attention to the student's diction and language. Furthermore, ADHD has been linked to low academic achievement, as the following two recent reports show.

These reports also seem to corroborate your observations about ADHD as a leading culprit in these cases of massive underachievement. Zoega and colleagues reported that among children with much later-treated ADHD versus ADHD treated by fourth grade, test performance scores from fourth grade to seventh grade declined by 73% in mathematics and by 43% in language arts. And the math decline was even worse among girls than boys.

Furthermore, Scheffler and colleagues reported a notable positive influence of ADHD medication upon mathematics and reading test scores during elementary school. With medication use, the academic gains were 0.19 and 0.29 school years, respectively, as early as the fifth grade alone. The authors pushed for the need for long-term studies regarding the influence of medication use in children with ADHD on academic achievement.

Treatment

After you discussed your appraisal of the 15-year-old's condition with both the patient and her mother, you felt quite comfortable that with successful ADHD medication treatment, her grades would likely show a profound improvement, likely into the A-B-C range. You also thought her reactive depression might also abate soon, as her academic struggles subsided; school was the unhappy situation where she spent the majority of her waking hours. You discussed the implications of treatment and the more common possible adverse effects, in particular, weight loss, appetite suppression, headaches, abdominal discomfort, and insomnia.

Regarding your medication selection, you told them that you did not want to be a policeman for drug diversion or prescription theft, a common problem for many stimulant drugs that you have observed for teen patients, even in "good" households. Therefore, you rarely prescribed the easily on-the-street-marketed Adderall products or short-acting methylphenidate. First line, you were going to use only longer-acting, difficult-to-divert first line stimulant drugs such as Concerta (Jansen), Vyvanse (Shire), or Focalin XR (Novartis), which would last 8 to 12 hours and could be used intermittently; or non-stimulant drugs such as atomoxetine (Strattera, Eli Lilly) or Qelbree (viloxazine, Supernus), which would last all day but required daily usage.

A urine drug screen would need to be obtained every 4 to 6 months or so. Any positive tests for illicit drugs would require you to abandon any further use of stimulant therapy. You also require follow-up every 3 to 4 months to monitor for dosage adjustments, pill usage, academic performance, and weight loss, etc.

Course

Within 3 months of initiating generic Concerta 36 mg daily, her grades have risen to the A-B honor roll category. Her irritability and bad moods have mostly subsided.

You have just experienced one of the more rewarding aspects of adolescent medicine—helping to totally turn around a bright young lady's academic and emotional life.

A Tale of Two Cities: Family Warfare and Global Warming

(Adapted from Block SL, A Tale of Two Cities: Family Warfare and Global Warming, *Infectious Disease in Children*, January 2006)

The protagonist of Charles Dickens' novel, *A Tale of Two Cities*, proclaimed: **"It was the best of times; it was the worst of times."** Dickens' era was marked by competing and contradictory attitudes toward government and rules. The era of adolescence is also similarly marred by this same attitude of contradictions—especially for a teenage girl toward her own form of government, specifically, her own mother.

Let me tell you two stories depicting this same "I hate you, I love you" attitude, as it was expressed by two memorable teenage girls. Just like the narrator of the Dickens novel, when I encounter a troubled adolescent girl in the office, I too must "ponder the secrets and mysteries that each human being poses to every other." And just like the theme used by Dickens, every troubled person in each room that we encounter likely possesses some dark secrets. Some will never be revealed. Others can be cajoled into divulging. Compressing all of this information into a single visit is daunting, but this may be our only opportunity to help.

The Worst of Times

"It was the spring of hope, it was the winter of despair."

On a typical busy November afternoon, I walked into the examination room to be greeted by Britt, a pert, smiling 14-year-old young lady, who had a subtle look of mischief in her eyes that only an experienced observer could detect. Her pleasant demeanor and affability were charming and disarming.

As is my custom, I initially listened to the parents' account of their teenager, with both parties present in the room. Her mother wanted to know if Britt needed counseling because she was caught sneaking out of the house late Saturday night, walking down a major thoroughfare in Nelson County. She added that Britt did not want to follow rules and "screamed and yelled a lot at her siblings, mother, and stepfather. She used to be on the honor roll at school, but now she had one C grade with A or B grades. A problem?" Her mother tearfully claimed that her defiance was "driving her crazy."

Finally, Britt blurted out, "She is being a stupid 'B'..." *Whoa, Britt. Give your mother a chance to tell her story, then I will give you your turn to explain your point of view while we are alone. Let's try to refrain from any mean words.* She cordially smiled at me and allowed us to continue.

Mother explained in detail that she had grounded Britt from the telephone, television, and activities for a month.

"So, how are other things going at home, Mom? Is everyone else getting along?" Britt interjected that "her mother is a perfectionist and over-controlling," which her mother did not deny. Her mother shifted in her seat and looked downward. She had forced the stepfather to leave the household last week due to his alcohol problems. She further admitted that she has not been very happy lately. I noticed that she looked somewhat despondent and even slightly disheveled.

I then asked to speak with Britt alone. Britt's smile returned, and she readily opened up about her situation. She enjoyed school, performing very well. She has had trouble sleeping, averaging about five hours of sleep nightly. She had a steady boyfriend of one month, but she denied a physical relationship, as she was not allowed to date yet. She also denied any recent depression, although last year she was cutting her arm, which she said she has not done for over a year. Her emotional outlet has been drawing and writing, as she did not like athletics. She further denied any sexual intercourse, rape, molestation, or bullying problems.

During the conversation, she appeared to possess an amazing wisdom and insight beyond her age as she discussed her family life. She said she was actually quite happy, as long as she was out of the home or with her friends—"and away from that alcoholic!"

What initiated your idea to run away this weekend?

This weekend, her stepfather had rejoined them, and she "really despised him." Then the trouble began. Challenging her curfew that night, her defiance led to a screaming argument, which escalated to the point where her stepfather had accidentally pushed her back. She immediately bolted out of the house and began running down the street.

I noticed multiple light bruises on her arm. So, I pointed them out to her. She said matter-of-factly: "Oh, I had refused to get out of the car to go into school yesterday. So, Mom was trying to drag me out of the car. I guess I resisted too much."

Later, I had the mother rejoin us in the room. With Britt's permission, I discussed the multiple issues with the two of them present.

Let's look at the global picture regarding Britt. Britt is actually doing quite nicely outside of your household issues. She is actually doing well in school, has many friends, gets along with her teachers, and her mood is generally good when not arguing with her parents. She has a delightful, spunky personality, which, although a challenge for a parent, and is quite bright and keeps up her attractive appearance. She isn't doing drugs or running around with a worrisome crowd. She loves her mother and siblings. Her attitude is sometimes challenging and often approaches that of a 2-year-old with a tantrum. But that was commonplace at her age.

Then I discussed some approaches to Britt's behavior, including continuing with the good limits her parents had already set, more negotiating with her on some minor limits, using a modified "time out," or going to separate rooms when arguments escalated, praising her good deeds, and avoiding any physical discipline. Unfortunately, I had to warn the mother (with the daughter listening) that any further physical discipline issues with the daughter would likely result in a protective services visit. She was much too old for this form of discipline to have any beneficial effect. I asked that this message be relayed to all caregivers as well. They both agreed that this was totally uncharacteristic of him. I would be happy to help them get counseling, which I highly recommended, particularly for the mother, who seemed so stressed and anxious. She actually had the heaviest burden, dealing with an alcoholic spouse.

Britt also agreed never to "run" again, with its inherent dangers in the middle of the night for a young girl. Instead, she would seek a safe haven from a relative or go to her room and contact help. I asked the family to return in a few weeks to update their progress. Sadly, she did not show up later. During a follow-up telephone call by our nurse, Britt said, "Things were somewhat better. No problems with the stepfather so far." The upbeat nuance was still in her voice. The nurse asked her mother to arrange for a follow-up appointment. None was ever obtained. Hopefully, "the winter of [maternal] despair" had not squelched "the spring of hope" in Britt.

Britt's situation is a common complicated example, and it shows again that adolescents can have emotional and behavioral problems, especially when they grow up in a stressful environment. For Britt, the issue at hand is to ensure a steady support system that gives her emotional outlets while working on her behavioral issues. I advise that we continue exploring family counseling for both Britt and her mother, as it seems that her mother is also in need of support for her anxiety and stress. Also, having a trusted adult or therapist to talk to about her feelings of anger and frustration will go a long way in helping her in the long run. The stepfather must agree to our terms as well.

The Best of Times

"It was the age of wisdom, it was the age of foolishness."

The very bright-eyed, somewhat obese, petulant 18-year-old young lady, Kate, was sitting beside her mother, as I casually introduced myself to both her and her mother. She was neatly groomed with a somewhat gothic appearance, dressed in black. She had a moderate, productive cough, but was otherwise healthy. I inquired as to why Kate was here. The mother said that Kate was failing two of six courses in school. Kate immediately began to contradict her mother about the level of failure, with her voice rising 20 decibels.

The mother continued, "Is there anything you can do to help her with her academic problems?" Kate was not turning her work in and failing most of her tests. Her grades were entirely As and Bs last year. Her mood was generally upbeat outside of her mother's interactions with her. "Does she have attention-deficit disorder, a learning disability, a drug problem, or depression? She is going to fail this semester."

Using a little academic "CSI": So, how did she score on her ACTs (or achievement tests, etc.)? *She scored a 28.*

Really?!?

"She still wants to go to college," Mom acknowledged quizzically. Yes, getting two Fs does not endear oneself to the college admissions person, I suggested.

Any outside activities?

No sports. However, she had the second-leading role in her school play, which, by the way, received a second-place award in the state high school competition. Kate's mother worked as a teacher. Her father had just opened and was managing a new restaurant. His dream finally came true. He was working mostly nights there as well. Her 12-year-old brother was usually at home with their sister, while Kate watched over him very carefully.

Kate's case is a common problem for older adolescents who are desperate for attention, but might not know how to ask for it appropriately. Kate's academic problems are probably a reaction to her mother's absence because of work and her feeling of being overrated, although reasonably capable and smart. I would advise that Kate and her mother attempt to re-establish an emotional closeness, and to seek better balance between family time and work responsibilities. An important part of what will help Kate is also providing her with a healthy way to satisfy her emotional needs, i.e., the continuing therapy or family counselling that will help Kate resolve her need for attention and minimize the dramatic expression of these feelings in the form of failure in studies.

It is equally important for her now to receive treatment for her pneumonia and advice regarding her contraceptive choice properly. Nothing is ever simple with teenage girls, it seems.

Alone with Kate...

Smiling, she said her mood is good, she thoroughly enjoys her thespian roles, and she actually loves her mother and father. So, what other problems are going on? No boyfriend issues, no drug use or experimentation, only recently sexually active.

"You won't tell my mom, will you?"
"Between you and me only. What kind of contraception are you using?"
"*Condoms alone. But my current period is normal.*"

Showing slight tears, "My mom is never home, since they took over the restaurant. She is always at the restaurant six days a week, and I even have to go up there and wait for them often. She never has time for me. Dad even missed my play."

Ouch!

So you are telling me that a bright young lady like yourself, who can easily do her schoolwork, is actually failing on purpose. Just to get your mom's attention??? She agreed to allow me to discuss the family time issues with her mother.

Mother was shocked that Kate had created this academic mess for herself. As the true "drama queen," this was her theatrics for help and for much more time from her mother. *But at age 18?* Mom grilled me. Yes, having raised four teenage daughters, even older daughters often really do still thrive on your undivided maternal (and paternal) attention. They still need their Mommas, I explained. But this was a positive sign, actually, as it indicated that her daughter loved her deeply and still valued her.

I complimented them both for her successes, as Kate was actually well-adjusted, capable, and avoiding most of the common potential teenage troubles. I suggested that the two of them work out a plan for "daughter time" and less restaurant time for Kate's sake, and eventually, just as importantly, for their upcoming adolescent boy, who was going to need more than cursory supervision after school these next several years.

"What about her cough, Doc?"

Time is pressing, now.

Yes, she did have pneumonia on my quick examination. She will need antibiotics for a few days, and a follow-up visit for this illness (and an ethically standard confidential plan for contraceptive counseling) next week.

The mother thanked me profusely, along with her daughter, as they shuffled out the door, warmly hugging each other.

It is a far, far better thing that I do, than I have ever done...

Humpty-Dumpty and the Hidden Agenda

(Adapted from Block SL, Humpty-Dumpty and the Hidden Agenda, *Infectious Disease in Children*, September 2005)

> Humpty-Dumpty sat on a wall.
> Humpty-Dumpty had a great fall.
> All the king's horses and all the king's men
> Couldn't put Humpty together again."
> —children's Mother Goose rhyme

Some things are just not learned in medical school. Like how to age gracefully. I am not getting older. That, my friends, is the truest fiction that my mind can concoct. But it seems as though lately, I often see the children of my former patients.

Some could misconstrue this as my aging process. But I look at this "glass half-full" phenomenon as the ultimate compliment a physician could receive, and I ignore the derogatory chiding. I also interpret this to mean that I had treated these former patients so well that they want to bring back their own special progeny to seek my sage advice, my superb clinical acumen, and, well, let's be honest, to hear me crack my inane self-deprecatory jokes and make fun of my goofiness again. And since our practice has a stable population base, I may see parents who are my former patients for about two-thirds of the day.

This phenomenon also provides me with some incredible rapport, which may be used advantageously sometimes.

Two Sisters with Unexplained Nosebleeds

Two sisters, ages 3 and 10, presented to my office with moderately severe nosebleeds, respectively. They were both asymptomatic otherwise. As I routinely do in these common bleeding issues, I inquired about other bleeding problems, such as bruising, gum bleeds, easy bleeding, swollen joints, fevers, cough, "knots", aspirin or frequent ibuprofen use, allergies, nose picking, family history of bleeding, and other medications. All were negative.

My physical examination was completely negative, including any tiny "spider hemangiomas" on the skin, except for some raw, scabbed mucosal tissue in the anterior nasal septum area. In fact, as I was finishing my exam, blood started pouring out of her right nostril, which required me to pack it with some gauze in the office. It was quite an alarming amount of bleeding that happened spontaneously. We discussed how to compress the soft part of the nose (alae) for 5 minutes to stop the bleeding and to "paint" the nasal septum twice daily with some Vaseline.

Due to mom's frustration and the transient copious bleeding I witnessed, I referred her to the ENT doctor and to the hematologist for further evaluation. First, I obtained the usual blood work and only found a mildly elevated PTT. This is one of four major laboratory hematology parameters that we initially obtain by venipuncture to evaluate for bleeding disorders, such as severe bruising or nosebleeds, in children. However, this is the rarest bleeding parameter to find abnormal, as it signifies some very rare clotting deficiency down the pathway to clotting or coagulation, unlike the more commonly uncovered platelet deficiency or elevated protime (think Coumadin or Eliquis anti-clotting drugs).

Further History

The girls' grandmother was from Romania, where herbal therapies are rampantly used in everyday home remedies. I never did find out which home concoction she had been feeding the two girls, and Mom would not reveal it either. However, Mom made her stop the next day after our discussion, and the problem was resolved within a few days.

An Unusual Encounter

The story doesn't end here. This family is the same as the one I encountered on a late evening visit to Walmart. As I was walking with my daughter by the women's clothing department, I heard a beckoning: "Dr. Block, how are you tonight?" she excitedly exclaimed. "I just had my knee surgery 3 weeks ago for my severe knee tear. And my scar looks great. Do you want to see it?" Before I could respond, she turned around with her back to me, flipped up her leg sleeve, and revealed her surgical scar. "It looks great," I replied. "They did a really good job on you. Most impressive. I'm glad you did well." Meanwhile, her prepubertal children were fidgeting and toying with some of the dresses hanging from the racks, but overall behaving well.

And I was left in a somewhat embarrassed state of shock. In the middle of open racks of women's dresses, I just commented, "How nice it was to see you," and continued pushing my cart, hunting for motor oil for my lawnmower.

Beaters and Cutters: The Underworld of the Teenage Girl

(Adapted from Block SL, Beaters and Cutters: The Underworld of the Teenage Girl, in *Infectious Disease in Children*, April 2007)

Today, a year later, while she was in the office, I joked with her that she was one of my more memorable and favorite patients. As unpredictable as a seething cobra, I joked to myself.

Undergarments

On a cold, dreary February morning last year, in a very common scenario, the agitated 14-year-old girl presented with her three-month history of headaches, presumptively migraine in origin. I have visited with her in the office since she was a newborn. She was well-groomed, slightly overweight, and was wearing the typical youth "beater" shirt, sometimes worn by her sex and age group—an Archie Bunker-style half tee shirt/tank top.

She had called the office numerous times in the last few months, asking for pain medications and some form of relief from her multitudinous migraine headaches, one of which was precipitated by an episode of streptococcal pharyngitis in December. The headaches were often associated with nausea, vomiting, photophobia, and phonophobia. She obtained some relief with zolmitriptan (Zomig, AstraZeneca) 2.5 mg tablets. The thought of narcotic-seeking behavior had entered my mind.

But I am still concerned about the possibility that her latest prescription for birth control patches for her dysmenorrhea and irregular menses may be exacerbating the problem. So last month, I tried to switch her to the etonogestrel/ethinyl estradiol vaginal ring (NuvaRing, Organon), which she must insert intravaginally. Normally, I would never suggest this formulation for such a young teenager, but this young lady is fairly mature and comfortable with this concept, as I had already fished around for her willingness to try it as an option.

Once again, she is in the office complaining of frequent headaches occurring once or twice weekly.

Cardinal Rules for Superman

Cardinal rule one (pediatric neurology): Unexplained recurrent headaches always deserve a thorough funduscopic (back of the eye) examination. Voila, spontaneous venous pulsations on the sharp optic nerve disc are visualized. The remainder of the cranial nerves is normal, as is the remainder of her brief neurologic examination.

Cardinal rule two (Jimmy Simon, MD): Always perform a thorough physical examination. I finally cajoled her to remove her sweatshirt over the T-shirt for my complete examination.

"But why, Dr. Block? Can't I just lift it up?"

As I teased her: "I am a super-doctor, but not Superman! I do not possess X-ray vision! So you will need to remove your heavy, tight sweatshirt and put on the gown, or you can just leave on your polo and 'beater.'" (Note that the beater has no psychological or sociological meaning for these young girls, so do not try to read much into this fashion undergarment statement.)

Under the Garments: Cut to the Quick

Underneath the garment sleeves, this hides: She had multiple small linear 4 cm to 6 cm old healing cuts on her left forearm-palmar aspect. (They are never on the right forearm, unless she is ambidextrous or left-handed.)

"And how did this happen?" (The usual girl response is: "The cat or dog scratched me," or "I just scraped myself on the door, trampoline, pipe, etc.") With this simple query, she promptly and unexpectedly popped up and stormed out of the room, hissing and fuming like a cat confronted by a barking dog.

Alone

So there I sat, alone with my chart. Decision time: sit alone, move on to the next patient, or search for a hormonally self-hijacked patient? I will usually wait about a minute to see if the girl will return. Then I will peek out into the hallway to determine whether she has vacated the premises.

And yes, this type of patient vitriolic exodus may happen to me about once or twice a year, usually whenever the topic becomes too uncomfortable for the teenager. In this case, as is the usual sequence, she was standing just outside the doorway, and I merely re-invited her, in an affable tone, to come back in and visit with me.

Despite my reassurances and calming demeanor, during this visit, she again became upset and stomped out of the room for a few seconds. Finally, I cajoled her that I just needed to ask her a few simple questions. I was trying to help her. She adamantly denied any sadness or depression, school or family problems.

Cardinal Rule Three: Never discuss "cutting" with the parent in the room—initially. These young ladies really appreciate the opportunity for confidentiality and to be treated as adults. Nothing alienates them more than when a physician "exposes" them in front of their parents. But they are eventually warned that their parents must be notified if the girl is a danger to herself or suicidal. And yet, most cutting events are considered major signs of depression or dangerous impulsivity.

I explained to her that I often see teenage girls who try to cut themselves when they are in pain emotionally, depressed, upset with a boyfriend or parent, or tormented by a previous rape or molestation. She said she was not suffering from any of this, but she did admit she was rarely happy lately. She denied any suicidal thoughts or attempts. I then moved on to my next topic for the self-tormented.

Fortunately, although denying any alcohol use, I was able to get her to discuss her recent marijuana dabbling. Her brother, whom I also have taken care of, was a somewhat nefarious drug peddler in the area.

Cardinal Rule Four: Whenever a teenager admits to using marijuana, quantify the frequency of use. For instance, a declaration of once a month often means weekly usage; once a week, most days use; and only on weekends, daily use. This is some kind of teenage exponential mathematical equation to rationalize that the real frequency is not as bad as they would have you think.

I then discussed the negative impact that marijuana was likely having on her mood and her grades. It was making her more depressed, sad, and irritable. She was bickering constantly with her mother, who was once her best friend. And this very bright young lady, who was previously on the honor roll, was barely passing academically this year. Her short-term memory was zapped. The lack of a stable father figure was further exacerbating her cloudy judgment. I figured she was, in part, with the highs, trying to escape the pain of this hole in her life as well.

I further attempted to explain to her that her father's absence was not her fault in any way... to buffer the egocentric magical thinking so common even in this age group.

Tempest in a Teapot

I have dealt with way too many young teenagers during their mercurial rages, both in the office and at home. So being a battle-worn veteran of many youthful estrogen eruptions, I always remain calm and, in Pollyanna fashion, anticipate the best will happen for my young patients if only I am patient too—for days or months.

Nonetheless, in too much of a funk, I decided to cut my losses here and have her return in a few weeks under the guise of checking on her headaches and to consider possibly starting her on some beta-blockers daily for her migraines, and MAYBE even a selective serotonin reuptake inhibitor antidepressant like zoloft, if the mood was a persisting problem. She seemed to comprehend much of what I explained earlier and shockingly gave me a hug at the conclusion of the visit.

Denouement

The headaches did not abate over the next few days, and I suggested by phone that we go ahead and start some daily beta blocker atenolol prophylaxis (no history of asthma) daily to see if we could prevent the attacks.

Much to my pretentious shock, when she returned in the next month, her teenage sparkle and joviality were evident again. Her headaches were much improved with the daily atenolol. She admitted that she had abandoned all her marijuana smoking. She was not having outbursts at home, and she actually said that she and her mother were getting along quite well. And proudly, her grades were rising to the A and B range since she had discontinued her illicit smoking habit. She even now laughed at dumb Dr. Block's wisecracks.

I still see this young lady frequently in the office and even out in public, and she always goes out of her way to talk with me and is quite affable. Today, in the office for her recurrent vomiting and abdominal pain, she continues to show impressive maturity with her perceptions of her schoolwork and her special relationship with her single mother. She is a survivor. And she is one less victim of that "recreational" drug.

Now, as for that recurrent vomiting and lower abdominal pain precipitating today's visit, I had to inform her that all indicators point toward the estrogen in her patches, in light of her negative mega-workup thus far. She may need to change to a non-estrogen contraceptive. But no fit was triggered today. Rather, she just said, "I hate you, Dr. Block, for making my life miserable again." And she giggled.

Marijuana Use: Adverse Effects

In my practice, I often explain the following to the teenage boys and teenage girls.

First, we need to inquire about his frequency of marijuana use. Is it once a month, weekly, or weekends only? As opposed to the hardcore user, rare recreational use is a cause for monitoring him in your office with repeat drug screens and simple counseling and questioning. I triple the rate of frequency that he may tell me, in order to get a better estimate of the actual use, which they really downplay. How long has he been using it? Even though he will often tell you that his friends "just give it to him," he is very soon going to need to start stealing and shoplifting to support his habit if he is smoking regularly. Some girls will barter their bodies in exchange for drugs, especially if they graduate to the harder drugs.

MJ is about 4-6x more potent than it was 3 decades ago due to modern farming hybridization techniques, so that a typical joint has tremendously more pharmacologic and brain effects, accentuating the following:

Even short-term MJ use is highly associated with a high rate of academic decline and school failure. It markedly impairs short-term memory so that simple academic memorization efforts become laborious and unmanageable.

A recent study from Australia showed that chronic MJ users who initiated before age 18 y.o., dropped their overall IQ scores by about 6 points compared with controls. This is a significant loss. Very few of us can afford to become stupider. This chronic group also suffers from long-term brain changes, which often lead to an "apathetic syndrome" that I called "burned out whoopers." And long-term use has also been associated with a notable increased risk (4x) for chronic schizophrenia—an extremely mentally crippling disease. Lastly, chronic use is highly associated with decreased libido, decreased sperm counts, and male gynecomastia (or growing breasts). Heterosexual boys may even start losing romantic interest in girls.

Finally, MJ is definitely a gateway drug into all sorts of other, more dangerous, more expensive, and more socially detrimental drugs, as the youngster's addiction escalates and becomes more costly. Now you have to become the drug dealer, the drug distributor, and deal with an extremely dangerous criminal element. We have had several boys shot to death in our community in "drug deals gone wrong" over simple $25 negotiations or claims of inferior MJ.

And two clinical pearls for us: suspect MJ use as a major culprit for vague anterior chest wall pain unrelated to costochondritis or pleurisy, for example. It is related to the tachycardia created by this higher potency MJ, and possibly some "lacing" by your non-FDA-approved, dirty-fingered MJ dealer. Thus, any unexplained chest pains in adolescence bear confidential questioning about recent or frequent MJ use by the patient. And chronic MJ use in adults has been recently reported to be associated with a significantly increased risk for heart attacks.

When one encounters a patient with chronic severe recurrent vomiting, one should be very suspicious that they have become a victim of MJ-induced hyperemesis. Ask questions and get a urine drug screen. The only cure here is to stop MJ use totally, and it takes weeks to return to normal.

For the higher than "recreational" user, I really suggest additional screening for chronic depression, anxiety, family discord, academic failure (especially ADD untreated), and sexual abuse.

The Hurried Pediatrician Versus 'The Hurried Child'

Pediatricians are all inundated with all the normal checkups at this time of year, but they can also have serious health issues that warrant attention.

The Power of the Human Spirit in Our Youngsters Never Ceases to Amaze Me

Much has been written about the problems with raising the "hurried child," as first written by David Elkind in 1981. Parents often feel pressured to have their child become the "top dawg" or "Superkid" in their child's class. This elite thinking has fostered classical music in utero, Baby Einstein TV for infants and toddlers, parents spending fortunes for kindergarten classes, boarding prep schools for middle and high school, multiple AP courses, and, of course, the obligatory expensive SAT preparatory classes with a goal for admissions to the penultimate college of choice. But, this is so far removed from the reality for over 90% of the children and teenagers in my rural practice that they may as well be referring to the physics of aerodynamics, or the neurotransmitters of the amygdala.

MYWorld.com

I practice in rural Kentucky, where we are proud of the many children who go on to attend a state college (who do a fine job by the way, as 3 of my daughters proved) or technical school; still, some may go on to high-powered colleges as well. And proud happily, for instance, of the two hundred teenage girls annually who decide to go on birth control and prevent premature pregnancy (some with a 20-year-old controlling boyfriend), or of those who have troubled backgrounds and who attend advanced school without first passing through a detention center or running away, or of the neglected boy who decides to avoid his drug-using cohorts, or of the depressed teenage girl with attention-deficit/hyperactivity disorder who finally stops "cutting," or of the borderline intellect 13-year-old trying to fit in with her classmates.

With almost one-half of our young patients on Medicaid, we are talking about a slice of a more mainstream America. Yes, welcome to a large part of my world, which is not quite "Wayne's World—One world, One party!" as Dana Carvey has exhorted.

Sure, in my world, we also have the many child prodigies, the well-balanced adolescents, the aspiring artists, the hard-working middle schoolers. We take care of the full representative spectrum of socioeconomic status, psychological personalities, and intellectual abilities.

Perhaps this new patient today lisped, or she walked with some noticeable knock knees. Ok, a lot. We can handle that. But I have a more urgent caveat at hand for my colleagues—the "hurried child" in a pediatric office.

I will assume that your pediatric practice is friendly and provides typical first-rate care to all of your patients. Yet, you are now dealing with not only all the normal children and checkups, but the conundrum of "caregiver casualties. " For instance, the co-sleeping, the nighttime bottle-feeding, and toddlers' or teens' out-of-control tantrums; the sicker, time-consuming babies during the multiple epidemics of respiratory syncytial virus, norovirus, enterovirus, or influenza virus. Thus, it becomes quite easy to make many of your patients a "hurried child" during your daily clinical schedule.

My Triple Play

It is a dreary, rainy January day. The influenza epidemic has hit. You know this because school absenteeism far exceeds the school threshold for fiscal sustainability, and they have closed some schools in your area.

You are seeing almost five to six patients an hour, which is really burning your tile floors. This is sustainable, as long as it is not interspersed with your typical behavioral or an ADHD child who is more problematic than usual. You begin drifting down the hallway to see a "triple."

You are currently two patients behind in the schedule, and the previous mother let you know that her time was as valuable as yours. The audacity of making her wait for half an hour with a fussy infant!

Moving along, and somewhat brow-beaten, let's get through the "triple" and make up some time here.

Cutting Corners Just Does Not Feel Right. Can you be so cursory?

The "directed examination" for an acute illness is a godsend to the "hurried pediatrician." This means you can forgo many of the finer examination details, if needed, such as the heart, the abdomen, and the partially exposed skin.

The Ill Toddler

You pick the sickest of the three children first.

The first sibling you quickly examine is a 38-month-old boy with a fever and cough. He looks ill, but more like influenza than bacteremia. He has a bulging acute otitis media. His lungs and heart are normal. His abdomen is non-tender, skin is without rash. Still, you want to obtain a CBC on him in light of his 103.5°F fever. You have been "burned" before—by the missed occult bacteremia in a febrile toddler.

You are not quite satisfied with all that you surmise about his condition. You have two other siblings to evaluate, and so you will still have a few minutes to mull over whether to intrepidly order the chest radiograph, the blood culture, and heaven forbid, the rare urine culture in a toddler boy. (Most guys hate to think about the trauma of a male catheterization.) You try to explain your complex line of thinking to the mother. Exasperated, you explain that you will obtain the CBC first and then order more tests as indicated.

"Rales" Against the Wind

Second, you graduate to his 15-year-old sister, who has a fever of 102°F and looks wiped out. Her examination reveals normal ears, mildly reddened pharynx, and mild non-tender anterior cervical lymphadenopathy.

She has some lung crackles, or "rales", in his left base, along with a normal heart and abdomen. His skin is also clear of rashes.

You explain to the mother that she has "walking" pneumonia, which may be related to one of the following: the influenza itself, a secondary serious bacterial infection from the influenza, or a primary mycoplasma or *Chlamydia pneumoniae* infection. You would like to order a CBC on her as well, and perhaps a rapid influenza test. You will likely still treat her with azithromycin to cover for the atypical bacteria commonly causing milder pneumonia. (Now, with all these complicated issues, you feel like you are drowning in a sea of diagnoses and tests, as you will still have to later explain the results for both children.)

The Hurried Child

Third, you begin to examine the 18-year-old sister, who is smiling and teasing her younger brothers. Finally, some relief—let's make up some time here. You realize that you are upset with the nurse who put all three patients in a single room. Your policy is always to separate the teenagers by gender, and for each teenager, a private room. Still, it is a wild flu day.

The young lady promptly asks you, before you can even pick up your otoscope, about her 10 pimples on her face, which she says "really bother her." A brief acne discussion ensues about the three classes of topicals she could use. Finally, on to the examination of this healthy-looking girl! So far, her examination is normal except for the clear rhinorrhea, and she has no neck lymphadenopathy. Her lungs are clear to auscultation, so you make the subconscious decision to forego examining her heart and abdomen. You begin to discuss with the mother and daughter that she looks fine. She merely has a mild upper respiratory infection, and she can just use over-the-counter cold medications. (You ponder, "So why is she really here, with all these sick kids?")

Better to Be Lucky Than Good

Something gnaws at you. It is the twinge of the beastly OCD that made you a good medical student, resident, and clinician.

But in your very early career, you never had to examine more than 15 to 20 patients in a day. The specter of your vigilant former attending, or your chief of service (i.e., Jimmy Simon, MD), and your guilty conscience, raises its troubling head. You should really complete the full "directed examination." Cutting corners just does not feel right. *What would your superb, respected chief of service say about you being cursory?*

So you ask the young lady if you can quickly examine her heart and abdomen, as you mumble an excuse about getting distracted with all the family commotion in a triangle of sibling rivalries. She throws you an "ice queen" stare as you apologize profusely.

"Does this mean that THEY are going to stay in the room?" "No, we can pull the curtain and make them stand behind it." (Meanwhile, you mutter to yourself about your nurse not separating them in different rooms per your custom.) After a Shakespearean thought of "much ado about nothing," you proceed to find a normal cardiac examination.

Your face turns pale, however, as you palpate her abdomen. Both the liver and spleen edges are about 8 cm below each respective costal (rib) margin. (Very enlarged.) You start sweating.

Having practiced pediatrics for more than two decades, you realize that now you are really in for a lengthy and critical discussion. This is serious. You sit down and ask the mother if you can also obtain a CBC from her daughter, while remaining as calm and collected as possible. (Your office lab is now threatening a strike.)

The obligatory why, and what does this mean, and what could it be, all confront you.

"Let's get all the lab results first." Your office schedule is now doomed.

A half hour later, between two acute illnesses, you sit down with the entire family and discuss CBCs. The middle girl's CBC is normal, but the younger sibling has a high WBC of 22,000. So you explain the need for a "traumatizing" blood culture and an injection of ceftriaxone for the possible occult bacteremia and certain severe acute otitis media, and a child who fights oral medication, too.

The list is as long as your arm!

Dreading the next finding, the daughter's CBC, you explain the findings and that you need her to see the "blood specialist" immediately. Her total WBC, hemoglobin, and platelets are very low (1,500 cells/mm^3, 8.5 mg/dl, 45,000 cells/mm^3, respectively).

Then the ultimate question emerges: "Could this be cancer, Doctor?"

You always preface your response with the following: "Whenever I encounter a really abnormal CBC and physical findings like your daughter's..."

"Hope springs eternal," some poet (Alexander Pope) once wrote (1733).

The guardian/parent usually acknowledges with body language the seriousness of the possible diagnoses, and tends not to want to pin you down for the ultimate diagnosis. The possible diagnoses causing the problem constitute "a list as long as my arm." (Show your long arm) "...I just do not know for certain. Perhaps, since you mentioned it, cancer is possible, but further tests must be performed first. That is why I intend to send your daughter down to my good friends, the blood specialists at the children's hospital, for definitive testing. I will make certain that you get the evaluation started TODAY," you emphasize.

You say this for three semi-selfish reasons: First, this type of result probably warrants immediate in-hospital observation for possible secondary sepsis, bleeding, etc. Second, the parents are entirely and rightfully freaked out by the possibility of cancer. The quicker you get going, the sooner the angst is settled. The wait becomes interminable. Third, you do not want to be the bad guy with the final bad news, because you do not know with certainty. You are not always correct, either, with overwhelming evidence, as you will soon read. You are also letting them know the urgency of the situation.

Sitting down face-to-face, you allow the shock to settle in and some tears to flow. Amazingly, most mothers are able to restrain their total terror, for the sake of not horrifying their child again.

A year later, her mother thanks you again for "saving her life." She knows that you likely knew all along that day.

And today, a year later, the elder daughter has a simple URI again. Her entire examination is basically normal, except for some rhinorrhea. You do not complain in your mind about her eating up your time with a minor illness. You are proud of her indomitable spirit. You do not hurry today, and you sit and chat for quite a while to catch up on her progress. She is a special young lady. Now, what was I saying about raising "super kids?"

Let's hope that "A.L.L." ends well, like a Shakespeare play. Yes, she had acute lymphoblastic leukemia (ALL) as you suspected, which is now in remission. You are proud to be a part of her life.

The Well-Child Checkup: Bright Futures or Dim Economics?

(Adapted from Block SL, The Well-Child Checkup: Bright Futures or Dim Economics? *Infectious Diseases in Children,* May 2005)

The well-child checkup is the bread and peanut butter and jelly of pediatric practice.

Although both things are often sticky and messy, without checkups, general pediatricians would become like the proverbially advertised Maytag repairmen—twiddling their thumbs a lot.

As their primary care pediatrician, we perform a host of valuable services for each of our patients—advocating and providing immunizations, along with dispensing sage advice about safety, child development, and lifestyle. However, like my wife's daunting "to-do list" for each Saturday, the laundry list of 20 to 30 items for discussion advocated by the AAP (American Academy of Pediatrics) "Bright Futures" policy for preventive care has become overly quite time-consuming.

Within the span of about 15 to 20 minutes, we are supposed to allow parents to ask multiple open-ended questions about child care and dispense a laundry list of advice, which must usually be learned on the job, as an editorial by Stein and Stanton in the April 2005 *Journal of Pediatrics* surmises. Next, what will the Medicaid cuts do to your bottom line with all this time spent counseling?

So, what can we do? Should we skimp on the physical examination? The open-ended questions? The litany of advice? The exchange of pleasantries? I can emphasize firsthand that we had better not shortcut or relinquish the physical examination, even for seemingly minor problems or healthy children. "Artificial intelligence" will never replace the pediatrician. Never.

Case Vignettes

A) The Time Crunch

In my allotted 15 minutes for a newborn check-up, I was discussing the routine issues about breastfeeding, later introduction of solids, importance and safety, and adverse effects of vaccines, sibling rivalry/jealousy, "back to sleep," etc., with the mother of a growing 1-month-old infant. Winding down, time had become quite short, so I wondered if I should just examine the "major" systems?

In the case of our 1-month-old infant under discussion, the otherwise normal exam did reveal that the abdomen had some significant hepatosplenomegaly. Oops! My face became drained. I feared something dreadful was wrong, and this perceptive mother, as a health care worker, sensed it. She asked me, "What could it be?" Taking my usual non-alarmist position, I answered with my customary, "I don't know. The list of problems is as long as my arm. Let me perform some more tests." So, then I asked her to submit her child to a venipuncture for CBC and serum chemistries and an abdominal ultrasound. (Trust and rapport are so critical.) So, my "routine checkup" may have saved this child's life. The incidence of this disease is about one in 500,000. Yes, you read that correctly.

B) Famous Last Words

Last month, an intelligent, charming 13-year-old female, who is active on her high school soccer and softball teams, returned for a check-up because one of her knees was still bothering her. On her routine sports exam eight months previously, she was complaining of bilateral knee pain, and her otherwise normal knee examination revealed an obviously painful unilateral tibial tuberosity, consistent with **Osgood-Schlatter's** disorder— a diagnosis we probably observe twice weekly in our heavily adolescent-populated practice. She was instructed to rest her knee when needed, and to use NSAIDs (Aleve) as necessary. But she was also asked to return if the problem worsened or significant changes occurred.

Although her father thought that she had the same problem of atypical gout as he suffered from in his youth, the daughter had normal serum uric acid and no other pattern suggestive of gout. After a two-month interlude of near-normal sports activity, the mother again became worried about the recurrence of her daughter's knee pain. But my cardinal rule is always: **listen to the mother**. The daughter's current examination revealed a complete resolution of the findings of Osgood-Schlatter's disorder. Now she had mild pain with compression or motion of her patella and a slight knee effusion. We concluded the visit, in which I had discussed her presumptive chondromalacia patella, but also her acne flare-up, her oligomenorrhea, and her dysmenorrhea—each of which required prescriptions. At the end, she implores, "But Doctor Block, this week she has begun crying whenever she straightens her knee." My antenna perked up.

Hysterical teenager? Manipulative teenager? I observed that when her knee was fully extended, tears rolled for the first time. This was not my usual case of chondromalacia patella. Spooked by a gut reaction and a healthy respect for adolescent female lacrimation (in the office!), I ordered a radiograph of the knee. The incidence of this disease is one in 200,000.

C) A "Spinous Process" or Medical Process?

A family friend of mine—a quiet, athletic, attractive brunette—saw my partner for her soccer sports physical. She is one of a minority of students in our area who sought her sports physical from her regular pediatrician, rather than the cut-rate "quickie" physical by the chiropractor in the school gymnasium. Yes, chiropractors have been granted the privilege to perform sports physicals by many state legislatures, including Kentucky and California.

Her rapid but thorough examination here revealed just a few too many bruises for our pediatrician's comfort. The CBC was abnormal, and as uncovered, he may have saved this girl's life from either hemorrhage or infection.

Do you suppose the clinical acumen behind a chiropractor's spinous evaluation and adjustment would have the same outcome? The incidence of this disorder is about one in 200,000.

Answers to Case Vignettes

A. Congenital leukemia. Her initial induction chemotherapy failed, but she received a successful bone marrow transplant in infancy. During the procedure at age 8 months, she also had an episode of asystole and was resuscitated fully. (Almost a miracle in itself.) She has been tumor-free for over twenty years. I still get overjoyed when I see her in the office. WOW. A stolen angel.

B. Osteosarcoma. Chemotherapeutic regimen induced a long-term remission.

C. Aplastic anemia—idiopathic. Successful bone marrow transplant received from her older sister.

Pediatric Patients: The Gray Zone Versus The End Zone

Exploring the age limits of pediatric practice

(Adapted from Block SL, Pediatric Patients: The Gray Zone vs. The End Zone, *Infectious Disease in Children*, July 2006)

It's Thursday afternoon at 3 p.m. I amiably saunter into room No. 6, which is filled with a young mother and her two children.

"Good morning, Gail. From my nurse's notes, I see that your baby has been coughing and cranky. Well, let's get a look at the young man."

I proceed to examine the 9-month-old, who seems quite skeptical of my examination initially, but quickly warms up to my charm and funny-looking nose. Although the cursory auscultation of his lungs is initially clear, I proceed with the gentle but firm chest compression, or as I like to term it, the "squeeze-a-wheeze" tactic, which I perform on any child with clear lungs and a significant history of cough. They almost never breathe deeply without help.

Aha! That is why the baby is coughing so vigorously. The lungs are full of wheezes and rhonchi when the chest wall is compressed. Then I bring out the otoscope, and somewhere in the recesses of his short-term memory, he remembers this thing may be more ominous than the stethoscope. He begins to struggle and cry. As the mother restrains his arms and legs, I firmly press his head against her chest and begin my diligent search for a possible acute otitis. Both tympanic membranes are indeed full of pus and slightly reddened.

"Gail, today John has some wheezy bronchitis and both ears are infected. Since he has wheezed two previous times—each time responding nicely to the nebulized albuterol and steroids—I would like to prescribe him a nebulizer with albuterol again, along with some steroids for five days and antibiotics for 10 days. Your medical card will cover them. We may have to label him as a mild asthmatic. He appears to have the usual infantile form of viral-induced wheezing, which is reversible. By the way, your other son sure has been behaving very well while I examined the baby."

Something is bothersome about the mother's own appearance, though. Between glances at the baby, I noticed that the mother had a reddened, angry skin boil on the zygomatic process of her face, just lateral to her eye. While trying to assimilate the degree of illness in her baby, the antenna also begins beeping in my cerebrum. This young mother appears to feel bad and looks somewhat ill.

I inquire: "I noticed you appear to have a boil on your face. Are you feeling bad? Has any doctor examined you recently?"

"Oh yeah, I went to the free clinic the day before yesterday, and the doctor gave me some capsules that begin with the letter 'K'."

"Do you mean Keflex?" I query.

"Yeah, that's it."

"Well, are you any better than yesterday?" I asked, certain that the answer was no. If she looked any worse, she would be in the hospital. "Your infection seems to be causing some peri-orbital edema of your eyelids. Have you noticed any puffiness in your eyes?"

"No, but I feel like I have some low-grade fever now."

"I think that you need to see the doctor again, and real soon. That skin abscess on your face looks as if it may be festering worse, and it may be traveling into the first stages of an even more serious infection we call periorbital cellulitis."

"But Doc, I do not have a regular doctor. And I have no insurance. I cannot afford to go to the ER. That would cost me $400 or $500." (We need more Medicaid budget cuts for young adults, eh???)

"How old are you now?"

"19."

"Perhaps, maybe I can help you get to see your last doctor that you visited. Who might that be?"

"It was you, Dr. Block. About 6 months ago." Oops.

"So no one since then?"

This is one of the perils or graces of practicing pediatrics for 40 years in the same small rural community as I have. I have probably seen most of the parents as patients themselves in the last 3 decades.

Her Personal War-Zone

Yes, I remembered her quite well as my patient during her rebellious teenage years. Her father was never available to her, and her mother worked in a factory. Her mother was often working too much. Left alone frequently, she found the ephemeral "love" in the bed of an adolescent male. She also frequently fought with her younger brother and even moved out at age 16 in a rift of anger and hostility toward her mother.

I could not convince her to use any contraception reliably at age 16; thus, the 3-year-old son of this 19-year-old mother. But at least she would come into the office to see me for her routine illnesses; pre-pregnancy and in-between pregnancies, and—I remember now—even post-pregnancy. She was temperamental, often reticent, and occasionally hostile in the office as well. But having raised four adolescent daughters in my own household, I had a healthy respect for the forces and stressors weighing upon any young lady—even in a stable, intact household. Not to mention one as tumultuous as hers!

So she was currently one of the 45 million Americans without insurance. She was not a statistic. She fell through the worsening Medicaid health insurance crack. She was a nice young lady previously working and struggling to survive along with her two children. She had a sick child at home needing her attention and care, no regular doctor recently, and now no job. She felt bad and was on the verge of a major worsening of a facial abscess unresponsive to cephalosporin. As is typical in our area, probably less than 30%-40% of abscesses seen in the office are Keflex antibiotic-responsive.

She could not afford a visit to the emergency department, and was in desperate need of incision and drainage and a switch of antibiotic to cover methicillin-resistant *Staphylococcus aureus* (MRSA).

Gray Zone of Pediatrics

I had encountered the gray zone of pediatrics: the upper age limit of our population. Often, I must examine a young mother during the same visit with her baby. This means if she does not bring a car seat, I must hold the baby or toddler while I examine the mother's lungs and abdomen. For me, it is just another real fun excuse to hold a cute baby.

At what point do we relinquish the care of our patients? Most certainly, the answer is during the pregnancy state, except for respiratory infections. But what about post-pregnancy for adolescent or single mothers? After all, they are still teenagers or young adults.

I surmised the following:

- She was still young enough for my practice.
- I had quite an expertise in the problem she was dealing with—MRSA and drainage. (Our office medical policy: all outpatient

moderate or worse abscesses require I&D and MRSA antibiotic coverage. Forget the I&D alone—nothing but failure these days.)

- I had an excellent rapport with the mother.
- I could make extra time for her visit.
- She was definitely in need of immediate medical care.
- Her medical options were limited due to the cost and the availability of a capable physician.
- And I could afford limited or no reimbursement from someone in true need.

Otherwise, as I explained to her, she was likely to wind up in the hospital within 24 hours with at least a $10,000 bill if she did not obtain appropriate treatment.

"Let me see what my schedule looks like for the rest of the afternoon. Never mind. If you do not mind waiting a bit or going to get your child's prescriptions filled, I will make sure that you are taken care of promptly. Today."

"How much will it cost? I cannot pay you today."

"Don't worry about it. Our most important rule is: take care of the sick patient first. Worry about the bill later. You just pay when you can, and only if you can. I will only charge you a 'brief visit' reduced charge anyway. The office manager in the billing office may have a fit, but I have the luxury of being the boss today." Owner practice!

I found a spot in the schedule for her that afternoon. I warned her that I would need to make a small incision of about 5 mm to release all the pus built up in the abscess. "It may scar a tiny bit."

End Zone of Pediatrics

Sterile prep and drape, 3 cc of 1% lidocaine injection superficially, small nick with a #11 blade, gentle firm squeezes, oozing of 5 cc of pus, probing and breaking of the adhesions with an instrument, bandage.

"Can you get this prescription for a different antibiotic filled?"

"No, I have no money."

"Not even borrowing it from your mother? (Too estranged still.) I have some samples of trimethoprim-sulfamethoxazole for free. However, I have major problems with this drug failing when the abscesses are this deep and involve some cellulitis. It just does not penetrate that well. I would prefer to use clindamycin, but it is somewhat expensive, and you would have to obtain it at the pharmacy immediately. You cannot wait to get it later or tomorrow. Any delay could put you in the hospital."

"I think I can talk my boyfriend into getting me some cash."

"I need to know for sure."

"Oh, he will give it to me, or he will be in trouble!"

"You must come back tomorrow, and so I do not want you to worry about any charges for that visit. I must ensure that your wound and abscess are improving."

When she returned the following day after promptly obtaining her clindamycin, the periorbital cellulitis had now become apparent, but the swelling and redness of the abscess had dramatically improved. The culture appeared to have an MRSA organism, which I asked the lab not to report and to toss it to avoid incurring any additional cost for her. By the way, the baby had also improved dramatically.

When she returned the following day, all signs of the periorbital cellulitis had dissipated; the skin over the abscess was slightly pink, and her malaise had resolved. Some days, it is downright nice to be able to practice like a country doc. Yet one must keep up-to-date with the continuing evolution of medical care to successfully reach the End Zone.

One wonderful aspect of practicing medicine is in the healing, not the money, for some of us. Saving the government more than $10,000 by avoiding her hospitalization and her subsequent Medicaid requirement reminds me that, in rural pediatrics, offering free care when needed has its own rewards.

As Sister Christine Lesousky, my English teacher, portended to me as a senior in high school: "Block, *noblesse oblige*."

A Simple Test?

Tread carefully when discussing seemingly routine matters with adolescent patients.

(Adapted from Block SL, A Simple Test? Infectious Disease in Children, February 2007)

I try so hard to entertain, yet not offend my teenage patients. I attempt to be quite cognizant of their need for both modesty and praise. But do you ever get the feeling that you just inserted your foot in your mouth, without even recognizing the width of your shoe size? The following encounter reminds me of the ultimate impossible "girlie question" from my wife: "Do you love me more now than when you first married me?"

Now listen, guys, there is NO right answer to this query. Think about it. I've been around girls (five of them) too long to realize a doomed response is inevitable. An old proverb stated, "A drowning man will grasp at a straw." You are trapped. It was one of those days. I just thought it would be prudent to order an additional "simple test."

The 'Hoarse' Is Out of the Barn

Amy came into the office for a simple upper respiratory tract infection. She was running a low-grade fever and suffering from hoarseness and rhinorrhea. She was still taking her Advair and occasionally her albuterol. She was worried that her asthma was flaring up. The cough was antagonizing her sleep at night.

Upon a careful physical examination, I determined that she was afflicted with a mild case of the parainfluenza virus and croup that was circulating in a mini-epidemic in our community.

I reassured Amy that her lungs were clear and devoid of any wheezing. "Nope, your asthma is doing just fine, Amy. Your continued use of preventive medications has worked wonders for keeping your asthma under control."

I have known Amy since she was about 5. Having seen her through numerous significant wheezing episodes and other respiratory conditions, among our six partners, she always asked to see me when she was ill or needed help.

I had even helped her through her most challenging problem in her life—her unintentional pregnancy at age 17. Believe me, I tried numerous times to get her on a stable regimen of oral contraceptive pills. But she continued running out of medication or forgetting to take her pills. She did not want that shot or implant. I begged her just to call the office when she was in short supply—we could always get her a temporary prescription to tide her over until her appointment.

A Long Track Record

On numerous occasions, I have even seen Amy in the office simultaneously with her baby when both were sick. Because she had no one else to assist her, I sometimes had to hold the infant while I examined her. ("I forgot the car seat, Dr. Block.") I consider that an honor, actually.

I had also seen Amy through some awful years during her mid-teens. Her father had essentially disowned her and refused to have any contact with her or her mother. The relationship had become so volatile that her father even threatened that "he would disown her" if she ever came around his house again, especially with that "no-good boyfriend of hers." Talk about a "Montel Williams" moment! Scary!

I attempted to console her through this heartbreaking tumult, with calm words of reassurance and by trying to emphasize that her father owned the problem, not her. I explained that he was just not accepting her recent pregnancy and was extremely distraught about the entire situation. We often discussed her multiple problems in her relationship with her mother as well. In fact, over the last year, Amy had become so depressed and unsmiling that I had elected to initiate therapy with a selective serotonin reuptake inhibitor. This worked its usual magic within a few weeks, and she had become more resilient to the everyday pressures of school, a baby, and an estranged father.

She had regained her teenage girl sparkle again. The simple smile and gleam in her eye that had been lost for a while returned. It is hard to define, but if you look carefully at the reciprocating smile, the eye contact, and the ability to laugh at your dumb jokes and self-deprecation, most of your content teenage girl patients emanate a certain glow. So in essence, she trusted me.

But at the end of this examination, there was one of those "oh, by the way" moments.

No Horsing Around

"Dr. Block, by the way, my urine is bothering me again, sort of like last time," she said. "I had a urinary tract infection three weeks ago, and I am starting to feel the same sort of urgency to pee. I finished my medicine a week ago. It's not really burning, it just feels sort of funny?"

"Well, let's just check your urine again to see if your UTI has recurred. Have you had any sores or vaginal itching or a change in the nature of your vaginal discharge?"

"No."

With the urine analysis results in hand, I explained to her that her urine had 5-10 white blood cells and no other findings. The urinary symptoms were most likely related to a mild yeast infection, and less likely to be early cystitis.

"We will need to wait for the urine culture to return tomorrow. And I will need to order one additional "simple test" on your urine. Your problem might be an occult urethritis from chlamydia or even gonorrhea."

Then came the mercurial adolescent meltdown. The tears began to flow, and she appeared quite distraught. I could not have anticipated the cascade of emotions that followed over the next 15 minutes. Once I calmed her down, she explained that she could not believe that I thought she was being promiscuous. She had not been with anyone else but her current boyfriend. I had betrayed her confidence in some manner.

"How many years have you known me? I would never do that sort of thing," she said.

It was easy for me to look at this adolescent girl with the baby in her arms and think that she would be extremely unlikely to be monogamous. Boy, did she let me know differently.

Changing Horses in "Midstream "

I tried to explain that possibly her boyfriend may have had sexual contact with someone else in the last year or two and infected her. But that was met with more anguish. "Never."

Backpedaling, finally, I explained to her that her obstetrician over the last few years performed these same tests on her with every PAP smear. This simple test was not an accusation, but an important precaution. "But you should know that I would never do that sort of thing." I told her I still respected her and appreciated her high standards and the fact that she had trusted me so much as well. The simple test was performed. And it was later negative, just as she had predicted.

Now, I "cannot wait" until we try to institute the mandate for everyday practitioners to perform yet another "simple test" on **every** adolescent. A venous HIV test at that! I have never seen a case of HIV in our large rural Kentucky practice in more than 40 years. Talk about a contentious proposition and some necessary billing and backpedaling with our parents and our adolescents! Like I said, I try not to offend my adolescent patients.

The Story of Romeo and Juliet: Never Was a Story of More Woe

(Adapted from Block SL, The Story of Romeo and Juliet: Never Was a Story of More Woe, *Infectious Disease in Children*, November 2005)

As we grow older, I realize we may not be fully able to understand the impetuous, vital self-importance and irrational exuberance of youthful love.

Five years ago, the 16-year-old athletic young lady from Lebanon, KY, entered the office with her tearful mother.

Growing up in a small suburban house with one younger, very boisterous sibling, Juliet was a star athlete, and she achieved in academics—mostly—taking advanced classes in her high school. Her parents were happily married, both worked steadily in professional jobs, and they cared deeply for their children, by all indicators that I witnessed, both in the office and what I saw of them in the community. And yet, her father rarely attended any of her athletic functions.

"O Romeo, Romeo, wherefore art thou Romeo? Deny thy father and refuse thy name" (Shakespeare).

She began to use illicit drugs by age 15, "hanging out with the wrong crowd." My daughter, a contemporary of hers, told me later. Family arguments became the norm, escalating to slammed doors, screams of contempt, and running away from home a couple of times.

"Is love a tender thing? It is too tough, too rude, too boisterous, and it pricks like thorn..." (Shakespeare).

When she turned 16, Romeo, the 19-year-old high school dropout, who also happened to be a convicted felon, impregnated our Juliet. He was somewhat domineering, always demanding to know her whereabouts, and they argued frequently. Her parents vociferously disapproved of this young man. Her pediatrician discussed her options regarding a pregnancy. Within four months of conception, she later said that she miscarried spontaneously.

She returned to the office eight months afterwards for a paronychia and uneventful ingrown toenail removal. Volleyball season had created great pressure on her time, and on her great toe, but she needed to return as soon as possible for the team's big game this week. "Tell me, how is everything?" I asked. *Fine.* "And your grades?" *Doing really well.* "Any problems?" *No*, she said, *I'm doing fine.*

"Is there no pity in the clouds that sees into the bottom of my grief?" (Shakespeare)

Five months later, she was brought into the office after cavorting for an entire weekend night, driving nearly 100 miles away from home with some of her new "friends." The same evening after the nocturnal escapade and threats of suicide and quite a hateful attitude, her mother drove her down to the local children's hospital, where Juliet was evaluated. She had a negative drug screening and was deemed to be reactively depressed due to her circumstances, and not at high risk for suicide. She was released home that night, and they were instructed to follow up with her local pediatrician the next morning.

The good news—she had been seeing a counselor for the last two months for her depression and family problems. The bad news—she was apparently not responding. Her mother said they never discussed her depressed mood or her miscarriage.

During my interview, my mouth went agape, for I noticed she had nearly 50 fairly deep, acute, and chronic slices/abrasions on her left forearm. She was despondent, avoided eye contact, and claimed she did not want to live. Her mother said the daughter constantly yelled epithets at her, argued with every request, and frequently screamed that she "hates her."

"Alas, that love, so gentle in his view, should be so tyrannous and rough in proof" (Shakespeare).

Upon further interrogation, she immediately denied to me that she had any lingering issues with the miscarriage, any recent drug or alcohol use, or boyfriend issues. She still "loves him," she said, as he only yelled at her a few times weekly, and he rarely hit her anymore. Since Juliet was now "grounded forever," she could only talk with her "lover" on the phone, during which time they usually argued and cried.

As some consolation, she was still faithfully using her weekly contraceptive patch. She also freely discussed her contempt for her mother. She said she was now failing several courses and had no desire to play sports.

Clinical Exam

Her examination revealed a pulse of 102 and blood pressure of 110/80, a flat affect, frequent tears, and she appeared to be otherwise physically normal. Except for one detail, her eyeballs appeared somewhat prominent, and the pulse rate was actually quite elevated for a volleyball athlete. Add these findings to the chronic mild tachycardia (for two years—I looked at our office chart) and some really erratic, tempestuous, and out-of-character behavior, and I subsequently checked her thyroid function, urinalysis, and complete blood count.

As we often see in our practice, her T4 and free thyroxine index were 17.6 and 5.8, respectively, which were way too high. Perhaps her thyrotoxicosis and early Graves disease (with slight exophthalmos) were exacerbating her alarming self-destructive behavior and depression. Perhaps?

Clinical Treatment

I elected to initiate therapy with methimazole (anti-thyroid medication) and fluoxetine (Prozac), along with careful monitoring for worsening suicidality and mood disorder, and elimination of access to any possible weapons and risky medications.

Within three days, a frantic phone call for some mild abdominal pain, nausea, and hot flashes or fever ensued. Hopefully, this was merely the gastrointestinal virus that was circulating in her high school, of which I had observed several cases that week. This event mercifully passed uneventfully.

It does not end here. An utter transformation—or is it?

Now she was pregnant. The thyroid options were almost nil. She was not a true candidate for surgery; radioactive iodine was out of the question. And methimazole was considered the safest fetal option with her flaming thyrotoxicosis. I could not get her into the endocrinologist for months, but in a phone conference with him, he agreed that at this point, oral methimazole was the best compromise. Could this medication affect the newborn and cause it to develop cretinism—brain damage and malformations? All the safety data in the literature said no. Who said pediatrics was easy?

During the follow-up visit the following week, I observed a happier, smiling, garrulous young Juliet—an utter transformation! She could even talk and interact with her mother in a peaceful tone. After a month of increasing doses of methimazole and stable use of her fluoxetine, all suicidal behavior had resolved, her grades had skyrocketed back to A's, and she once again appeared to be contentedly heavily involved with her sports. She was living at home without problems, she reported. I patted her on the back and congratulated her. Next, I patted myself on the back and sighed in relief.

"Thy head is as full of quarrels as an egg is full of meat" (Shakespeare).

A few days later, I discovered that the thyroid function had not improved. She had run away from home again. Old Romeo, the boyfriend, had entered the picture again a week ago, and he broke her feeble heart again by "dumping her." A tirade to the family ensued, and she ran away from home for several days in an absolute tiff, only to wind up at her grandmother's house as a safe haven. Playing "phone tag" with her mother, her counselor said she needed "more antidepressants."

I finally caught up with the mother a few days later, spotting her car as she was leaving my parking lot in the morning, while I was ready to stroll into the office out of my Ford F-150. Window down, we exchanged the latest news, plan of action, and medication adjustment for her contentious daughter.

Without her chart staring at me, these specifics were retrieved in my ancient mental computer very slowly while standing in the bright sun.

"I may need medicine for my nerves more than she does," she pleaded tearfully.

"You and me both," I agreed. Will our Shakespearean "Juliet" survive? Next, will she, I and the baby all survive this Romeo and Juliet romance?

"This is not hard, I think, for men so old as we, to keep the peace" (Shakespeare).

Her household

I always cringe when starting many medications with out-of-control female adolescents for fear of teratogenicity, no matter how benign the medications allegedly are. Thus, my routine emphatic emphasis on continued contraception monitoring by the parent, if at all possible. As we grow older, I also realize we may not be able to fully understand the impetuous, vital self-importance and "irrational exuberance" of youthful love. (Much like Federal Reserve chairman Alan Greenspan said about tech-blinded traders in the stock market.) How can a talented and lovely young lady turn into a "star-crossed lover," a victim of such a brutish Romeo, and a sheer menace to herself, and in such woeful proportions?

She showed up at school again this week with an ecchymotic eyelid. Just wrestling with him allegedly? However, her thyroid functions had finally normalized the next week, and she had "allowed" her parents to live in "her" household world again.

Let me tell you a secret.

Could my gut instinct have been wrong about her tumultuous history for the last two years, as I may have been seeing her world through my own rose-colored glasses? Clearly, insidious Graves' hyperthyroidism could explain it all. But...

Too many times, I have witnessed the utter despair that follows a teenage abortion. Could it be that she was not actually a victim of uterine spontaneity? Perhaps earlier, it was an intentional "miscarriage or other trauma?" In my lengthy experience, a few external tragedies in any Juliet's life will certainly drive a young lady to this depth of despair and anger, namely abortion, rape, or sexual abuse, particularly in the community in which I reside.

I then realized that I am like Friar Laurence in *Romeo and Juliet*, as I repeated his mantra:

"Care keeps his watch in every old man's eyes."

This old man will keep his post, monitor the thyroid, and be caring and available to this tormented family and Juliet, for "Parting is such sweet sorrow."

Well, after the next seven months of careful obstetrical and thyroid follow-up, she delivered a healthy, full-term, normal infant. His thyroid function was normal on newborn screening. For the next two years, whenever I saw her child, I held my breath at each visit. Was there any intellectual deficit detectable? I knew that his thyroid tests were all normal at birth and for several months after. Still, that now irrational fear lingered. A few years later, she is bringing her children to see me as their pediatrician. She is always so pleasant and gives me a hug in acknowledgment of helping her through her past crises. The child is excelling in elementary school. She had her thyroid ablated by radioactive iodine, and she is still on replacement thyroid and doing well.

Each quote was excerpted from Shakespeare's *Romeo and Juliet*.

The Blind Squirrel Finds a Nut

The very reticent, petite, short-haired, dark-haired clerk was discussing specific metal nails and galvanized Phillips screws with me in the local hardware store where she had been working for a few months. "Do you remember me, Dr. Block?" she said when she spotted me.

I was attempting another DIYer project, fixing my aging swing set for my grandchildren. Carpenter bees were wreaking havoc on the lumber. Destructive little critters!

Two years earlier, this young lady from Elizabethtown, KY, had presented to my office at the age of 14. with notable shortness of breath, some tachypnea and tachycardia, and mild distress and anxiety regarding her illness; hyperventilating too, due to her left-sided chest pain. She had no fever and minimal cough. She relayed a pattern of moderate pleurisy, with some chest pain on every inspiratory breath in the last 12 hours. Her examination was otherwise unremarkable, including clear lungs, normal heart, and no swelling or pain in her legs or abdomen. Her pulse oximeter reading was 92% and she was tachycardic (HR = 110), which are borderline readings in a previously healthy adolescent. Her chest X-ray and ECG were normal.

Reviewing her medical history again, I discovered that she had been recently placed on a course of antibiotics for bronchitis and wheezing a few weeks ago. Incidentally, the earlier prescriber also uncovered that she was experiencing heavy, crampy menses. Thus, he elected to place her on a course of routine oral contraceptives, with the usual warnings.

Over the next 30 minutes in the office, her diaphoresis, chest discomfort, and shortness of breath were somewhat worse. I suspected, AT THE TOP OF MY LIST OF PULMONARY AND CARDIAC MALADIES, that she needed a diagnostic CT scan of her lungs to check for a pulmonary embolus (PE)—a highly life-threatening blood clot to the lungs, which would not typically show up on chest radiographs. But as mitigating evidence for a PE diagnosis, she had no evidence of any deep vein thrombosis (DVT) or swelling or pain in her legs. Now, PE is rarely encountered in young teenage girls, even much less so without any signs of leg DVT. Never say never in my patients. Nonetheless, she had been recently receiving oral contraceptives, which have a minuscule risk of triggering blood clots or particularly DVT.

To get a venous D-dimer blood test (abnormal with a DVT) and a CT scan of the lungs at the local rural hospital, I thought, would only delay the diagnostic time to the discovery of the possible PE. This was too life-threatening an issue for any delays. So I thought!

I told the mother explicitly that she very likely had a PE, and that she needed an immediate CT scan of her lungs in order to start the life-saving anticoagulants to prevent sudden death or even a brain stroke. I sent them with a copy of my office notes, the ECG, the chest radiograph, stating such as well. I also thought that the ER could obtain her D-dimer blood test for PE, as I did not want any delays. I also had directly notified one of the ER physicians.

With an oxygen tank and tubing to a mask on her face, the ambulance was called, and they then delivered her to the emergency room at the tertiary care hospital. After a few hours, the pediatric resident eventually examined her and could find no obvious reason for her distress. After checking with her attending ER physician (her boss), she told the mother and patient that she was ready for discharge home.

Oh no!

(Typically, 98% of the time, our emergency room referrals go extremely well, and lives are often saved. Not so much here—anybody can have a bad hair day.)

"But Dr. Block emphatically stated that she needed a CT scan of her lung to look for a pulmonary embolus. He said not to leave without this test," so the mother asked the ER docs to reconsider.

The ER doctors thought the CT scan and D-Dimer tests were unwarranted in light of their findings. Her pulse oximeter was slightly low at 93% and her chest pain seemed to have improved somewhat. After further discussion and mom's pleading to test for PE, they agreed to perform the tests, despite PE being very rare in a healthy, non-smoking younger teenage girl with no signs of DVT (no leg clots or swelling). In fact, it is almost unheard of. I guess they were thinking the girl was "probably just a histrionic adolescent female," which is a common scenario in the ER. Her D-Dimer was only marginally elevated.

OOPS.

The scan showed an obvious small PE in the left lower lung. The attending physician then sent in the pediatric resident to explain to the mother that her daughter would need to stay in the hospital for blood thinners for a few days after all. That the hematologist would be consulted and that heparin would be started immediately.

After three days in the hospital, she recovered uneventfully and was placed on long-term anticoagulants and was told to never take estrogen products again. Genetic blood testing also uncovered that she had a rare homozygous (2 of the 2 genes) gene for MTHFR gene deficit—(i.e., really prone to blood clots and spontaneous miscarriages with certain triggers).

Meanwhile, I was so happy to see her now in the hardware store, doling out important information to her patrons, and holding down a great full-time job post high school. She looked content as well.

My philosophy: Even a blind squirrel finds a nut once in a while. And always listen to the mother.

Why Do Bad Things Happen to Good People?

Late Sunday afternoon after church service on a warm spring day two years ago, I was summoned to the local hospital delivery room for an emergency caesarean section for a baby who lost her heart tones. The busy pregnant 34 y.o. G5P4 mother from Cecilia, KY, had only received sparse prenatal care, and she had no previous fetal ultrasounds performed. The baby's gestational age was unknown. The actual delivery went smoothly. But...

When the baby was handed over to me by the obstetrician, I noticed she was quite small, covered in vernix, and seemed rather dysmorphic (unusual appearance). APGARS were 1/1. I started bagging her with 2 liters of oxygen flowing, but the lungs were extremely stiff. I then began using more tactile stimulation due to no respiratory effort. Her minimal heart rate did not improve. The lung sounds were distant and muffled. A typical premature infant. Or was she? More like a stillborn baby.

But on my more complete inspection after trying to resuscitate her for a minute, she was more than the usual dysmorphic child, as she was actually malnourished-looking as well. She had very short extremities. Her thorax was severely narrowed, her forehead and her abdomen were quite protuberant, her eyes were bulging. I suspected much more than the usual dysmorphic syndrome. We bagged her with oxygen, and then I proceeded to intubate her with a 3-0 endotracheal tube within a few minutes, and her lungs were extremely stiff (indicating almost no aeration). Still, almost no air was proceeding to the lungs. I promptly obtained a chest radiograph and leg/hip radiographs. Yes, her long bones were severely bowed. Her chest radiograph showed a total whiteout of the lung (confirming no aeration at all, despite adequate bagging). The radiologist had confirmed my suspicions about the diagnosis.

She had the diagnostic classic features of a specific, lethal chromosomal abnormality, which mostly results in stillborn or miscarriage.

And if born, this condition is uniformly fatal within hours or at most a few days. But we continued the bagging and warming of the infant to give me some time to talk with the parents. She remained cyanotic and not perfusing her body, with imperceptible pulses during the entire resuscitation. I needed to promptly have a discussion with the parents about the baby's lethal condition. She would never even make it until the transfer ambulance arrived, even if we wanted to.

This is awful timing (this was supposed to be a time of celebration of a wonderful newborn), and instead necessitated a depressing, devastating talk. I conveyed the findings, then showed them the textbook and her findings, and then relayed the prognosis to the mother and father. "There is nothing we can do for the baby. I cannot aerate her lungs at all because they never developed in utero, and they never will. She has a lethal chromosome disorder. You possibly have a few minutes to a few hours to be with her alive in her current condition. No additional medical intervention is worthwhile or helpful. That would be futile and painful. Just hold her and keep her comfortable for her short time with you."

I further explained: "Although I had seen several similar cases in my career, nearly always this disorder is a spontaneous gene mutation. The defect just happens, and it is not foreseeable or preventable. It will almost never affect any future pregnancies. It spontaneously occurs in 1 in 50,000 births. No one is to blame for this."

In agreement with the parents, I then removed the futile ET tube from the airway.

I held their hands for a few minutes and stayed for the prayers with the on-call chaplain. The nurses had her swaddled up neatly and tightly. The cyanotic face peeking through the covers was obvious, though. The breathing was now agonal. Without the mother's placental support and despite medical intervention, the baby's mild bradycardia and cyanosis rapidly deteriorated after birth. I updated the obstetrician on her condition also. The funeral home was notified to pick her up.

Sometimes, there are no words worthwhile on this horrific occasion.

Adolescent Chest Pain

The older teenage girl from Mount Washington, KY, was mixing paint cans at the local hardware store on this pleasant spring day. I needed some touch-up white paint for my bathroom.

She blurted out: "Hi, Dr. Block, so good to see you. " I had taken care of her since infancy. And I had actually been the doctor to her mother many years ago as well.

Her story: the 18-year-old pleasant Black female was complaining of right side chest wall pain for 4 days. The pain seemed to radiate in an anterior thoracic 5-6 dermatome distribution. She had minimal cough, no fever, and seemed very healthy otherwise. She had a 2-year history of juvenile-onset diabetes mellitus, which I had diagnosed for her.

Her examination was normal with normal vital signs, except: she had some slight pain on palpation over her right lateral anterior ribs.

My gut feeling was that she was suffering from a mild case of shingles known as *zoster sine herpeticum*—herpes zoster without a rash. It does rarely occur without any rash. She was fully immunized with the varicella vaccine, but vaccine recipients can still rarely erupt later in life into shingles.

Consequently, I started treatment with Valtrex twice daily. But I warned her to absolutely return in 4 days if the chest pain persisted for a chest radiograph. Well, 4 days later, she returned, and her pain was somewhat worse. I obtained her chest radiograph, and it showed the large, round opacification seen in the chest radiograph below.

I referred her to my superb pediatric surgeon, Dr. Foley, who said that it was the smallest and earliest bone sarcoma that he had ever seen. Almost always, the pain is ignored by clinicians, and patients have massive bone abnormalities by the time he sees them, he said. Typically, they are undiagnosed for so long that weight loss and anorexia are problematic. It usually occurs in White patients and in the second decade of life, unlike this case.

She had normal spleen, liver, brain, and lungs on MRIs. The biopsy confirmed that she had **bone sarcoma** of the rib, which is only observed in 1/500,000 patients and is termed an "Askin tumor." (Another case. Can we get any rarer?) She underwent chemotherapy first for several weeks to prevent metastasis. Then he surgically removed the remainder of the tumor. She has been tumor-free for years now. And she is fully functional. She had some of her eggs frozen for her future childbearing as well. And she is a good store employee. She continues to be very successfully diligent with her endocrine problem.

College was not for her, she said.

We chatted for a while about her life and her mother, who always insists on seeing me with her in the office, as we go way back in both their lives. Then I checked out at the cashier.

Good follow-up in private practice is so essential in pediatrics.

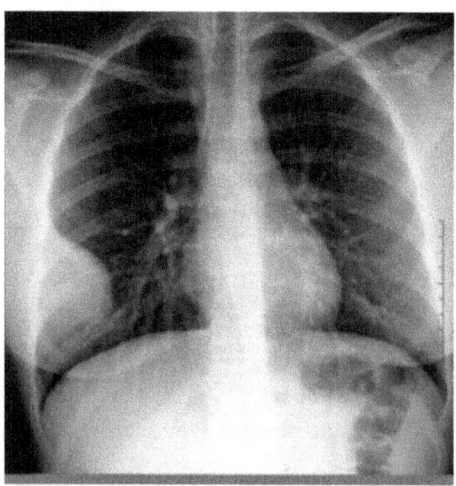

Figure 17. X-ray of chest of 18 y.o. female. Note the white mass in the right lower lung.
Source: Dr. Block

Letter of Recommendation: Dr. Ken Zangwill

I am a pediatric infectious disease specialist and am well aware of Stan's accomplishments in the field. Stan always claims that he is "just a country doctor," but his professional output begs otherwise. This country doctor has, while tending to the needs of Kentucky children in a busy general pediatric practice for >21 years, established himself as one of the premiere primary-care-based pediatric researchers in the United States. He is a recognized expert in several areas of interest to pediatricians, most especially otitis media, influenza infection, and ADHD.

These efforts have been recognized by several national organizations, including the American Academy of Pediatrics (Researcher of the Year Award), the American Society of Pediatric ENT, and the Society of Pediatric Infectious Diseases, each of which awarded him highly coveted awards. His national influence and name recognition are confirmed, especially when one considers that he is often asked to give Grand Rounds lectures all over the country, reviews scholarly articles for several international journals, regularly writes folksy yet informative medical columns, and has and continues to publish scores of research articles in peer-reviewed journals. A breadth of output rarely seen from any researcher, let alone one who, every day sees many pediatric patients in the office!

Most directly, I have had the pleasure of working with Stan on a national Education Council, which completed a large effort to educate clinicians about influenza disease and vaccination. This included many flu experts and resulted in the creation of an informative interactive website, development of a teaching slide set, and formal Symposia given at national meetings, compilation of a newsletter sent to all pediatric practitioners, and other efforts. His input was always practical, informed, credible, and I dare say often hilarious. Again, all of this while continuing to practice general pediatrics in Kentucky! Stan is truly a credit to the

Medical School, our shared profession, and to children who have benefited from his clinical practice and research findings.

We all should have the breadth of talents and energy that Stan has. He is most deserving of the Distinguished Alumni Award.

Sincerely,

Ken Zangwill, M.D. Professor of Pediatrics, David Geffen School of Medicine at UCLA

The Wizard of Oz's Unveiling of the Most Complex Humans in the World: The Teenage Girl

A Dad's Thirteen Rules for Raising Teen Girls.

Managing the Estrogen Tempest in a Teapot!

As my family's patriarch, even the slightest change of voice or minuscule indifference to the adolescent daughter's utterances or problems can bring a deluge of tears or an avalanche of irrational verbal assaults. It's just one of those great mysteries of life to men, and it's more than just an issue of *Men are from Mars and Women are from Venus*. As the only man (and father) in my household of five young women (which includes my wife, of course). I am perpetually reminded that: "You just don't understand, you're just a dumb boy!" Well, no truer words have been uttered.

The trials that women and young girls must endure while growing up are quite amazing and unfathomable after all.

Think about it, guys.

Female Metamorphosis.

The torturous road begins during middle school, when an abrupt metamorphosis from a naïve, undeveloped little girl into a full-grown estrogen-enhanced woman occurs in less than 3 years. During this miraculous transformation, a girl's body and mind must endure incredible wrenching weekly or monthly growth, hormonal and mood surges—enough to make even the Father dizzy watching it unfold. I have personally observed this female molting unfold 4 times in my household. Bad hair days and Chernobyl-like meltdowns frequently became more common than good ones. And with each of four daughters born three years apart, I rarely received a respite from this estrogen tempest in a teapot for decades.

During her pubertal years, your daughter will likely face the following challenges: monthly menstruation often associated with a few days of miserable cramps; dealing with "mean girls" and taunting and cliques in middle school; navigating the perils of dating and boy-girl relationships in high school—sometimes as early as middle school; selecting the "perfect" outfit for school or work daily; achieving the ideal makeup, hairstyle and "look" daily; changing clothes sometimes four times a day, depending on the occasion. Then most importantly, the teenage girl pinnacle faces the bi-annual angst—the preparation ritual for the senior (and freshmen, and sophomore and junior) "Prom" and Christmas dances. So many hairstyles! And how many dresses do we have to buy and return to the department store—only to skip out of prom 30 minutes later after making her grand appearance? This is the reality of your blossoming young lady.

Male predators.

Now, the one thing during this developmental stage that these incredible, wonderful female folks do not need is some bullying, blustering, or mean-spirited male mistreating or domineering them.

As the father of four daughters and as a pediatrician caring for thousands of young ladies over the last several decades in our delightful agrarian community, one aspect of our community's life I particularly dread: the male predator.

Of course, our rural town is not particularly different from any other community in America in this regard. But I have witnessed firsthand the devastation and hopelessness that this most dastardly problem fosters. I am not talking about drug or alcohol problems (although their correlation is high), but rather about domestic violence and abuse—the male-bullying-female variety. It is much more commonplace than most of us realize or recognize. It can go on for months or decades. Although it frequently rears its ugly head in marriage, the pattern most often festers during the teenage daughter's dating relationships—just visit my office on any day. I have even witnessed this egregious meanness perpetuated by fathers upon their own daughters and step-daughters.

Listen, Fathers, our preteen and teen daughters have it rough enough just trying to navigate the perils of puberty, dating, fashion, and mean-spirited same sex peers. The last thing that these young ladies need from someone who they are supposed to trust and love is the verbal assaults upon their esteem, or the belittling running commentary, or repeated emotional or physical traumas to their bodies. Paradoxically, these ladies often try to protect their brutish nemesis from discovery.

In the case where she develops a relationship with an "enchanting" dating partner—who just happens to enjoy demeaning or pulverizing her—the ladies frequently say that he "just got mad" or that "he didn't mean to" or that "he is always so nice to me **most** of the time."

Thus, one must ponder the question as to why any young woman would tolerate this pugilistic treatment from her "Romeo." Sometimes, there appears to be no answer as to why they fall into this trap. Most think: "I can change him." (See commandment #8.)

But as one father to another, I can emphatically state that **your** certain particular attitudes or treatment of your daughters can have long-term beneficial or devastating impact upon their future perceptions of male to female relationships, and their ability to recognize a perilous choice of boyfriend. (Think: John Mayer's song—*Fathers be good to your daughters*.)

A Father's Thirteen Commandments

I believe the following 13 commandments for fathers raising teen daughters or step-daughters may help prevent them from heading toward this self-destructive relationship. (Of course, many of these rules would be appropriate for raising boys as well.) These rules should foster a more resilient, self-confident young lady, and hopefully reduce the likelihood of dating a slick, manipulative predator. Always expect respect; stick to your principles and morals.

1. Thou shalt adore, nurture, and discipline thy daughter as long as she lives in your household through the teen years. Sincere praise is good. Your one-on-one companionship is always more important than any purchased goods.

2. Thou shalt treat thy daughter as you would like to be treated. (Compassion and respect come to mind.) Provide a shoulder to cry on, a body to lean on, an ear to listen with thoughtfully.

3. Thou shalt keep sacred some exclusive time every day for your daughter, especially during the teenage years. (Include a daily hug, a kiss good night, a stupid self-deprecating joke, and an "I love you.")

4. Honor and respect thy daughter's predilection for: occasional emotional meltdowns, an intense sensitivity to your commands, a need for privacy, and her occasional misdeeds and failures. Were you ever perfect, Buster?

5. Thou shalt not spank, slap, insult, belittle, or insult her. Ever. (If, while growing up, she is the recipient of this type of behavior from her most trusted male, the seeds for tolerating future male aggression in a relationship have been planted.) Discipline by denial of privileges, curfew, and time out, which works even until high school graduation. (See below.) And never bluff. Teach them the art of negotiation—when "grounded", allow the possibility for an early parole for extra good behavior. Eliminate words like "fat" and "stupid" from your vocabulary. You will pay royally in the long run for any utterance of such words.

6. Thou shalt not steal thy daughter's youth by asking her to grow up too fast, by granting her a television in her room, by allowing her to watch sexually advanced television and movies. A PG-13 rating is basically the old R rating anymore—do you really trust the

judgment and morals of those in Hollywood with your most prized progeny? Screen the videos, movies, and internet sites! Just say no, despite her lacrimations and lamentations. Social media is the stealthy monster in the room.

7. Thou shalt not covet thy neighbor's wife, or mistreat your own wife for that matter. A daughter does not need to witness a role model for a male demeaning a female (or for your own drug or alcohol problems, for that matter). Those two innocent little eyes are absorbing every move (good or bad) that you make.

8. Thou shalt intervene in her disastrous dating relationships, and preemptively tell her that you forbid dating of males 12 months older than she is while in high school. (Controversial, yes, but trust me!) Intervene in any subsequent really dastardly choice after a few weeks if she does not recognize it. First by reminding her: how unhappy she is, how badly he treats her, etc., and then civilly ask that she move on. If cajoling for a week or so fails, then "for her own good," remove her driver's license or car keys or cellular phone (the real torture!), a week per week she insists on continuing the self-destructive relationship. Inertia on your part will only increase the intensity and the impact of her impending collision with the harsh reality. The wailing and tears may seem endless, but the offending agent must be forbidden. Protect her innocence. Purchase some earplugs for this one.

9. Thou shalt not nag or nitpick thy daughter over the small stuff. Remember the big picture—is she doing well outside the household academically and socially, and non-addicted and non-pregnant? Well, there you go! If she falters, you will still need to support her—forever emotionally, and hopefully temporarily economically.

10. Thou shalt not take personally her insults in anger, her whining, tantrums, and snideness either during the terrible twos or terrible teens or 'tweens (12 to 13 year old). Civilly and calmly remind her

that she is yelling, and that you DO NOT appreciate it. **Never confront irrationality with irrationality.** If overwhelmed, resort to showing her the door to her room, or show her your trusty phone's video camera that surreptitiously just might record her outlandish behavior. But always try to avoid embarrassing her in front of her friends and other family members. Take all confrontations to a private (soundproof?) room. But remember, the more tears she sheds, the more likely your request or denial is on target. If she chooses rather to negotiate a change, always listen carefully for common ground.

11. Try not to leave your sexually mature daughter alone at home for more than two hours during the teen/high school years. Longer duration of parental absence may require supervision from a trusted adult. Or, always double-check on her whereabouts when she is "just going out" or "spending the night." Do you really know where your daughter is? One-third of teens will sneak out in the middle of the night—my own included.

12. Thou shalt help her get involved in any reasonable form of extracurricular activity—sports, music, horseback riding, etc. Afternoons actively watching soap operas or seeing "that boy daily" only count as "kindling for pregnancy or premarital activity."

13. Thou shalt commit her to attending school daily, completing homework, and achieving her academic potential. Accept what she is capable of. Expect courtesy toward others of all ages.

OMG. You might even wind up for a week without your wife in Panama City during Spring Break, alone with your 12-year-old daughter to "supervise" your 17-year-old's beach activities for a few minutes each day. (Wife will be on a cruise ship.) A week of your total sacrifice with your intermittent presence is again worth the avoidance of "a permanent reminder of a temporary feeling" (Jimmy Buffett).

I am a battle-weary, testosterone-challenged member of the species who has endured four endearing, but periodically (no pun intended) challenging daughters. Fathers, your patience, acceptance, love, and *A Dad's Thirteen Rules for Raising Teen Girls* will pay off in the end game.

Surviving Ophelia: Saving the Fathers of Adolescent Daughters

Fathers, note well: the years 13 through 16 for the adolescent female are merely a phase of what I loosely term a temporary emotional "psychosis." Interludes of bizarre, unpredictable, or snippy behavior are commonplace. Lots of eye-rolling. Speaking of "eyes," you will go from being the "apple of your daughter's eye" during pre-adolescence to becoming the disgusting worm in the apple in the eyes of your teenage daughter. Not only will you frequently be told how uncool and stupid you are, but because your daughter has always been so brilliant and perceptive, you will become self-doubting and totally unsure of whether you even want to enter the same room with her royal highness. Don't fret, it seems to be part of the divine plan to ensure that parents gladly wean their "chicks" from the nest in later teen years.

I was raised as the youngest of 5 very athletic and competitive sons, and as an elder sibling to two younger sisters, whose comings and goings were basically ignored. For me, testosterone-challenging activities and boy-things reigned and were role-modeled. Now, as the proud father of 4 vibrant, beautiful daughters, I must admit that, similar to most fathers, when it came to the psyche of the adolescent female, initially, I was a total moron, so much so that if ignorance is bliss, then I was ecstatic.

Nonetheless, I have discovered several helpful insights over the battle-scarred years while dueling with these metamorphosing estrogen-enhanced persons that I would like to share with similarly basically clueless fathers.

Mary Pipher's treatise, ***Reviving Ophelia: Saving the Selves of Adolescent Girls,*** is a must-read book for fathers (even more important than *Sports Illustrated*). Pipher thoughtfully explores and explains many of the foils and pitfalls for the adolescent female. As her title implies, the angst of the adolescent female has been described as early as the 1600s. To paraphrase adolescent vernacular: Ophelia, the "clueless chick of the stuck-up Hamlet dude in Shakespeare, is in desperate need of an emotional makeover." Her entire self-worth is based on whether Hamlet accepts or rejects her as a lover. When scorned, instead of moving on or lashing out at him, she drowns in her own self-pity, both metaphorically and physically. As Pipher wisely explains, many adolescent female woes (anorexia nervosa, depression, and extreme rebellion) are commonly metaphorical expressions of their inner pain. Just listen to Taylor Swift's song "Fate of Ophelia."

In order for fathers to remain relatively unscathed while raising teenage daughters, both self-discipline and a Kevlar outer hide are essential. The home can be like a tempest in a teapot. "Don't look at me!" or "You just don't understand!" are favorite bylines. Akin to the weather, the moods of these young ladies can change in seconds. One minute, a gale-force wind of anger is being unleashed on the household after a thwarted demand to stay out till 4 a.m. at the Christmas dance. (The imposing guilt-trip: "But all my friends are.") However, should the phone ring during her tirade, an entirely new weather front of bright, cheery skies and pleasantly calm winds will instantaneously be encountered by the caller. (Anticipating the boyfriend, I guess.) Whoa. Turning that emotional spigot off and on in seconds?

In the long run, how we raise our adolescent daughters during their "stormy" years directly correlates with how much damage they will inflict upon the household, and is comparable to the probability of harm from tumultuous, dangerous weather. The young adolescent female may levy damage equivalent to a thunderstorm, a tornado, or a hurricane.

I consider myself youthful and in tune with the times. Yeah, right? LOL.

Alas, I am getting old, though. Having raised four teen/pre-teen daughters can prematurely do that to you. My then 10-year-old daughter proclaimed at one point that my clothes were so "last season" and that I was no longer a "butt."

Like a fool, I glanced into the mirror, and I saw nothing more than a clown in the metaphorical Jimmy Buffett's "gorilla disguise."

But with age comes wisdom. A minuscule consolation.

Funny. Despite my authoritative ways and the incessant downward spiral of my appearance, my four sprightly, lovely daughters still love me. It is apparent in the way that my then 21-year-old lays her head on my shoulder during 10 o'clock Mass—the same girl who, at 16, snarled at me while she was peeping over her cereal box of Trix during every breakfast. (Apparently, it's a family rite of passage, still yet unbroken by her three next of kin.) Apparent in the way my 12-year-old cackled at her Daddy's hijinks and bear hugs—the same girl who refused to hold my hand while walking beside me to the same 10 o'clock Mass. She said, "her friends might see me," yet she routinely jumped on my lap after supper at home or when dining out. I suppose girls go through much of adolescence fantasizing that they were hatched and reared by reptiles, not actual parents.

I am constantly reminded that, as the boy of the family, "you just don't understand" and "you could never understand." Having been raised with four older, bellicose brothers who made the WWE seem like ballerinas, they may possibly be right. I cannot fathom the "abyss of despair" inherent in the daily crises of my daughters. What color khaki pants to wear in the morning to school, the un-ironed shirt, the boyfriend who forgot to call back last night, the mismatching nail polish, the broken curling iron? Traumatic.

In the Byzantine convolutions of the female adolescent cerebral cortex, why do the higher functioning synapses hibernate during this phase of endocrine estrogen surges? Whirlwinds and whirligigs. Giggles and haggles. Left in the dust, that's me.

Ah, but despite the obtuseness of me as a despot in the perpetual tempest in a teapot of my girls, I do understand they are quite like the stormy weather.

You see, raising adolescent daughters is like forecasting the weather—seldom right but never in doubt. Many days are fortunately bright and sunny, with calm winds—well, at least no gusts over 30 or 40 mph. But it is the magnitude of the turbulent weather that sends any sane father seeking shelter.

Unfortunately, it is critical that the father be stalwart and squarely face the plethora of storms unleashed by adolescent daughters, no matter the rantings of the rebellion or the torrent of tears. However, the magnitude of these storms commonly reflects the degree of paternal involvement. Working as a pediatrician in a small rural community, I witnessed firsthand the pivotal role that the father plays in raising our "Ophelias." When your daughter metamorphoses from a cute little pig-tailed girl to a full-grown, responsible, mature woman, it is **awesome**. But you must endure some of the **awful** moments as well.

Thunderstorms: These include mostly well-adjusted daughters who have been raised with mutual respect, love, and acceptance, as well as discipline and earned privileges. These daughters will more likely create much innocuous noise and bellowing, along with many beautiful, brilliant, but often scary lightning flashes. Minor damage may occur: occasionally, family circuits are mildly shocked, or viewing appliances that would ordinarily allow a glimpse into their personal turmoil can become totally destroyed by the high voltage. And exceedingly rarely, the lightning will strike only a single household in the community directly and instantaneously with its full fury, due to unpredictable circumstances (wrong peer group, chemical abuse, rebellious temperament, surreptitious school failure), and devastate it. No matter how superbly the parenting is performed or how well "grounded" the home is, we are unfortunately all at risk for a very rare, damaging thunderstorm.

Tornadoes: These daughters have been raised in very permissive or poorly supervised but caring households, with ineffectual discipline, dysfunctional parents, acrimonious divorce, or parents who want to be "friends" instead of parents. The frailer egos of these girls are similar to surviving a storm in a trailer with its weaker foundation and little support. Even during a *tornado warning*—without a direct tornado hit—the high-velocity winds associated with their severe storms often blow the entire household off base. Windstorm and emotional damage from their verbal tirades are frequent. Less commonly, when the scourge of an adolescent "tornado" actually hits and wreaks havoc, although short-lived, it damages a long but modest swath of homes in the community. Its toll takes many years to rebuild.

Hurricanes: these are daughters who are caregiver casualties and neglectfully brought up in chaotic, alcoholic, or drug-using, abusive, or uncaring homes. The damage inflicted on a household by these massive forces of destruction is widespread for miles and quite extensive. Many daughters and families become awash and may sink even with professional intervention.

More Cardinal Rules for Weathering the Stormy Weather of the Adolescent Female

- Do not hurry the child into adulthood.
- Daily hugs and genuine displays of love.
- Courteous responses to questions, regardless of her attitude.
- Frequent humor, but never sarcastic or denigratory.
- No "dissing" (disrespectful comments) by either party.
- Avoid many of the teen magazines.
- Limited makeup until after 15. (Except for acne.)
- Phone: cut off after 9 to 10 p.m., depending on age and homework burden.
- Curfew: Nothing good happens after midnight. Senior (or junior) year: Limit to 2 later weekend nights (11 to 12 p.m.) per week.

- More on Dating: Not until age 15. To avoid sexual predators, no romantic relationships with a male 12 months older than daughter, until high school completed. (Many young girls will become sexually active with an older male within 6 months into the relationship.) Get to know and always meet the date. (A father's presence is key to preventing mishaps such as controllers, date rape, promiscuity, and pressured unwanted drug use.) Assess the daughter's breath (alcohol and cigarettes) and demeanor (marijuana) after the date.

- Driving: Seat belt must always be used. Any drinking in the car forfeits license for several long months.

- Smoking/vaping: Never allowed. (Smoking teens are at increased risk for early promiscuity, chemical abuse, and school failure.)

- Be skeptical of the daughter's whereabouts by double-checking with an occasional phone call or unexpected visit. Network with other parents if possible. If someone says your 13-year-old daughter was driving her friend's aunt's VW Beetle in the neighborhood, believe it. Denial is dangerous—never say your daughter would not do such a stupid thing! Do not directly confront the perpetrator, but rather gather as much evidence as possible and circuitously interrogate about the incident. Again, note: sometime during adolescence, almost one-third will sneak out of the home in the middle of the night.

- Discourage PDA (public displays of affection) and encourage modesty in clothing styles, a never-ending battle for fathers, particularly. This is a fine balance between prudishness versus fashion-consciousness.

- Poor or declining grades always warrant careful, thorough evaluation, particularly for surreptitious drug usage. Simple solutions include reduced television/**phone**/dating time.

- Allow for the every third week shopping addiction or "mall madness." It often soothes their verbal savagery.

- Reminder on Discipline: Never physical; always commensurate to the crime—deny privileges, such as earlier curfew, grounding, reduced phone time (girls would rather be grounded than have the phone denied???); or add extra chores.

Grounded. Grounding. The dreaded essential tool of corralling the wayward behavior or "heinous" crimes of a normal adolescent. "Guess what, dear? Because you have committed XXX offense, you now get to bond with daddy for the next x weeks." (Ouch!) I am not sure who suffers more, you or the teenager? "Grounding serves to plant on the ground the feet of daughters who think that they can soar too high or become too adventurous to prevent them from incurring a mythological meltdown like Icarus. Grounding is etymologically derived from the word, foundation, and is part of the foundation for reducing rates of troubled teens and teen pregnancy. I like to tack on an extra week initially to teach them the art of negotiating early parole in exchange for chores or other barter. It also prevents much mischievous activity, because the teenager can use the excuse: "If my father finds out, he will lambaste me, ground me, be pissed off (jokingly), or lecture me."

All potent deterrents.

Persistent strange withdrawal behavior or prolonged tearful psychosomatic complaints should be carefully assessed for the possibility of school failure, pregnancy, rape, or sexual molestation.

Sexuality: If you suspect your daughter is sexually active, discuss the issues and then seek medical help immediately.

My hair is a little grayer. But my purgatory and penance have been performed, so that I am assured my spot in heaven, as my daughters have finally left the fold.

Christmas Letter—Family Time

Three down and one to go!

Christmas 2008

Well, another year has passed since we last conversed, and it has been a doozy financially for all of us. Bah Humbug! Foreclosures. Abysmal stock drops. You can thank Macroeconomics U.S. Fed style 202: 1), the greedy big banks with their usurious and slipshod lending practices and balloon mortgages and whimsical adjustable to the sky's-the-limit rates and no down payment loans and thus no vested owner; 2) the greedy big banks and their 25% APR credit cards (yet they need a $600 billion government bailout at a low interest rate??? And still not a single foreclosure has been stopped) And you think Poppa is stupid!; 3) the avaricious investment banks/brokers and their fictitious "derivatives" (or trust me—I am not greedy!) and "reinsurance without any assets" of incredibly shaky loans; and 4) 10 billion dollars a month for 5 years for another untenable war in 2 Muslim countries in Mess-o-pot-mania, er, Mesopotamia, where tribal fighting is a new thing—for the last 5000 years! Man, are we smart or what?

Oh yeah, it's a Christmas letter.

Micro-Economics 101: Over the decades, thank goodness our 4 girls have been taught well on how to handle a credit card. You just pull it out of your wallet, insert it into that little thing-a-ma-jiggy (with the magnet strip down, of course, dummy), put a signature of someone on the little paper or on the nice little LCD machine, and save the little receipt for whenever you might want to return it. Or just wear it once and be really nice, and then donate it to Goodwill next year. There are needy people out there after all. Oh, and be careful not to spend too much, or Daddy will explode in a tirade. Or at least one better have the excuse: Mom said it was OK.

Ellen Goodman, a syndicated columnist, wrote today that thrift was in, and, by god, retail therapy was out. Whatever! That credit card still is cheaper than a psychiatrist weekly. Oh my gosh, and the sales at Macy's (who rarely ever sends out coupons, eh!) can save a boy so much money. You cannot afford to NOT shop. "But my Daddy did teach me to never use double negatives in a formal paper, a not uncommon oversight by the less informed."

So as not to get carried away, let's review the family year in a nutshell. We are all still in good health—just Poppa is a little crazier.

Numero uno daughter, demur Mindy, remains the shining star and main troubleshooter of her computer advertising firm, and the firm relies on her heavily to sell the product. She could sell snowshoes to Caribbeans. Her hubby, Evan, is having an incredibly successful impact on his new medical practice in Frankfort as an internist. Baby Jake is now 3, full of boyishness, and loves to visit his poppa and mimi. So adorable; garrulous; intense about playtime. We are learning how little boys perceive the world—cars and trucks. Jake #2 (March EDC) is healthy in the momma hatchery, and all are excited.

Numero 2 daughter, loquacious Misty, works the local real estate market as best she can, but too many greedy and incredibly stupid big bank lending practices have decimated this market (see above). She will be going back to teaching real soon, and will put her wonderful way with kids and her master's in education to work. (See, the old man was right about college education and contingencies.) She also has a little hatchling in the hopper (June EDC), and all are excited. Danny, her hubby, is steadily working at Marathon Oil as general go-to-it guy, whose work is sorely appreciated there, and here too, as they have acquired and thoroughly refurbished a new large house here in town—which is none too close for her momma. He is nearly finished with his college degree from WKU. Two dogs, Elle and Jed, are their surrogate children for now.

Yes, daughter numero 3, industrious Lindsay, was married this summer to her dentist man in a lovely, lavish affair here in B-town. (Although no one else does, Poppa loves eBay's wedding gown section, where you love 'em and leave 'em.) Josh is marooned in the army for another 1.5 years as a dentist in Fort Benning, GA, but doing very well. She is in the midst of her 3rd year of med school at U of K, and her daddy had the pleasure of her company on a med student rotation in his office this summer. Most patients figured out the relationship, except they could not fathom how she could be related as she is so smart and pretty—qualities the old man lacks. The medical school likewise thinks that she must be adopted also, for she is achieving smoking hot grades. The long distance is a strain for the lovebirds, still they are thriving.

Numero 4 daughter, studious Mollie, is finishing her 3rd year at UK, and was recently accepted into the UK pharmacy program—a highly competitive school. Studying and working amazingly hard in her schooling. She loves her gadgets, especially the iMac and blueberry, er, blackberry phone. She is extremely adept at handling her finances—see the credit card recipe above—but admits that her 2007 Ford Escape is not likely to hold her through one more year of college. Time to trade up! She is enjoying her 3 roommates in their apt. (Yes, they are female, duh.)

What does all this mean? A truly merry xmas. We now have 4 daughters who have succeeded to become independent and to embark upon highly gainful careers. Perhaps, 4 daughters soon off the payroll entirely, you surmise, eh? Certain Old habits wane too slowly.

Melinda, the proud pulchritudinous matriarch, still has her world revolve entirely around her little chickies. Not a day goes by (or is that buy?) without hearing from the chickies. Nor a weekend without seeing her chickies. Girls never leave the nest—they just bring back hungry boys with them. And sometimes with a really cute little baby boy. She is quite busy with the Certified Nursing Assistant program—testing and teaching for the state, and works more hours than her lazy husband anymore.

Poppa gripes but continues to be busy with his general pediatric practice, his national speaking and advisory boards, and his office pharmaceutical research, mostly in new vaccines. His group has had a huge role in the development of new meningitis vaccines, new expeditious production methods for flu vaccines, improved ear/pneumonia vaccines, cervical cancer vaccines for teens, etc. Prolific, he has been a first or co-author on about 10 nationally published medical papers this year. His office staff of peds is fairly stable, and he actually looks forward to seeing his patients daily. He hopes that his medical daughter catches this *joie de vivre* of pediatrics, but who knows.

Hope you are well and have a merry Christmas.
The Bardstown Blocks, daughters et al.

Pediatric Annals Articles—Tweaking Conventional Wisdom: Part 2

For each article that is the "first of its kind" to report a novel approach or finding, a gold star will be placed beside the title to indicate it.

More Pediatric Annals articles

Put Some 'Teeth' into Your Pediatric Preventive Counseling, and The Fluoride Hoax

(Adapted from Block SL, Put Some 'Teeth' into Your Pediatric Preventive Counseling. *Pediatric Annals*, September 2012)

In my own experience, the number of general dentists capable or willing to see Medicaid-insured children younger than 4 years of age is significantly limited. However, dental caries caused by the bacteria, *Streptococcus mutans,* are among the most common chronic bacterial infections found in early childhood.

Consider the following: only 14 of 39 states had more than 50% of dentists who treat Medicaid-insured children, 33.3 million children live in an area with a shortage of dental care professionals, and about 10% of all children, regardless of insurance coverage, never see a dentist. Pediatric dental surgery is now the most common outpatient procedure in many Canadian pediatric hospitals.

Early childhood dental caries (ECC) also creates a tremendous demand on our nation's resources for pediatric restorative and dental surgical care. In addition, the costs of ECC, such as for general anesthesia, a dental surgeon, outpatient services, etc., and the months or even years of horrendous daily oral pain are considerable.

Pediatrician's Role In Preventive Dental Care

From 1999 to 2002, as many as 11% of children in the United States, ages 1 to 3 years, and 41% of children ages 2 to 11 years, had ECC in their primary teeth. The two best predictors of ECC in a child's primary teeth were parents with lower educational achievement and lower socioeconomic status. However, in the last few years, I have seen the local rate of patients on Medicaid soar from 30% to nearly 55% as a result of recent economic hardships; thus, socioeconomic status may not be as relevant a risk factor.

In pediatric offices, most children between the ages of 9 months and 36 months are seen an average of five to six times annually for their well-visits and a multitude of other complaints. These patients all have or will soon have teeth. These visits provide an opportunity to start our patients on the road to a lifetime of good dental hygiene and the habits they will likely teach their own children.

To do this, doctors should consider adding routine dental counselling to most well-visits after age 6 months.

The 'Root' of Dental Caries

ECC is a consequence of the interaction between normal bacterial oral flora and dietary fermentable sugars. The oral flora creates a sticky biofilm, known as dental plaque, that ferments sugar into an acidic substance that erodes the dental enamel over time (Figures 18 and 19). Although only a few oral bacterial species are highly associated with dental plaque, the major culprit is *S. mutans*. Chronic consumption of sugary foods and liquids will continually recharge the plaque matrix.[2]

---

[2] Marshall TA, Levy SM, Broffitt B, et al. Dental caries and beverage consumption in young children. *Pediatrics*. 2003;112(3):e184-e191

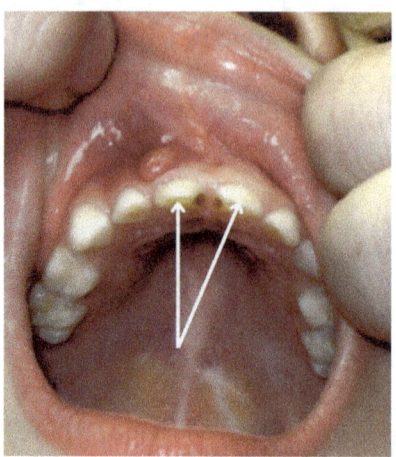

Figure 18. Gum boil due to ECC. Note the moderate dental erosions on the central aspect of the two frontal dental incisors. The girl had a history of sleeping with her bottle until she was 18 months old. Dental caps were placed on the teeth by age 2 years. Therapy with oral amoxicillin was initiated along with a prompt dental referral for extraction or root canal. **Source:** Dr. Block

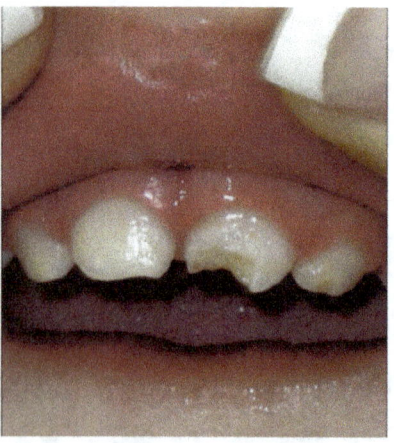

Figure 19. A 2-year-old girl who was given a bottle in bed up to age 15 months. Note the erosion and nontraumatic chipping of the dental enamel of the two left incisors. The start of further ominous teeth rotting. **Source:** Dr. Block

ECC Prevention

Based on the latest recommendations from the American Academy of Pediatrics (AAP), which this original article helped influence (2013), and 40 years of my own pediatric practice, the following are my cardinal rules of pediatric (and adolescent) dental care once primary teeth have fully erupted.

Modification of Diet

The following three practices will greatly reduce the incidence of ECC in children: 1) avoid all juices and sugary beverages, except for on special occasions; 2) avoid day-long "grazing" on starchy cereals (Cheerios) and first foods; and 3) always have the child sit at the kitchen table to eat or drink; this reduces the temptation to over-indulge on sweet drinks and foods.

Good Oral Hygiene Adherence

A child's teeth should be brushed twice daily, **particularly at night before bedtime.** Beginning this ritual before the child is 12 months old will spare most parents a nightly battle. Using an electric kids' toothbrush confers distinct advantages over manual brushing because it more thoroughly covers all dental surfaces, even if the child does not cooperate. An electric toothbrush is also an interesting "toy" and a good distraction for the toddler. I recommend an electric toothbrush that has a distinct on/off switch. I also recommend that, immediately before or after the child brushes their own teeth, an adult should brush the child's teeth until the child is at least 6 years old. Dental flossing of children's teeth is advised, but I pick my "battles" with young children, and flossing is less important than nightly and morning brushing of teeth.

Once the teeth are brushed at night, never allow the child anything to eat or drink, except water, until the next morning. This applies to breast milk as well, because "it may become cavity-causing when combined with other carbohydrate sources." If the child ingests anything besides water at night, the teeth must be brushed again. If the child sneaks food at night after everyone else has gone to bed, the parent should lock the refrigerator and/or cabinets at night.

Remember that saliva, which is highly protective for teeth, is minimally produced during sleep. A morning teeth brushing is optimal, too, according to the American Academy of Pediatric Dentists (AAPD).

Fluoride Administration-Somehow Now Made Controversial!!

At home: I still advise the supervised use of fluoride toothpaste for all children older than 12 months. For those children between 12 and 24 months, I suggest using merely a tiny smear or rice-sized grain of toothpaste on a soft (electric) toothbrush. For children older than 24 months, use a pea-sized amount of toothpaste. These are the current recommendations by the AADP and the AAP for children on Medicaid and for "high-risk" children (I say all children).

Although this advice may seem somewhat controversial for toddlers (because of concerns over ingestion of too much fluoride), in my opinion, the "high-risk" dental caries state is nearly universal. Most toddlers consume fruit drinks, soda pop, and sugared and non-sugared high-carbohydrate cereals more than three times a day, and many also have parents or siblings with cavities.

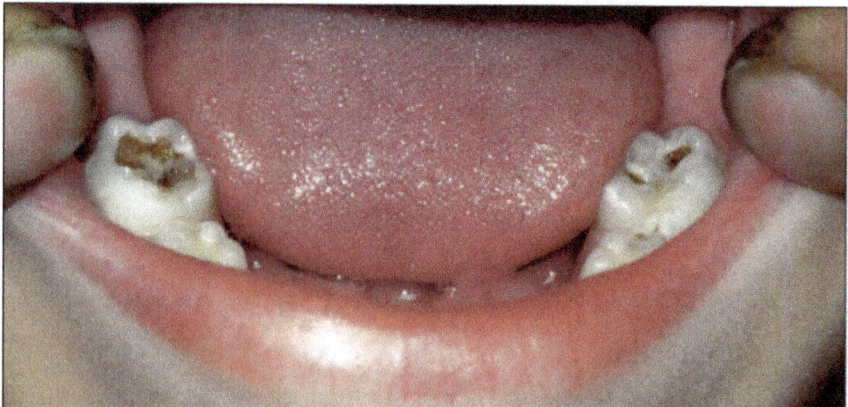

Figure 20. Severe erosion of the two posterior molars in this 5-year-old girl. She required extensive caps and dental restoration, along with prolonged general anesthesia for the dental procedure.
Source: Dr. Block

This "grazing" on snack food during the day is now the apparent norm. Just look at the sweet-drink "sippy cup" spills and the crumbs that accumulate on your office's waiting room floor by the end of the day.

In the office: This has now become controversial for many dental **non-experts**. Fluoride varnishes may be applied twice annually in the office by the pediatrician's staff for all children who have teeth who are 9 months to 3 years old and covered by Medicaid. These applications are associated with a **17% to 49% reduction in ECC**, are easy for office staff to perform, and the Medicaid payments are worthwhile. Even though the CDC recommends it, commercial insurance may not reimburse medical offices for this procedure.

You have surely heard some non-medical politicians recently proclaim that we should no longer fluoridate our community water. This was based mostly on a very faulty recent multi-site analysis study in 2025 *JAMA Pediatrics,* which apparently found that in some communities, higher fluoride levels in the water were associated with a 1 to 3 point lower IQ score on intelligence tests in some children.[3]

The devil is in the details. (I dare say that a one-point difference in an IQ of 100 versus 99 is clinically insignificant as well.) Careful reading and analysis of scientific articles is essential to combat misinformation based on faulty conclusions, like in this article.

First, the standard fluoride levels in the U.S. water sources are 0.7 mg. No higher. (Except for on-property wells occasionally, which means all well sources should be checked for fluoride levels.) The only children in the *JAMA* study who showed decreased IQ scores had been exposed to community water fluoride levels of 2.0 to 4.0 or higher! In the study, those with community **levels of 1.5 or less showed NO decreased IQ scores!** Regardless of any other environmental fluoride exposures.

---

[3] Taylor KW, Eftim SE, Sibrizzi CA, Blain RB, Magnuson K, Hartman PA, Rooney AA, Bucher JR. Fluoride Exposure and Children's IQ Scores: A Systematic Review and Meta-Analysis. *JAMA Pediatr. 2025 Mar 1*;179(3):282-292.

Secondly, most of the studies were conducted **in China (45/74 studies)**. Since this is most likely the group with the higher fluoride levels, I have real problems with this. Two other well-known environmental CNS toxins to children must be assessed—**lead and arsenic—in all study sites, in my opinion.** In China in 2018, the average blood lead levels uncovered in children in several areas were 37.5, totally neurotoxic!!! And the majority had levels over 50! Now, in my office, we panic when our routine blood lead screening in patients 1 and 2 years old is discovered as over 10. We immediately send out the health department team to search for the environmental sources (paint, soil, toys, etc), because of the extreme neurotoxicity of lead. The CDC says that any levels above 10 are poisonous to the child, no exceptions. Without assessing the lead levels in populations with already known high lead levels, one could never directly point to the low or even high fluoride levels as a toxin. And these high lead level exposures have likely been ongoing for years in these Chinese communities!

Thirdly, this type of IQ study must assess arsenic levels as well, especially with the known association with rice and uptake of arsenic in this major childhood food source (see above infant feeding chapter). **What is one main staple of the Chinese child's diet?—rice!** Even low levels of arsenic are a well-known neurotoxin in the U.S. It must also be excluded as a source of lower IQ scores in any community study.

Furthermore, when a Canadian province discontinued its routine water fluoridation a few decades ago, rates of dental caries shot up by 35 to 40%. Thus, I still strongly recommend routine low-level community water fluoridation as a supplement, which is: "Much ado about nothing!"

Role of Nutrition

Reducing both the amount of sugar a child consumes and the frequency of its intake is critical for better dentition (and obesity reduction). For that reason, I also recommend that children have no juice, but if they do, then no more than 4 ounces of juice once daily.

Instead, children should have 16 to 32 ounces of milk daily and some fluoridated tap water daily. If parents balk at being told not to give their child juice, you can also inform them that juice is a notable culprit in the obesity struggle, even if the label says "fruit juice, which parents often think means it is "healthy." Low levels of arsenic have been found in some fruit juices as well (see infant feeding section).

For instance, ingestion of 32 ounces of juice daily may comprise nearly 400 calories—or about 40% of a younger child's recommended daily caloric intake. Thus, depending on their metabolism, these extra empty sugar calories can increase the child's risk of obesity if the child still consumes a typical caloric diet. Or on the other hand, it may create a very finicky eater, as the child might forgo other, less sweet essential calories and nutrients.

According to the AAP, sucrose (table sugar) is the most cariogenic sugar because it can form glucan, which enables bacterial adhesion to teeth. Cereals and starchy chips are also cariogenic. The child who frequently "grazes" or eats carbohydrate-laden snacks is definitely at increased risk for ECC.

I have parents check the cereal labels carefully for the percentage of calories due to added sucrose.

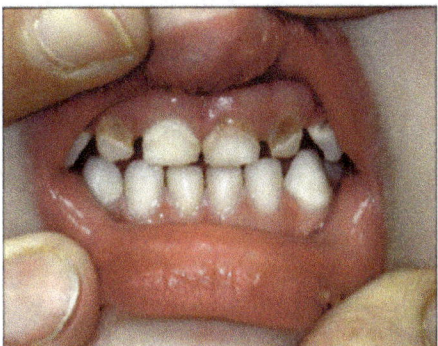

Figure 21. This 3-year-old boy had severe ECC of the upper frontal incisors, characteristic of his receiving a bottle or a "sippy cup" nightly, despite brushing his teeth. Also note the white chalky appearance on the enamel of the right front incisor, which is indicative of ECC.
Source: Dr. Block

CONCLUSION

In most states, each child must see a dentist to enter school. However, here in rural Kentucky, my patients who are 9 to 36 months old have minimal access to a full-time pediatric dentist, as the closest one is at least 25 miles away. Thus, our practice uses the pediatrician-first screening approach.

Consequently, we refer any child younger than age 4 years who adheres poorly to any one of my cardinal rules of primary dentition, or has any hint of ECC from chalky white spots to small brown erosions to overt cavitations.

In my opinion, most ECC could be prevented if general pediatricians and family practitioners would routinely stress the vital importance of early routine teeth brushing and avoidance of sugary drinks and "grazing" on carbohydrates and most importantly, no nighttime feedings or drinks ever besides water. And, a recent economic projection from *JAMA Health Forum,* by Cho and Simon, demonstrated that elimination of fluoride in community water would cost the U.S. an excess of almost $10 billion in expenditures and 25 million additional dental caries (cavities) (7.5% more cavities per child) over 5 years.[4]

I have practiced what I preached. Even though they complained some when younger, my four daughters with an accumulated dental exposure of over 160 years have experienced only two cavities in total.

---

[4] Choi, S. E., & Simon, L. (2025). Projected Outcomes of Removing Fluoride From US Public Water Systems. *JAMA health forum, 6*(5), e251166. https://doi.org/10.1001/jamahealthforum.2025.1166

✹ Improving the Diagnosis of Acute Otitis Media: "Seeing Is Believing"

(Adapted from Block SL, *Pediatric Annals*, December 2013)

[Since this is the most common respiratory bacterial infection that we see in children, and generates the most questions and myths, I am giving my readers most of the article.]

Acute otitis media (AOM) should remain an entirely visual diagnosis for all of us. A much-improved guideline on the diagnosis and management of AOM was recently published in *Pediatrics*. The new diagnostic emphasis in AOM is now the presence of infected middle ear effusion (MEE), as it appears with different levels of a bulging or convex (eardrum) tympanic membrane (TM). In the guidelines, the child with moderate to severe bulging TM or otorrhea is definitely considered to have AOM, whereas the child with mild bulging TM (once termed "fullness") should also have concomitant recent ear pain or intense TM erythema. Remember that straightforward "otitis media with effusion," or serous otitis, should not be treated with antibiotics, but rather followed up over several months.

As every pediatrician is keenly aware, AOM is the most common reason for prescribing antibiotics in every general clinical practice. In fact, before routine PCV7/13/15/20 vaccination, an AOM episode developed in 94% of all children in a non-inner-city population by the age of 24 months. So, one would assume that probably the most important aspect in the entire discussion of AOM and its treatment would be how to correctly diagnose AOM and the optimal methods needed to obtain its diagnosis. However, one would be mistaken.

We in pediatrics are all painfully aware of how poorly diagnosed or misdiagnosed AOM can often be. Just ask any otolaryngologist or general pediatrician who sees patients in follow-up from many of their own less-experienced health providers, community emergency rooms, urgent care centers, and even from other too-busy pediatric offices.

Unfortunately, for such an everyday problem, the amount of time spent on teaching the correct diagnoses and management of AOM in medical school is negligible. Even in most pediatric and family practice training programs, training is minimal. So, why do we give such short shrift to such an important, ubiquitous pediatric assessment that must be ascertained in nearly every young pediatric patient's well or sick visit?

Do not kid yourself; this is one of the most technically difficult tasks to perform on young children within a general pediatric practice. It requires a confident, firm parent to restrain the child, as well as your own extreme diligence, patience, a lot of upper arm strength, and a stable eye to perform this task in most children younger than 24 months and in many children up to 4 years old. To compound the technical difficulties, the TMs in nearly 80% of children under age 12 months are partially or totally obscured by wax. You may never adequately see the TMs in most of these children without some manner of cleaning the debris from the ear canals. Thus, it can often take a great deal of extra time and effort to obtain the correct diagnosis—hard to do in busy office practice!

For example, each of the following obstacles may become glaringly manifest as you examine the TMs of young children:

- Inferior instrumentation
- Tiny ear canals
- Too much ear cerumen
- Too much feistiness and pushback from the child toward either the parent or the pediatrician
- Poor practitioner training in assessment of TM markers of bona fide AOM

The remainder of this article addresses each of these issues from my point of view as a U.S. Food and Drug Administration preferred clinical investigator of AOM. I have previously written many treatises on the management of AOM, most recently touching on the diagnosis of AOM in the neonate in the June 2012 issue of *Pediatric Annals* and in the third edition of our book, *Diagnosis and Management of Acute Otitis Media*. For the last 31 years, I have examined bilateral TMs in more than 3,000 patients annually, performed tympanocentesis in more than 400 patients with severe AOM, and been a principal investigator in nearly 50 clinical trials involving AOM and approximately 10 clinical trials involving TM (normal and abnormal eardrums) instrumentation.

The "Stumbling Blocks" to Accurate TM Assessment: Inadequate Instrumentation

One of the most important and most overlooked areas of assessing the TM is the use of optimal instruments. I much prefer the new version of the MacroView otoscope because of its crisper optics and longer-lasting, brighter lithium battery. It is worth the price differential. Just be sure to line up or adjust the green line according to your own visual needs.

I cannot emphasize enough the critical importance of using the original non-disposable speculum for all children younger than age 4 years. These speculums are longer in order to get past the bend of the ear canal, more tapered, have a critically wider aperture, and reflect light better from the plastic onto the TM. You will need to wipe them down with an alcohol pad after each visit, and they sometimes require cleaning of the aperture with a cotton swab. The little bit of extra effort is well worth it, as the shorter, stubbier disposable speculum is simply inadequate for younger children.

Occasionally, you may encounter a child with such tiny ear canals that they may preclude the entrance of even the 2.5-mm speculum. Some may even have atretic (undeveloped) canals, and you will need to consider otolaryngology referral and probably a CT scan of the middle ear space to see if any functional TM remains. For the rest of these rarely encountered patients, the Welch-Allyn surgical otoscopic head and its 2-mm green speculum will frequently allow you to visualize the TM until it enlarges enough for the routine otoscope as the child matures over time.

Ear Cerumen (Wax)

You will often encounter children with significant amounts of cerumen obstructing the ear canal, challenging your adequate visualization of the TM. It is important to make sure that the debris is not pus and/or blood from otorrhea.

Cleaning the cerumen ear canals is the bane of pediatrics, without a doubt. You will need one or several of the curettes. Personally, I prefer the stiffer metal curettes like the dark-handled one, but it can pose the potential hazard of scratching the canal and causing subsequent secondary brief bleeding; however, this can be tamponaded with a portion of a cotton ball.

The key is the gentle but firm restraint of the child by the parent or, rarely, by your nurse. When cleaning ear canals in infants or obstreperous young children, I often use the technique of laterally positioning the child upon the exam table with the parent firmly restraining the arms while lying on the lower trunk and legs; I can then restrain the head with one hand. The cleaning often takes up to a few minutes, as well as patience and gentle strength on the part of the physician, as most of us know. This positioning technique especially pays off in children younger than 6 months. The less we aggravate the child, the easier the exam will usually be the next time.

For those many children who are too difficult or too compacted with cerumen, ancillary personnel are needed when resorting to the instruments; however, make sure the child does not have a history of recent PE tubes or TM perforation. Our techs pre-soften the cerumen by instilling several drops of peroxide for about 5 minutes. Often, young children can merely sit on a parent's lap during the process of gentle irrigation until the tech perceives that the wax has been flushed into the irrigation basin. The tech has to be keenly aware, however, and stop if the child seems to really be in pain—not just fussing—during the flushing process, as very rarely, a hidden tympanic membrane perforation or a patent tube may be present.

Three Criteria for TM Physical Diagnosis of AOM (without Otorrhea)	
Position	Bulging or "full" always means acute otitis media (AOM) vs. neutral (normal) or retracted (serous otitis media, or OME)
Opacification	Absence of bony landmarks, completely opaque, opaque air-fluid level (AOM or OME) vs. translucent (normal)
Discoloration	Mostly or entirely cloudy/purulent (green, pale yellow or non-scarring white fluid) or marked hyperemia indicates AOM vs. gray (normal) or amber/orange (OME).

AOM = acute otitis media: OME = otitis media with effusion: ™ = tympanic membrane.
Data from Block

Table 4. Three Criteria for TM Physical Diagnosis of AOM (without Otorrhea)

Feistiness and Pushback by the Child

This is truly the art of pediatrics. You must decide how much restraint, pressure, and calm reassurance to administer to each child. You should not "box" the ear, but rather use the gentle force of your thumb against the pinna and the child's skull to apply mild upward traction. Novices also tend to force the speculum too far into the canal, when it often only requires inserting a few millimeters or so. Being gentle but firm must be finessed. A minimally traumatic experience will often pay off, with quicker and more compliant future examinations of all body parts.

For those more common "ballistic" children, accept your losses for the TM examination and routinely place them on the exam table as described above. I suggest keeping your stethoscope in your ears when examining a "screamer," as, over time, this will prevent damage to your hearing, and this may also make you less likely to rush your TM exam at hand due to your own auditory "ear pain."

TM Characteristics of AOM

Fortunately, the 2013 AAP guidelines on AOM now emphasize the diagnostic importance of purulent or cloudy middle ear effusion (MEE), along with either severe redness or new-onset otorrhea. Symptoms plus a non-purulent MEE are no longer considered evidence for the diagnosis of AOM. AOM symptoms in young children "are mostly non-specific, variable, and not infrequently absent." The current AOM definition is now mostly synchronous with my previous delineations of AOM diagnosis over the last decade. However, according to the AAP guidelines, the presence of significant fever (102.2°F) or significant ear complaints will place the child into different categories of AOM severity, which will have implications as to how to approach antibiotic therapy.

Most pediatricians in practice can readily ascertain fullness or bulging of the TM within a clear ear canal. It is this positive pressure upon the TM that foremost assures the diagnosis of AOM, even as espoused by the new AOM guidelines.

Interestingly, the "true" mobility of the TM (a very difficult process for most of us to determine) or ascertaining the severity of otalgia rarely ever changes the diagnosis of AOM! Seven U.S. experts in AOM assessed 945 middle ear images; out of all AOM cases, bulging TM and marked redness alone were present in 93% and 2%, respectively. Otherwise, knowing the presence or absence of TM mobility altered their diagnosis of AOM in only three of 945 TM evaluations. Of these three cases, one each was changed from AOM to OME (otitis media with effusion), one from AOM to normal, and one from normal to AOM. Furthermore, knowing the presence or absence of "otalgia" changed the diagnosis of OME to AOM in seven (10%) of otalgia cases, and from AOM to OME in seven (0.8%) of non-otalgia cases.

The simplest and cheapest method is to use the handheld insufflator. However, this inexpensive auxiliary otoscope part also requires much bimanual dexterity, as well as the sufficient restraint of the child for a period of several "eternal" arduous seconds. This time may be better spent in pursuing the accurate position and color of the TM in the often unruly child. Also, if you are not careful, this blowing process and "jamming" the speculum into the canal to create a seal can be quite uncomfortable for the child, thus **jeopardizing future cooperation** with this and other simple examinations.

For those who still wish to pursue TM mobility, two ancillary instruments are available: tympanometer and acoustic reflectometer (SGAR). Note that each of these instruments requires a fairly clean ear canal. The first one is also not likely to be very reliable in children younger than 6 months due to the elasticity and tininess of the ear canal in this age group.

Of these two other options for the indirect assessment of MEE, we do not use either, as neither instrument will differentiate AOM from OME, and the sensitivity for either machine in predicting merely MEE ranges from 80% to 90%. SGAR is cheaper, portable, does not require a seal, and is simpler to use. By contrast, tympanometry is a stand-alone machine in a separate room and requires a canal-to-instrument tip seal. However, it is also considered the only adequate supplemental measure to determine MEE within the 2013 AAP AOM guidelines.

TM Characteristics for AOM

The best way to learn about the defining characteristics of AOM versus OME versus normal is to examine a plethora of variations on TM findings with oversight from a qualified mentor. An excellent initiation and training CME program for differentiation of the TM findings has been developed by the otolaryngology experts at the University of Pittsburgh. The website is located at www.pedsed.pitt.edu under the subheading "Enhancing Proficiency in Otitis Media (eProm)."

The diagnosis of normal TM and bulging TM is relatively straightforward, as seen in the first three middle ear samples. However, it is those TMs with more subtle findings, as shown in the remainder of the TM photos, that create the diagnostic dilemma for all of us in pediatrics. My evaluations for each of these TMs were corroborated by and totally harmonious with each of my three astute, highly experienced otoscopist general pediatric partners, James Hedrick, MD, Ron Tyler, MD, and Dan Finn, MD.

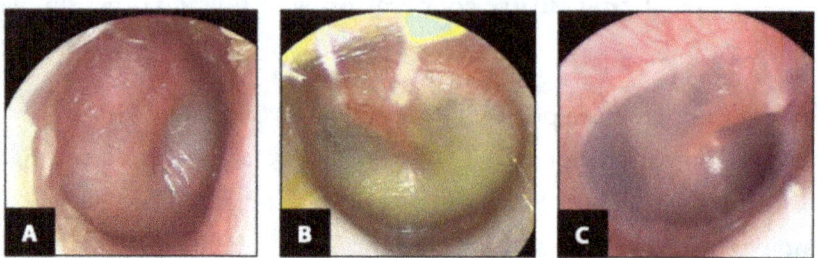

Figure 22. Obvious diagnostic tympanic membrane (TM) findings regardless of TM mobility and patient symptoms. (A) and (B) Examples of bulging, infected TM. (C) An example of a normal TM.
Source: Courtesy of Alejandero Hoberman, MD, University of Pittsburgh

In the group of TMs in **Figure 23**, the TM photographs in A to E were each considered by us to be definitive cases of OME, and therefore not treated with antibiotics. Photographs F and G were considered as cases of OME with early superimposed infection due to the "fullness" in F, and the notable hyperemia and fullness of the pars flaccida in G. Thus, we would prescribe antibiotics for these last two cases.

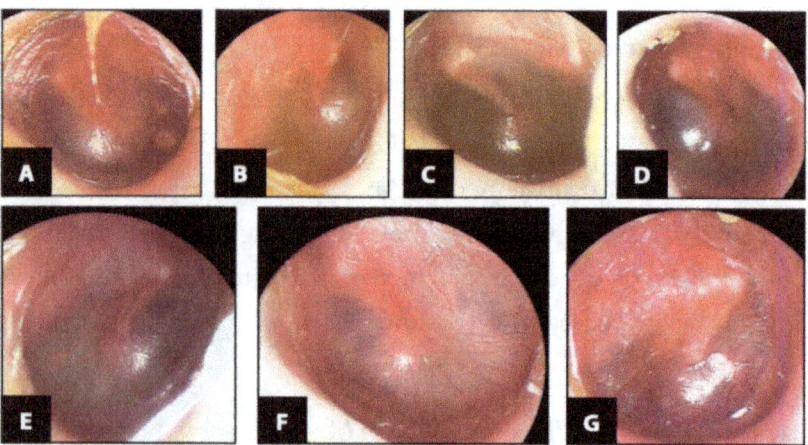

Figure 23. The subtler and more difficult diagnostic tympanic membrane (TM) findings, regardless of TM mobility or patient symptoms. Each one has an element of middle ear effusion: infected/treatment-worthy or not?
Source: Courtesy of Alejandero Hoberman, MD, University of Pittsburgh

Each of the TMs in **Figure 23** was considered to have a purulent air-fluid level and, therefore, we would treat them if they initially presented with significant symptoms of URI, fever, or fussiness. Over the decades, having performed tympanocentesis in numerous similar-appearing, mildly infected TMs (simultaneously with a contralateral bulging TM) as those in **Figure 23**, we nearly always observed the recovery of an identical bacterial pathogen from both ears. However, we would also not treat any asymptomatic children in **Figures 23B, 23C,** and **23D** if they had recently finished antibiotics within the last few weeks. We readily acknowledge both the common persistence of some MEE after an episode of AOM and the "post-antibiotic effect" or persistent low-level antibiotic concentrations after a recent course of antibiotics. Because of the fullness or mild bulging that we perceived in **Figures 23E, 23F,** and **23G,** we would proceed with further antibiotic therapy. Only one of us thought that the findings on insufflation of these particular TMs would possibly change our minds.

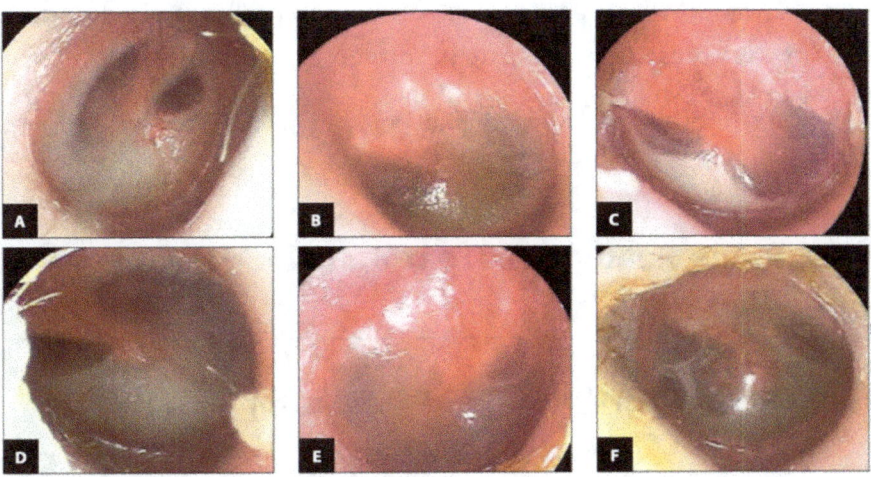

Figure 24. The subtler and more difficult diagnostic tympanic membrane (TM) findings, regardless of TM mobility or patient symptoms. Each one has an element of purulent middle ear effusion: infected/treatment-worthy or not?
Source: Courtesy of Alejandero Hoberman, MD, University of Pittsburgh

With all due respect to the AAP 2013 guidelines, the concept of "otalgia" and "ear tugging" or direct ear pain is much too infrequently observed, too vague, too non-specific, and too unreliable to be of much use in the infant or child aged younger than 36 months. And far too many young children with normal TMs constantly tug at their ears during any illness.

CONCLUSION

The diagnosis of AOM for clinicians continues to remain almost exclusively "what you see, not what you hear." New, improved 2013 AAP guidelines for management of AOM have refined the physical diagnostic criteria for AOM without providing many specifics about diagnostic techniques. Practitioners need to use the optimal instruments and approaches, particularly in infants and younger children, when attempting to differentiate AOM from OME and normal. With all the physical and time obstacles, as well as the major difficulties encountered while examining TMs of young children, I recommend a simplified and quick approach using my three criteria for the diagnosis of AOM: position, opacification, and discoloration. The plethora of subtle variations in TM findings when MEE is present will continue to challenge the diagnostic skills of every otoscopist and "parental diagnostician," as well.

For more information, refer to the book by Block and Harrison on *Diagnosis and Management of Acute Otitis Media.*

Should We Really Not Treat Bona Fide Ear Infections?

Controversy Over "Watchful Waiting" for Ear Infections

The American Academy of Pediatrics (AAP) issued guidelines several years ago stating that ear infections (acute otitis media) may sometimes be left untreated under a strategy called "watchful waiting." This means that instead of prescribing antibiotics immediately when observed by the doctor, with the parents' permission, doctors wait to see if the infection resolves on its own over several days.

Most importantly, three different AOM studies have documented bacterial recovery in 87% to 95% of children with bona fide AOM. AOM is a bacterial infection!!! (One definitive study was from me, which won a national award.) One to three rounds of antibiotics do work most of the time.

Furthermore, this earlier AAP recommendation is truly controversial for the *bona fide* (PUS-FILLED MIDDLE EAR) ear infection with any symptoms at all. Ear infections are typically painful and can very rarely lead to serious complications if left untreated.

A child with a *bona fide* moderate to severe ear infection often experiences intense pain for days, making watchful waiting an unnecessary burden on both the child and the parents. Delaying treatment may also increase the VERY RARE risk of serious complications, such as mastoiditis, a dangerous bacterial infection of the bones behind the ear.

Additionally, chronic ear infections may develop, often requiring surgical tubes to also prevent persistent fluid buildup and hearing loss. I think that if you could ask the child and if they could tell you, they would say, *Get me better as quickly as possible, doctor. It really hurts.*

By starting antibiotics upon presentation, an actual, accurately diagnosed infection can resolve faster, leading to quicker pain relief, better sleep, and a shorter duration of illness.

Also, guidelines on watchful waiting seem to contradict standard pain management principles in medicine. For example, adults with migraines receive immediate and often expensive treatment despite migraines being non-life-threatening and without any known sequela. Meanwhile, children with definite bacterial ear infections are expected to "wait and see," even though their painful condition involves an active bacterial infection that could persist or worsen over time.

Garlic, "similars," herbals, and chiropractic maneuvers have no business in otitis treatment.

✴ The Enigmatic Sacro-Coccygeal Dimple: To Ignore or Explore?

(Adapted from Block SL, The Enigmatic Sacro-Coccygeal Dimple: To Ignore or Explore? *Pediatric Annals 43(3)*, March 2014)

In everyday practice, pediatricians routinely encounter congenital midline coccygeal and sacral dimples (Figure 25). These cutaneous coccygeal and sacral stigmas, most of which are below the intragluteal (butt-crack) crease, occur in as many as 4.8% of all children. Yet the incidence of the "true" problematic lesions related to these dimples, such as spinal dysraphism, is only about 1 in every 2,500 births; spinal lipoma, which occurs in 1 of 4,000 births; and dermal sinuses, which occur in 1 of 2,500 births. More importantly, as explained below, the more common coccygeal dimples seem to be uniformly benign. So, what is all the fuss about? And why are so many babies undergoing expensive spine evaluations?

Unfortunately, another study of nearly 2,000 consecutive neonates found that as many as 3% were observed to have a significant paraspinal abnormality above the intergluteal crease. These findings are among the more worrisome observations and definitely require further evaluation. However, this high incidence of abnormal sacral dimples seems to be relegated merely to this one study from 40 years ago. Additionally, practitioners seem to be lumping together the rates from each dimple region—those above (worrisome) with those below (usually innocuous) the intergluteal (butt-crack) crease.

Therefore, apparently, many practitioners feel compelled to further evaluate the mere simple dimple in the lower sacro-coccygeal area, at least by ultrasound, in most of these children. During their training, they have been instilled with a persuasive fear that these sacro-coccygeal dimples may be the only manifestation of an occult spinal dermal sinus tract, tethered cord, spinal dysraphism, etc. Once they decide to perform the additional imaging, they must then explain their fear to the family in order to obtain permission to perform the test.

If as many as 4.8% of normal infants have this physical manifestation of the coccyx area, then these usually unnecessary evaluations can become very expensive for the family, as well as from a public health perspective. The potential clinical ramifications for the infant also become manifested by terrifying the parents and extended family of this potential newborn problem, once they learn your rationale for this evaluation. "You mean my baby could become paralyzed, never obtain bladder control, or require major neurosurgery on the spinal cord?" they'll ask.

We need to do a better job deciding when to further evaluate the differentiating features of sacral and coccygeal dimples and other associated cutaneous stigmas in this region.

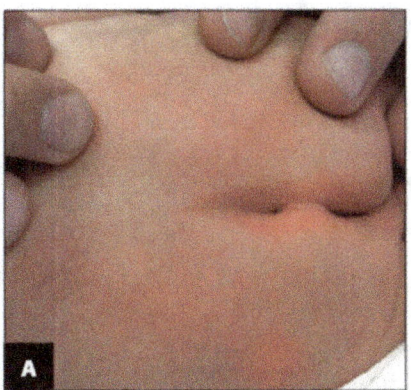

Figure 25. An 11-day-old white male with a very deep coccygeal dimple located within 2.5 cm of the anal verge. But is the most important characteristic the depth of the dimple, or the distance from the anus? Lower is benign.
Source: Dr. Block

Dorsal Spinal Sinus Tracts

These upper sacral dermal tracts can be associated with a heterogeneous set of five major problems in children:

1. Tethering of the spinal cord

2. Bacterial meningitis secondary to bacteria entering the connecting dermal tract
3. Aseptic (chemical) meningitis secondary to debris from the spinal tract entering the spinal canal
4. Compression of the spinal cord or nerve roots from a dermoid cyst
5. Diastematomyelia

Other than the very rare case of meningitis, the most commonly observed signs related to these "true" abnormalities include focal neurologic abnormalities, which may develop in 50% and 92% of children aged younger than 12 months and older than 12 months, respectively. In addition, these children may also develop severe constipation, scoliosis, back pain, and orthopedic foot abnormalities—**especially very tight heel cords and persistent toe walking**.

"Simple Dimple Rules" for Sacral Dimples

The following parameters define which sacral dimples are high risk:

- Larger than 0.5 cm in size.
- Located more than 2.5 cm cephalad (toward the head) to the anal verge.
- Associated with overlying cutaneous markers (see: blue tumor article).

True hypertrichosis, or hairs within the dimple, is distinctly different from the mild hairiness.

- Skin tags
    - Telangiectasia or hemangioma
    - Subcutaneous mass or lump
- Apparent aplasia cutis
    - Abnormal pigmentation
- Bifurcation (fork) or asymmetry of the superior gluteal crease

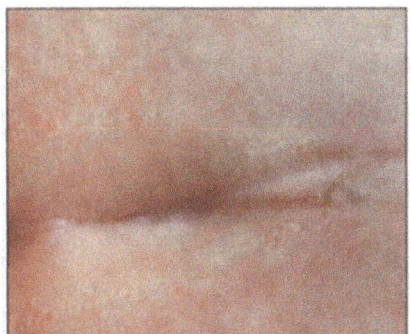

Figure 26. The photo reveals no other ominous dimple characteristics within the area except for a worrisome **intragluteal (cleft) fork**.
Source: Dr. Block

Kriss and Desai observed that none of the 207 neonates with a sacral dimple who did not meet any of the first three criteria above had spinal dysraphism or abnormalities.[5] By contrast, spinal dysraphism was present in 40% of the 20 neonates who met any one or more of the first three criteria.

As Drolet reported, "Most sacral dimples that fall within the gluteal crease are healthy." [6] Furthermore, the depth of the tract is also probably irrelevant. It is the associated additional cutaneous abnormality, such as a hemangioma or additional dimples observed more cephalad, that requires further evaluation. Overlying *café au lait spots*, flammeus nevus (stork bite), and Mongolian spots are not considered abnormal.

True Incidence of Abnormal Sacral Dimples

A more recent 2003 retrospective study of 5,440 neonates by Lee and colleagues[7] found that only 0.5% of 200 neonates had an abnormal finding with the sacral dimple confirmed by ultrasound. Note, however, that

---

[5] Kriss VM, Desai NS. Occult spinal dysraphism in neonates: assessment of high-risk cutaneous stigmata on sonography. AJR Am J Roentgenol. 1998 Dec;171(6):1687-92.

[6] Higgins, J. C., & Axelsen, F. R. A. N. K. (2002). Simple dimple rule for sacral dimples. *American family physician, 65*(12), 2435.

[7] Lee, A. C. W., Kwong, N. S., & Wong, Y. C. (2007). Management of Sacral Dimples Detected on Routine Newborn Examination: A Case Series and Review. *J Paediatr (new series), 12*(2), 93-95.

similar to other studies, this child also had additional overlying abnormal cutaneous findings and an abnormally cephalad dimple. The "Simple Dimple rules" continued to predict abnormal dimples.

Gluteal Clefts

Although the *Nelson Textbook* states that the imaging requirement is considered "uncertain" for gluteal fold deviations, several experts have said that an asymmetrical or **bifurcated gluteal cleft** may be a fairly good harbinger of occult spinal dysraphism abnormality. Albright, a neurosurgeon from Wisconsin, estimated a notably high association (approaching 30%) between tethered cord and bifurcated or angulated gluteal cleft. In fact, the above figure shows our lone recent case of ultrasound-documented tethered cord with a conus medullaris at L2 spine, which was related to this sacro-coccygeal finding. Note that this child had a bifurcated gluteal cleft. The child's condition will need to be confirmed by MRI and repaired after age 8 months, per our neurosurgery consultant.

Further Evaluation of the Abnormal Sacral Dimple

Ultrasound Screening

Early Ultrasound screening is the imaging evaluation of choice for most practitioners. It can be used to screen the neonate at lower risk or marginal risk for spinal dysraphism, such as those in the Figures—if you still insist on screening them. The procedure must be performed before the child is 4 months of age, and it does not require sedation. However, ultrasonography may miss smaller spinal cord lesions, many lipomas, and especially dermal sinus tracts. This technique is also highly operator-sensitive for accuracy, and I would recommend typically performing it inside a major hospital with higher-level neonatal capabilities. Our small community hospital, with its limited neonatal ultrasound experience, would not be a prudent choice for this procedure.

MRI Scan

For dimples that are higher risk, more suspicious, or with multiple overlying cutaneous stigma, MRI is the preferred initial imaging method. Any abnormalities on ultrasound should also be confirmed with MRI to determine the full extent of the lesion. However, MRI requires sedation, a significant issue with neonates and infants. It can also occasionally miss smaller lesions. If you have any lingering suspicions about the dimple, neurosurgical consultation is recommended regardless. And remember that if you also find an incidental, asymptomatic, or occult spinal dysraphism in any pediatric patient, the child may need further investigation of the entire spinal cord by MRI, as well. This lesion has been associated with more severe upper spinal abnormalities such as syringomyelia, diastematomyelia, and particularly tethered cord.

CONCLUSION

Entirely too many expensive and anxiety-provoking imaging evaluations for sacral and coccygeal dimples are being performed in otherwise healthy neonates. Almost no coccygeal dimple requires further evaluation, unless additional overlying dermatologic abnormalities are also seen, such as those described in the "simple dimple" rules. Furthermore, sacral dimples that do not meet the "simple dimple" criteria rarely ever need further evaluation. Be aware of the **high association of bifurcated or asymmetric creases with a tethered cord**. When imaging evaluation is undertaken, ultrasound is a reasonable screen for low-risk lesions, but MRI is preferred for either higher-risk lesions or for confirmation of an abnormal ultrasound finding.

If you are still uncertain or suspicious of the sacral dimple, consult your neighborhood neurosurgeon.

✴ Making "Lemonade" out of Lyme

(Adapted from Block SL. Making "Lemonade" out of Lyme, *Pediatric Annals*, *42*(2), pp.57-60)

(One physician letter claimed this full article was the best-ever discussion of Lyme disease)

Case 1

A previously healthy, white, 3-month-old girl presents to your office with a faint, concentric 3-cm ovoid rash in the posterior axillary area (Figure 27) that started yesterday. During a 3-day family camping trip at a Kentucky state park the previous weekend, the mother noticed a small black dot under the baby's axilla, which she scraped off with much difficulty. The baby's immunizations are up to date, she has been healthy, and is growing well. There are no other symptoms such as pruritus, fever, cough, rhinorrhea, or fussiness. Her physical examination is otherwise unremarkable; there is no fever, and the range of motion in her neck and joints is normal. The mother remarked that the day after the camping trip, she removed a lot of "tiny little dark ticks" from her 4-year-old son. Could a 3-month-old child develop an arthropod-borne illness?

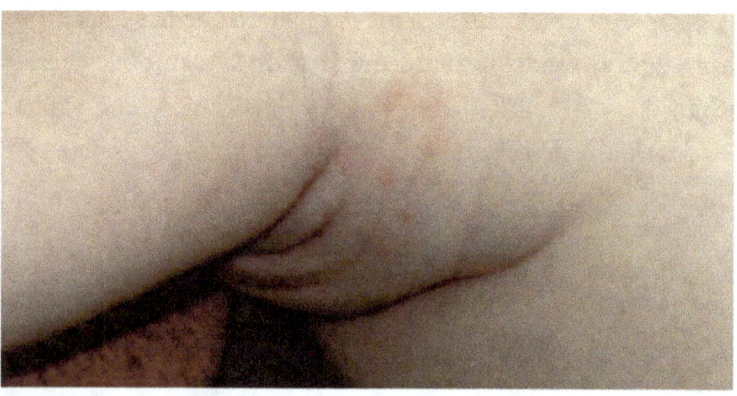

Figure 27. A 3-cm, faint, oval, maculopapular annular concentric lesion with some clearing in the posterior axilla of a 3-month-old girl. The small central papule, or "punctum," was the site of a tick bite.
Source: Dr. Block

Case 2

A previously healthy, white, 4-year-old boy from Central Kentucky comes to your office with a rash that has slowly progressed across his back since having a "tiny" tick removed. His mother reports the boy constantly plays outside on his family's farm, and that the tick was on the boy's back for 7 days before it was removed 3 days prior to the office visit. Since the removal of the tick, the annular rash has enlarged to 5 cm in diameter with central clearing, a maculopapular border, and a central punctum bite (Figure 28). The boy has been healthy recently and is fully vaccinated. He has no complaints of pruritus or pain with the rash, and also denies sore throat, other rashes, headache, fever, arthralgias, and gastrointestinal symptoms.

The mother demands that her son be tested for Lyme disease. Is this rash alone significant enough to be diagnostic of an arthropod-borne illness?

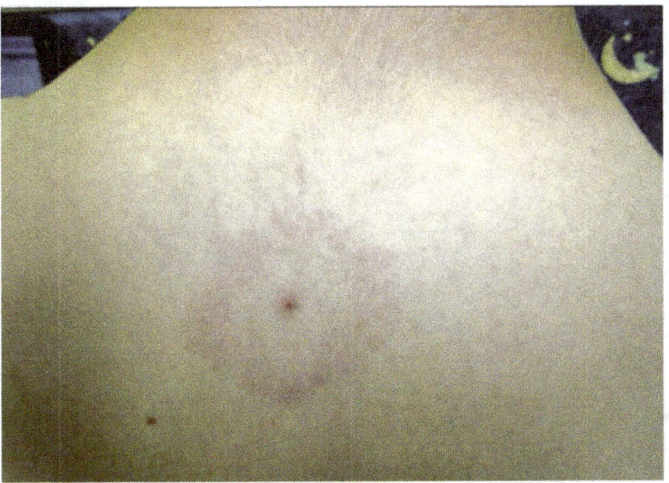

Figure 28. A White, 4-year-old boy with a 5-cm rash with concentric round halo of raised maculopapules surrounding a central punctum, deer tick bite from 10 days earlier. **Source:** Dr. Block

Case 3

A previously healthy, White, 3-year-old boy from Central Kentucky sustained a deer tick bite 8 days before coming to your office. When removed, the tiny tick was noted to be engorged and still barely visible. Six days later, an oval rash started on his left anterior chest region, which has now enlarged to 3 cm by 6 cm over 2 days (Figure 29). The punctum area of the tick bite now has some mild papular urticaria as well. The rash has a mostly flat border, some central clearing, and has recently developed a tail of lymphangiitis spreading posterior-laterally. The rash is not painful and only slightly pruritic. The boy has been fully vaccinated. He denies any sore throat, arthralgias, headaches, neck stiffness, fever, other rash, or gastrointestinal symptoms. His physical examination is otherwise unremarkable.

Does an arthropod-borne rash ever develop a mild lymphangiitis? Could there be two concomitant bacterial infections, such as lymphangitis from a concomitant staphylococcal infection?

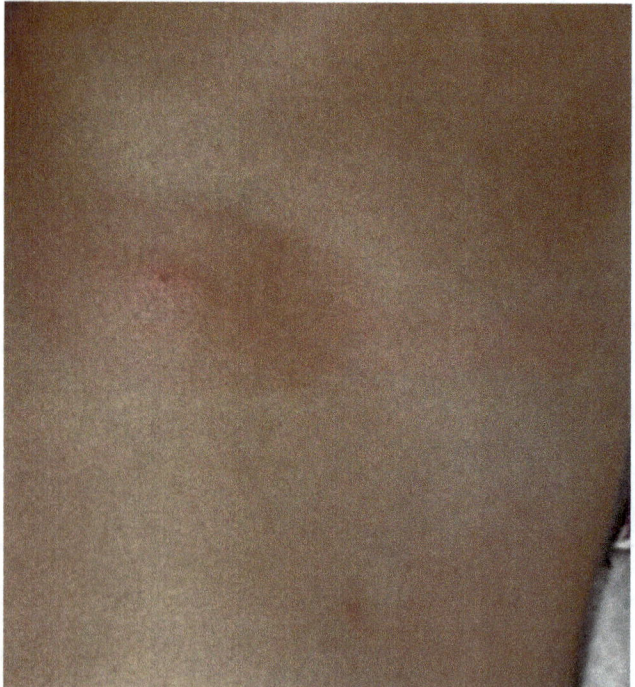

Figure 29. A White 3-year-old boy with a 3-cm by 6-cm, oval, 2-day rash with slightly raised rim surrounding a small raised papular-urticarial punctum deer tick bite from 8 days earlier. Note the faint 6-cm-long, flat tail of redness spreading posterior-laterally from the rim of the lesion. Slightly pruritic directly over the tick bite, the rash was not painful.
Source: Dr. Block

Discussion of Cases

Each of the 3 cases presented a specific diagnostic aspect of Lyme disease. All cases were treated with appropriate doses (50 mg/kg/day to 90 mg/kg/day, with a maximum dose of 1 g) of amoxicillin twice daily, and each patient responded rapidly and uneventfully to therapy. I did report a teenage girl who failed amoxicillin and was then successfully treated with doxycycline.

Case 1

You were perplexed by the very young age of this patient with an early erythema migrans lesion. But all other indicators pointed to the Lyme diagnosis, including the deer tick removal, the timing of the rash's appearance several days later and not immediately (tick hypersensitivity), the punctum, the central clearing, and the raised border. The downside of non-treatment was too consequential because of high morbidity, and the risk of antibiotic treatment was minuscule.

Case 2

Despite your objections and clear explanations to the child's mother that serologic titers were unnecessary for early localized Lyme disease, at her insistence, you obtained the serology. The acute *Borrelia* titer results were negative, and the child did fine, with total resolution of the rash in a few days.

Case 3

Despite a fairly typical solitary ovoid erythema migrans lesion, this child most likely also had a secondary bacterial infection of the tick bite with a mild ascending lymphangitis from either a staphylococcal or streptococcal infection. The most important factor in atypical cases is the careful follow-up over the next several days.

For initial antibiotic failures with early stages of Lyme, a repeat course of a different appropriate oral antibiotic for 14 to 21 days is recommended.

Finally, for early disseminated Lyme disease, appropriate oral antibiotics are still considered first-line therapy. In pediatric patients, oral doxycycline for 21 days has been shown to be as comparably effective as intravenous ceftriaxone for the same duration. Hospitalization and intravenous therapy with ceftriaxone are only indicated for symptomatic patients with meningitis, carditis, second- or third-degree atrioventricular (AV) block, or first-degree AV block with a very prolonged PR interval ($\geq$ 300 milliseconds)

One Final Point

The rates of reported cases of Lyme disease are extremely low in most Southern states due to the fact that the CDC will not accept a Lyme diagnosis unless blood titers are positive. The vast majority of cases present to clinicians in the early (or primary) Lyme stage, which is almost never antibody positive, especially in children. And because of Lyme dangers, they are antibiotic-treated promptly, thus not allowing for the development of a blood antibody conversion, which usually requires a month without treatment. The rash, history, and our judgment are not adequate for the CDC. Believe me, Lyme disease is still very common in rural KY!!

✸ Infant Gynecomastia—Baby Breast Lumps— Related to Lavender and Tea Tree Oil

(Adapted from Block SL, *Pediatric Annals*, February 2012)

(The first ever large series of reported cases)

For years, I was fascinated by the increasing number of cases of infant gynecomastia (breast lumps) past the age of 6 months that I saw in my office. Normal newborn breast lumps disappear by age 4 or 5 months old. I was observing this alarming finding in occasional children who were six-month-old, twelve-month-old, and eighteen-month-old babies—mostly girls—who developed noticeable breast lumps, sometimes so pronounced that they looked like pubescent teenagers needing training bras. For a decade, pediatricians and researchers across the United States were searching for the cause of these breast lumps in infants, with no definitive answers.

Initially, many of us believed that the culprit was soy-based formula and foods, given their known hypothetical estrogenic properties. However, upon deeper investigation, I discovered an obscure critical piece of research published in the *New England Journal of Medicine* (1997) by an author named Levi, which documented three young boys—aged four, four, and eight years—who had unexplained major breast development—way too young to be the typical male adolescent gynecomastia that occurs in about 20 to 30% of young teen boys. These three boys underwent exhaustive hormonal testing, including adrenal gland and central nervous system evaluations, yet no abnormal hormonal imbalances were found.

Their breakthrough came when researchers took breast tissue cells from adult female biopsies and placed them in a petri dish alongside various compounds the boys had been exposed to. Remarkably, only two substances caused the breast tissue cells to proliferate at an alarming rate: **lavender products and tea tree oil.** Nothing else triggered this reaction.

This groundbreaking study was published in 1997, but I did not come across it until 2001. Once I made the connection, I began asking parents of my patients with infant breast lumps whether they had exposed their babies to lavender or tea tree oil products.

The most common source? At least 90% of the babies with gynecomastia had been exposed to **lavender-based lotions, soaps, creams, and calming nighttime products.** Mothers adored these products, frequently applying them to their babies' skin. Even infant exposure to the mom's skin on which she had lathered lavender products seems to be a culprit in her skin-to-skin contact. The pattern was undeniable.

The next most common culprit was tea tree oil, mostly in Burt's Bees products. When I was confronted by the manufacturer of one major brand of infant topical tea tree oil products, they denied that their product could cause such an effect. I asked if they had tested it on infants specifically susceptible to this problem. Their answer? No. Until proven otherwise, I stood by my findings: **lavender and tea tree oil were causing excessive breast lumps in infants over 4 months old.**

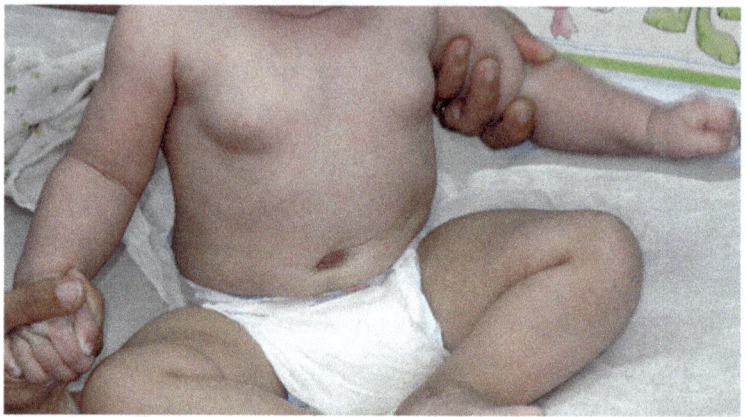

Figure 30: A 9-month-old infant with heavy topical exposure to a purple bottle of topical cream containing lavender.
Source: Dr. Block

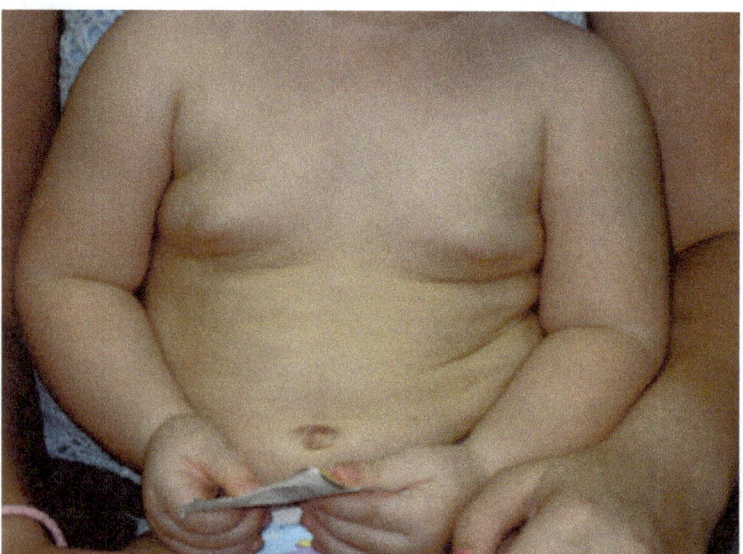

Figure 31: Precocious thelarche in a chubby 18-month-old female with daily lavender "calming cream" exposure.
Source: Dr. Block

To confirm my hypothesis, I advised parents to stop using all lavender-based and tea tree oil products on their children—especially those packaged in **purple and (yes!) pink baby bottles of lotion.** The purple color was a telltale manufacturer's sign of lavender-containing products. But the **pink colored** bottles had on the ingredient label years earlier—"contains tea tree oil." That ingredient was later re-labelled as "flower fragrance," I think, and the term tea tree oil no longer appears on the label of the pink bottles.

When these substances were discontinued in the child, I noticed within six months, and up to a year, that the breast lumps significantly decreased or disappeared entirely. However, in cases where parents continued using these products, the lumps persisted or even grew larger. This anecdotal potential cause-and-effect relationship was a likely explanation for my observations.

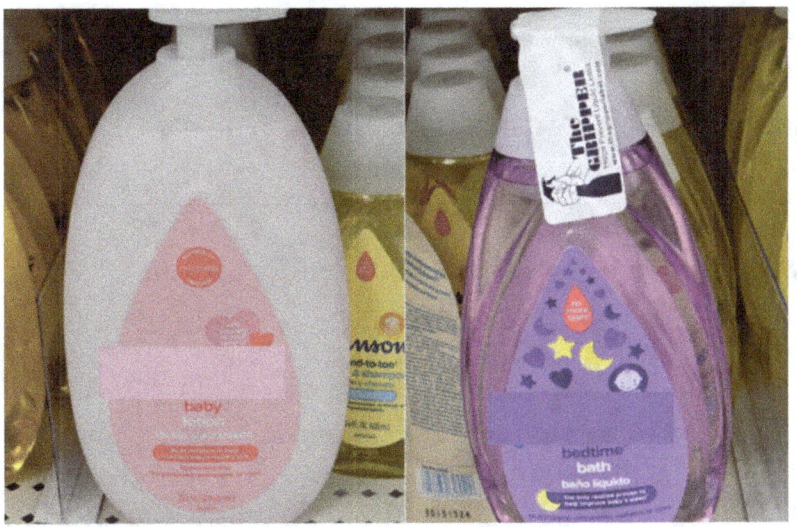

Figures 32 and 33. Pink baby lotion and purple wash/shampoo
Source: Dr. Block

In 2012, I published my findings, and the information quickly spread across the internet and in pediatric circles. Today, this knowledge is widely available, and my observations were the source, exposing the potential issues with these products.

I warn all my families: If you want to prevent persistent and worrisome gynecomastia in your babies and toddlers, avoid pink and purple colored bottles or labels for any topicals (lavender and tea tree oil products)—especially in the form of calming creams, soaps, and lotions, even when applied on the mother's skin. A simple step of avoidance would prevent the extensive and expensive laboratory evaluation of a baby/child with notable breast lumps after age 6 months.

The rare exception to watchful waiting of breast lumps is the concomitant presence of either pubertal or axillary hair, or massive breast lumps.

To further test the limits of lavender's estrogenic effects, a 21-year-old woman patient of mine who had very small breasts wanted to try using lavender lotion for three months to see if it would enhance breast growth. She laughed about it. Unsurprisingly, it did nothing. This effect only works on pre-pubertal breast tissue, meaning only infants may be particularly susceptible. (Years later, she chose breast implants.)

Can Bottle Mechanics Cause Infant Failure to Thrive?

※ The Unlikely Culprit: Baby Bottle Mechanism

(Adapted from Block SL. An Unexpected Cause of Infantile Failure to Thrive. *Pediatric Annals*. 2012)

One of the more worrisome cases I encountered involved a mother with three children. Her first two daughters were robust and healthy, but her third child—now a 4-month-old baby boy in my office—was becoming more frail, underweight, and struggling to grow. By seven to eight months of age, he was visibly emaciated and losing weight.

Failure to thrive is a serious diagnosis requiring extensive medical evaluation. I conducted a ~$10,000 workup, testing for heart disease, kidney disease, lung disease, cystic fibrosis, neurological disorders, inflammatory conditions, and gastrointestinal issues. Every single test came back normal. The caloric intake "seemed" normal. But, frustrated, I turned my attention to the most basic factor: feeding. As I spoke to the mother during my 3rd visit with the family, I noticed that she was feeding her baby from a baby bottle with an internal tubing into the nipple. The baby sucked on the bottle for 10 to 15 minutes, with meager amounts of formula actually coming out.

Curious, I took the bottle, shook it in my hand over the sink, expecting to get drenched, and as I watched the formula drip out painfully slowly—it flowed at a rate of about one drop per second. It was barely flowing. To my knowledge, two brands of bottles now have a built-in internal tube designed to slow formula flow in a theoretical attempt to reduce colic and gas. However, this so-called innovation had a major side effect for a weaker, less efficient feeder: they were struggling to get enough formula due to the too slow flow of milk. The baby was sucking for up to an hour just to consume a few ounces of formula, burning more calories in the feeding process than he was ingesting.

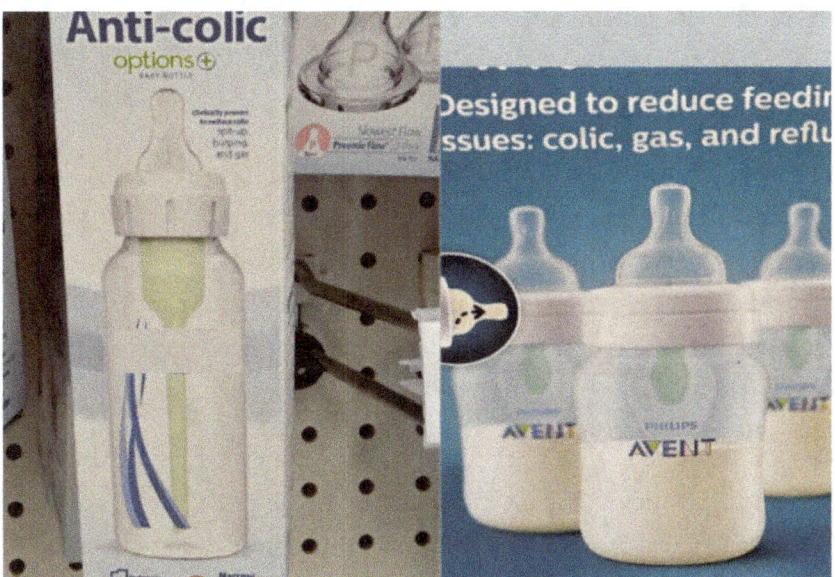

Figure 34. The too-slow flow anticolic bottles: related to some cases of FTT?
Source: Dr. Block

After switching the baby to a non-apparatus typical baby bottle with a slightly larger nipple hole, the transformation was dramatic. Within weeks, he began gaining weight, and within a month, he was thriving normally. I took before-and-after photos, which showed a frail, malnourished infant who later turned into a chubby, happy, well-fed baby—all because of a simple change to a different, typical bottle design.

The Hidden Epidemic of Bottle-Feeding Problems

Since publishing my findings, I have encountered dozens of similar cases of failure to thrive or poor growth caused by restrictive baby bottles. The problem extends to at least two companies, including the commonly used Dr. B....

Whenever I see an underweight or poorly growing or very fussy baby in my office, my first question is no longer about medical conditions. Instead, I ask, "What brand of bottle are you using?" Let me see it. If a restrictive version is being used, I immediately recommend switching to a traditional bottle along with a larger-sized nipple hole. This fixes the problem for nearly all of these infants, thus solving this iatrogenic epidemic of infant FTT.

A healthy baby should be able to finish a four- to six-ounce bottle in 10 to 15 minutes. If it takes 30 to 60 minutes, something is wrong. Babies should not have to fight against their bottle just to get fed. Pediatricians worry about failure to thrive being caused by serious medical conditions like kidney disease, heart defects, or neurological disorders. But now we must add a new, much more frequent modern cause to the list: restrictive baby bottles.

Many parents don't realize the problem because they assume that if their baby is sucking, they must be eating. But in reality, the baby could be sucking for 30 to 60 minutes with minimal milk coming out. These babies become frustrated, exhausted, and ultimately malnourished.

The key warning signs include:

- Babies taking **longer than 30 minutes** to finish a bottle.
- Baby frustration and fatigue while feeding. (Always check with your doctor first, as associated excessive sweating or rapid breathing may be a sign of cardiac or respiratory failure.)
- Poor weight gain or **failure to thrive diagnoses**.

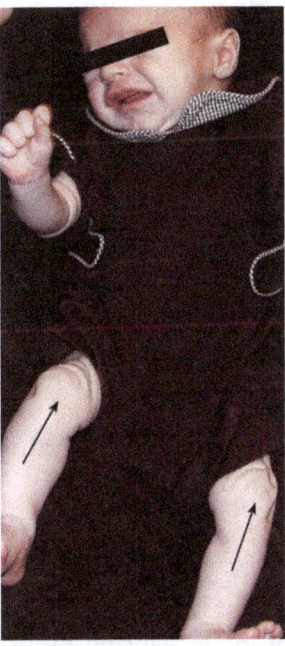

Figure 35. Crying 6-week-old infant with FTT; note his very thin extremities. Note the absence of subcutaneous fat and overlapping skin in his thighs and knees (arrows). **Source:** Dr. Block

✴ First How-to Photographic Article on Tongue Clipping

The issues about tongue-tie (ankyloglossia) and the need for frenulectomy (tongue clipping)

(Adapted from Block SL, Ankyloglossia: When Frenectomy Is the Right Choice, *Pediatric Annals*, 2012; 41(1):14–16)

Newborn tongue-tie (also known as ankyloglossia) is a hot topic in pediatrics today. Some practitioners believe it is overdiagnosed and overtreated. Most pediatricians will carefully evaluate the degree of tongue tightness on the first examination of the newborn, particularly in the newborn nursery, because it can severely impact breastfeeding success.

A "tongue-tie" occurs when the lingual frenulum, the tissue connecting the tongue to the floor of the mouth, is too tight. This can vary in severity:

- Mild cases may cause little to no feeding difficulty.
- Moderate cases can make breastfeeding painful for the mother due to abnormal infant sucking mechanics.
- Severe cases restrict tongue movement so much that feeding becomes difficult and very painful for the breastfeeding mother.

The University of Pittsburgh conducted a study on notable tongue-tied, dividing a group of infants into two categories: those who underwent tongue clipping (frenulectomy) and those who did not. Within a week, mothers who had not received the procedure were begging for it, reporting severe pain, difficulty breastfeeding, and frustration.

This can be a major issue for the breastfed baby. Mothers of babies with significant tongue-ties often stop breastfeeding early because they cannot tolerate the pain. Their babies struggle to latch properly, causing nipple trauma, frustration, and an overall poor breastfeeding experience.

For this reason, pediatricians should perform frenulectomy in their office or the nursery promptly when indicated. The procedure is quick, safe, and minimally painful at this age when done correctly. There is no need for anesthesia, but many of us use a lidocaine injection with a 27-gauge needle or a cotton-tip application of numbing gel to the frenulum. The next steps are simple—restrain the baby in a papoose board:

1. Clamp the frenulum using surgical forceps, which crush the tissue for 30-45 seconds to further minimize bleeding.

2. Clip the frenulum there using fine scissors (iris scissors are ideal).

3. Observe for more than just minimal bleeding, which resolves quickly if it does occur. Promptly use an infant pacifier for the baby. (Make certain that a newborn IM vitamin K shot was given previously.)

Within minutes of the procedure, the baby is often able to breastfeed more effectively and comfortably. Mothers report instant relief from pain and improved milk transfer.

Unfortunately, some dentists and oral surgeons have commercialized tongue-tie treatment by promoting laser frenulectomies. NO! This is an expensive alternative to the simple clipping procedure. While laser treatment is effective, it is also overboard in my opinion, causing a bit more burn pain and adding unjustified delay and costs for parents.

A **frenulectomy** performed in the pediatrician's office or newborn nursery is quick, effective, and far less expensive than a laser procedure. I think that there is no valid reason to send a baby to a pediatric dentist or oral surgeon for something a willing pediatrician can easily perform in under a few minutes.

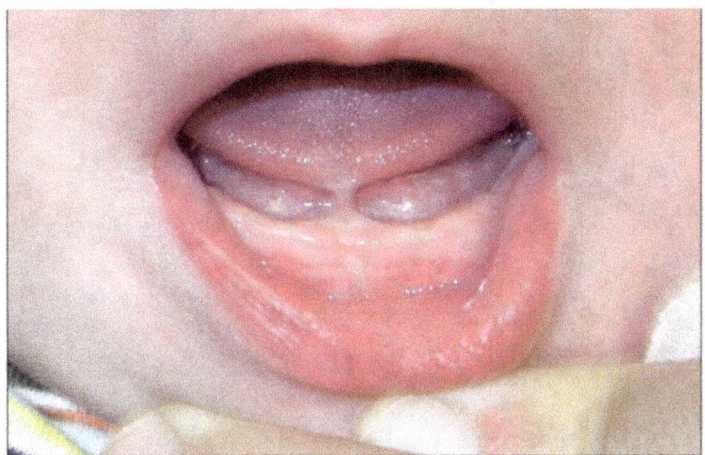

Figure 36. Ankyloglossia in 1-month-old infant. Note the thickened lower tongue frenulum.
Source: Dr. Block

Upper Lip Frenectomy: An Unnecessary Procedure

On the other hand, some practitioners, particularly lactation consultants, have started pushing for upper lip **frenectomy,** claiming that the tissue tightly connecting the upper lip to the gum causes feeding issues. This has not been an issue that I have ever seen in over 40 years of practicing pediatrics.

The American Academy of Pediatrics (AAP) recently released guidelines stating that upper lip frenectomies should never be done. NO, NO!!!!!!!!!!!! There is no evidence that the upper frenulum affects sucking, speech, or feeding. Most children naturally tear this tissue on their own between the ages of three and five when they fall or hit their mouth.

This procedure is:

- Unnecessary
- Expensive
- Ineffective

Parents should not allow their child to undergo an **upper lip frenectomy.**

Some may ask: why perform frenulectomy in the non-breastfeeding infant?

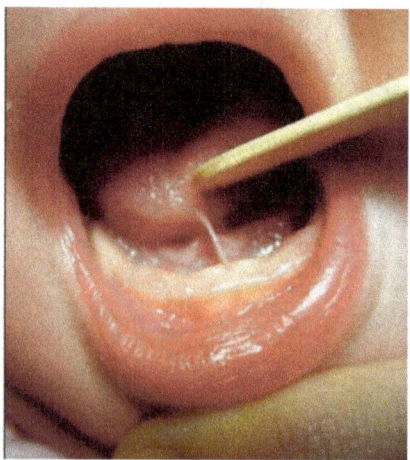

Figure 37. Ankyloglossia in a 3-week-old infant.
Source: Dr. Block

Children with untreated severe tongue-tie really rarely ever face speech difficulties as they grow older. But there is an unexpected but real cosmetic impact—tongue-tied children struggle with kissing. Many teenagers and young adults with untreated tongue-tie find themselves unable to "French kiss" properly, which can be socially embarrassing.

💥 Caloric Needs of Infants: The Reality of Feeding Large Babies—Is 32 Ounces Daily Really Enough?

(Adapted from Block SL, Delayed Introduction of Solid Foods to Infants: Not So Fast! *Pediatric Annals* 2013;42(4):143–147)

No rice cereal!!

Breastfed infants feed on demand, and their intake can vary significantly. Some larger babies consume between 40 and 50 ounces of breast milk per day if solids are not introduced by four months. Graphs (e.g., *Harriet Lane Handbook of Pediatrics*) show that babies in the 75th percentile or higher require more calories than can be provided by a rigid recommendation of 32 ounces of milk or formula alone. If they do not receive additional nourishment, they risk becoming failure-to-thrive infants.

Mothers of bottle-fed babies, on the other hand, often tried to follow the guidelines restricting formula intake to 32 ounces. However, frustrated and hungry babies led to frustrated mothers. I think that most mothers quickly realized that their babies needed more calories, and surreptitiously began feeding them some cereal or an additional bottle or two per day, which helped them grow properly. The concern over obesity due to overfeeding at this age was largely unfounded; rather, babies required these additional calories to support their normal growth and development.

By five to six months of age, 32 ounces of formula alone is insufficient for many babies, especially larger infants. The idea that limiting formula intake would prevent obesity was not supported by actual growth needs, and this guideline required reevaluation. I think that babies should be allowed, for the most part, to self-regulate their feeding per their vocalization and hunger cues.

Thus, my article further prompted later AAP guidelines to also allow for "solids" being introduced between 4 and 6 months old as the standard of care in all babies.

The Importance of Iron-Rich Foods, Particularly Boxed Baby Cereal

Another major misconception was that jarred baby foods, particularly the meat dinners, were sufficient sources of iron. However, jarred baby food meats or meat dinners contain very little iron. Babies must continue to eat iron-fortified cereals such as oatmeal (or rarely rice cereal—later discussion) until they transition to table food meats rich in iron, typically around 9 months of age when solid foods and table meats are introduced. If infants primarily consume jarred baby foods after 6 months old, without additional iron supplementation, they are at risk of developing iron deficiency anemia, especially in the exclusively breastfed infant.

Iron deficiency in infants is more than just a short-term concern. Research shows that babies who are iron-deficient by 12 months of age may experience long-term cognitive effects, including a significant reduction in IQ points. (Data that is 1000 times more convincing than the fluoride story.) This emphasizes the necessity of ensuring adequate iron intake through boxed baby cereals (jarred baby cereal is a poor source, too) and later, iron-rich table food meats.

Some countries start solids as early as three weeks to six weeks of age, which may be too soon. Early introduction of gluten-containing foods has been associated with a slightly increased risk of celiac disease, but the data is not substantial enough to be conclusive. I think that the optimal time for introducing solids appears to be around four or, at the latest, five months old for both breastfed and bottle-fed infants.

Scheduled Introduction of Complementary Foods

Introduce a single-ingredient food item one at a time, usually every 3 to 5 days, to ensure no reactions or intolerance. Food variety also helps the infant develop an important diversity in taste preferences. Delayed introduction of more allergenic foods until 12 months does not prevent atopic disease. Daily iron-fortified cereals are preferred due to their enriched concentration of protein and minerals as well.

Customarily, rice cereal has been the first food for the first weeks, but new data on detectable inorganic arsenic concentrations in infant rice cereal (including in one organic brand) makes me wary. Thus, I now recommend boxed oatmeal cereal routinely, as oatmeal and wheat tend to have lower detectable arsenic concentrations than rice. *Consumer Reports* recently reported low-grade inorganic arsenic contamination of the rice supply chain, including four different infant rice cereals (0.8 to 2.7 mcg of arsenic/serving).[8] The lower limit of the most protective standard in the U.S. for ingestion of inorganic arsenic is 5 mcg/liter consumed.[9]

One suggested approach to initial complementary feedings at 4 to 6 months is as follows:

- **Month 4:** Oatmeal cereal. Rarely, a few teaspoons of pureed applesauce or pears may be necessary to "jump start" the feeding process in reluctant infants.
- **Month 4.5 to 5:** Meat dinners like turkey/noodle or chicken/rice. The single-ingredient meat jars are barely palatable (taste them yourself) and only provide minimal iron or zinc. I prefer that you puree your own table food meats.
- **Months 6 to 7:** Vegetables. Introduced one at a time, four or more single ingredients as routine staples.

---

[8] Arsenic in your food. *Consumer Reports*. November 2012.
[9] Ziegler EE, Nelson SE, Jeter JM. Iron supplementation of breastfed infants from an early age. *Am J Clin Nutr. 2009;89*(2):525-532.

- **Months 7 to 8:** Fruits. Introduced one at a time, four or more single ingredients as routine staples. Fruits are started last to avoid developing a "sweet tooth" and a subsequent reluctance to eat vegetables and meats.
- **First year:** Liquids. Feed only breast milk, formula, or occasional water. I prefer infants to receive no juice at all, but if they are used, the AAP suggests parents use no more than 4 oz of pure fruit juices daily, and start only after 6 months old. I also suggest parents do not use "infant feeders" and that they do not add solid foods to bottles.

Based on some recent Scandinavian data, newer recommendations now suggest introducing peanut butter and eggs to babies as young as 6 months old. It may prevent a fair number of cases of later treacherous peanut and egg allergies. A small amount of peanut butter can be smeared on the spoon or stirred into the baby cereal.

Concerns Over Contaminants in Baby Foods—Dangers "Under the Boardwalk" Lumber! (a popular 60s song)

Another critical issue I reiterated in my article was the contamination of baby apple juice and baby rice cereal with **arsenic**. *Consumer Reports* Magazine had reported elevated levels of arsenic in baby juices and certain baby fruits. But the pediatric literature had not picked up on this baby cereal issue much at the time of my article. Based on these arsenic findings and my prodding, it was further recommended that babies avoid juice altogether for the first few years of life.

Additionally, **baby rice cereal** was found to contain significant levels of arsenic in the article. This was an issue across all major brands, including organic and non-organic varieties. The contamination stemmed from the use of arsenic-treated lumber in Louisiana and other rice-growing regions. The arsenic from treated wood in the posts and decks leached into the water supply, contaminating rice paddies. Since rice is grown in water-saturated conditions, it readily absorbs arsenic, unlike oats or barley, which are grown in drier environments.

Following my prodding, the American Academy of Pediatrics later revised its recommendations and advised against feeding babies rice cereal, rather suggesting oatmeal or barley cereal as safer alternatives. This marked another significant shift in conventional wisdom and improved infant nutrition practices across the country.

CHAPTER 7

The Perils of Refusing Infant Vaccines

Changing the AAP Guidelines for accepting families who refuse infant vaccines. After I published several articles (three included here) about the issues of continuing to provide care to non-vaccinating infants as of 2016, they changed the standard of care, which now allows pediatricians to have a choice in their offices.

2009 A Pediatric Treasure: Autism's False Prophets by Paul Offitt, MD

(Adapted from Block SL in *Infectious Diseases in Children* 2009 February: 1-3)

MMR does not cause autism! The autism scare related to vaccines was a medical hoax.

Rarely does a physician find a detailed, cogent explanation of an enigma in medicine that has plagued them for years.

Have you ever seen the television show, *Magic's Biggest Secrets Finally Revealed*? This show enlightens the viewer about the sleight of hand performed by the big-time magician. We now have a comparable exposé, in this case, a book that elucidates the mysterious appearance of the myths that have evolved around vaccines and autism in children.

The author, Paul Offit, MD, is the chief of pediatric infectious diseases at Children's Hospital of Philadelphia, one of the lead developers of the human pentavalent rotavirus vaccine, and, in the interest of full disclosure, a member of this publication's editorial board.

His book, *Autism's False Prophets—Bad Science, Risky Medicine, and the Search for a Cure,* is a compelling read that should be examined by every physician, nurse, or interested parent involved in the vaccination of children.

Vaccine Controversy

The book explores four recent vaccine controversies: 1) the measles-mumps-rubella vaccine and autism link, 2) the thimerosal and autism link, 3) the snake oil cures perpetuated by both, which prey upon the fears of desperate parents of children with autism, and 4) how the author's stance to shine a light on the nefarious underworld of vaccine innuendo and under-the-radar payments to a few key scientists had created a terrifying nightmare in his personal life. Shockingly, the antivaccine "mafia" sometimes resorts to incredibly threatening behavior against clinicians of science.

Dr. Offit admits upfront that he is not a developmental specialist and he is no expert in autism. However, it is clear that he understands the plight of families with autistic children and how they can staunchly defend their positions against vaccines. Coupling medicine's past mistakes and our current uninformed trial lawyer head of the human health services, and rarely our own experts' waffling about vaccines, each has created a challenge to medicine's credibility with journalists, politicians, and parents. For example, think of Guillain-Barré cases following one year of the Swine flu vaccine four decades ago.

Subsequently, for vaccines, we are no longer supposed to look at a risk/benefit ratio in preventing disease, but rather we must march to the new mantra: "We can accept NO risk at all for vaccines. *Primum non nocere,* or first do no harm, even if it does remarkable good." The morbidity and mortality that could be prevented with a particular vaccine have become inconsequential if one listens to the vaccine nihilists. And boy, with shock-talk radio, the internet, blogs, and non-medically trained leaders, it has become incredibly easy to scare people with **temporal** serious adverse events, which are rarely, if ever, *causal*. Most serious reported AEs by recipients are merely **background cases.** For instance, all children ride in car seats, but if your child develops a platelet disorder 2 weeks after the car ride, this faulty logic can lead you to believe that riding in car seats CAUSED the platelet disorder. It was temporally associated in time, but not causally related.

Although Vaccine Adverse Event Reporting Safety data can be helpful in possibly establishing **trends for a particular Adverse Event (AE), it must be interpreted in light of a critical background rate of the particular finding** in the general population, which seems to be an extremely difficult concept for many laypeople to grasp. And more worrisome, one pediatric publication showed that nearly half of these **supposed AEs were reported by plaintiff lawyers,** which were typically second and third-hand hearsay reports. These lawyers, even now in the top government positions, have a highly vested interest in promulgating class action and individual lawsuits against vaccine manufacturers and doctors. Unethical? You be the judge! But the pediatrician is left cleaning up the disinformation from many folks of what Google has termed: **"disinformation dozen."**

Grilled by Parents

Not a day goes by in my office that I am not grilled about the safety of vaccines. Do you really understand the actual objective threat of measles, the absence of any thimerosal (which is no longer contained in a substantial amount in any pediatric vaccine except for multi-dose vial influenza vaccines used for adults only), and the use of multiple vaccine antigens in causing autism in infants and toddlers? If a parent, scientist, or politician wishes to really understand how this all evolved, they MUST read this book. It will provide them with the arsenal to understand the origins of the mythical problem, along with the additional verbal tools and references to defend one's scientific positions more clearly. We all already know that the pediatricians, the Institute of Medicine, the CDC, and the World Health Organization have each found an abundance of **no evidence** for a link between vaccines and autism.

Remember, measles infection can kill about 1 in 250-500, recently hospitalized almost up to 20 % of children, causes brain damage from encephalitis about 1 in 500, blindness, and puts your child at major risk several years later for SSPE (subacute sclerosing panencephalitis, 1 in 1350 from California data)—turning the brain into a total non-functional mess.

NEWS FLASH: Measles also makes about ⅓ or more of infected children severely immunodeficient (highly susceptible to all sorts of other severe infections) for years after the infection. They become almost predisposed to infectious diseases, like a child cancer patient on chemotherapy. Measles infection is a wicked problem you do not want your child to experience.

And there is NO effective treatment available for any healthy child, even though the CDC has recommended two doses of vitamin A when measles is diagnosed "just in case," based on the benefits of vitamin A for those children living in a **third-world country** who have been chronically vitamin A deficient. Even there, it is likely to only occasionally prevent death or severe morbidity. Furthermore, longer-term daily continued high-dose vitamin A is very often toxic as well, causing its own set of problems, particularly intracranial hypertension (pseudotumor cerebri), which I have seen firsthand, and blindness.

Offit's book describes in succinct detail the incredibly sordid background surrounding this purported "scientific breakthrough," actually a hoax, by a group of British investigators. I had personally searched out some of the background on the MMR-autism panic created by Andrew Wakefield, a British gastroenterologist. Much of the material for the book on Wakefield's thinking can be confirmed by searching the website of Brian

Deer of the *Sunday Times* of London, or linking the keywords: Wakefield, MMR, and Deer.

Envision a real-life plot of a John Grisham novel with a boatload of money exchanging hands between lawyers and alleged independent scientists. These scientists were developing a patent application for a competing new MMR vaccine, which they even alleged could prevent autism. (Yeah, right, Pinocchio!) Duplicity abounds, as one of the 12 families with purported measles particles in their child was actually suing vaccine companies. (No conflict of interest, eh?) All this can be found in this book as well.

As Offit reveals, "Beginning in 1996, Chadwick (his lab scientist) was in the operating room during the collection of both intestinal biopsies and spinal fluids from autistic children." He had personally tested all specimens for measles RNA by PCR. The Lancet 1998 paper reports that all 12 patients had detectable MMR vaccine particles, yet the work could never be repeated by independent investigators. Apparently, the data was mostly fabricated. What then happened? Read the book.

Offit's book is a fascinating read, and it leaves no duplicitous stone unturned. He portrays in painful detail how and probably why a scientist misled his co-authors and co-investigators into believing his scientific discovery of an MMR-autism link. This falls into Offit's category of scientists "who choose to ignore the data," as I first mentioned. The cascade of events that followed from this bogus discovery by Wakefield is astonishing. The lay press dissemination of a single medical report from a mere 12 patients has continued to almost totally dismantle the developed world's vaccine program. Criminal science.

And it continues to conflagrate the factual scientific world.

Six years later, after the damage was done, Wakefield's publication in *The Lancet* was retracted, with nearly all of his co-authors recused from the original paper. But it was too late. This cat was really out of the malicious bag. Furthermore, some politicians, personal injury lawyers (guess who?), and parents "were angry and frustrated." They needed someone to pay for all the bogus vitamin injections, blood tests, antifungals, antivirals, mineral supplements, cranial manipulation, special diets, sonar depuration, hyperbaric oxygen, Lupron (puberty blocker), and chelation (metal vacuum in the blood)," Offit reports in his book. One by one, Offit provides the lack of science behind most of these purported "cures" for autism. (Check the background for autism treatments from our current head HHS investigator for autism's causes. OMG!)

Pseudoscience, False Prophets

The book itself is eloquently and clearly written and can easily be understood by most parents. So, as a pediatrician, one can recommend that some of your parental fence-sitters on the issues of vaccines should purchase and, of course, read the book. The book often cajoles parents to be especially mindful of all the false prophets and pseudoscience involved with management and cures for autism.

As is Offit's style, the book is painfully honest and credible, as it even takes to task a few of our own pediatric expert policy makers, a portion that made me quite squeamish. But overall, kudos to one of our best and brightest vaccine wonks for his valiant effort to explain the pseudoscience and the "false prophets" behind the nightmare of delayed and missed vaccines.

By the way, all of the proceeds from this book are being forwarded to research in autism. So, either way, you cannot lose when you purchase this book. If it does not turn out to be a true treasure for your pediatric practice or your bestseller book collection, you have at least contributed to an important charity.

✴ The Pediatrician's Dilemma: Refusing the Refusers of Infant Vaccines

(Adapted from Block SL, The Pediatrician's Dilemma: Refusing the Refusers of Infant Vaccines, *Journal of Law, Medicine & Ethics,* 2015:43(3); 648-653 (Autumn))

Introduction

A mother new to my general pediatrics practice says that she wants no vaccines for her infant because she says, "I have read on the internet...," or "I heard from a nurse...," or "So-and-so celebrity says they can cause autism, brain damage, poisoning, cancer, neurological disorders, and even death." Perhaps she has read about "the dangers" of vaccines in the first edition of Dr. Sears' *The Vaccine Book.* Or people on her Facebook page also say that the "preventable" diseases are just too rare anymore to ever take "the risk" of a vaccine with "known" risks. These vaccine risks are already clearly explained, and even sometimes overstated (such as a never-seen risk of death for *Haemophilus influenzae* type B (HIB) vaccine) in the routinely distributed Centers for Disease Control (CDC) Vaccine Information Sheet (VIS). On the other hand, the families typically overlook the risks of "omission," or non-vaccination, such as brain damage or meningitis, etc., which are also clearly stated in the VIS.

"So why should I take any risks with my healthy son?" she inquires. Despite your cogent and concise scientific explanations, your CDC handouts, and your American Academy of Pediatrics (AAP) pamphlets about the risks and benefits of childhood vaccines, she finally declares, "I still think that I shall forgo all vaccines for him." This paper will focus on this group of families, unless otherwise stated.

All of us in general pediatrics have spent at least 7 years of rigorous medical training, including learning about the vaccines and the immune system, which have saved more lives and prevented more morbidity than any other medical treatment in the last hundred years. We want to protect our newborns, our fragile, and our healthy patients. The scientific validity of the protection provided by infant vaccines is impeccable. But even outspoken trial lawyers have recently again challenged this verifiable body of scientific and epidemiologic work.

The Magnitude of the Problem

In the U.S., similar to the ongoing current pertussis epidemic, 48,277 and 24,231 incident cases of pertussis were reported to the CDC for the years 2012 and 2013, respectively, the highest levels since 1955.[10] We are on our way to this level in 2025. Nine deaths occurred in infants younger than 3 months. The CDC estimates almost 1.4 cases of pertussis per 1000 infants younger than 6 months. Over 40% of 5351 cases younger than 7 years old had received no vaccines or had "unknown" vaccine status. Many of these families understand the concept of **herd protection** incurred with high rates of vaccination by other families, and may feel safe because of it. Their reasons for refusal may include the belief that immunizations result from government conspiracy or pharmaceutical corporate greed; or that they are unnecessary because the target diseases are so rare; or that they provide too many antigen exposures for their presumably fragile (though healthy) infant; or that they are too toxic, based on pseudoscience. Illegal immigrants are not the source of the epidemics.

Historically, the earliest largest measles outbreak in Minnesota history alone occurred in 2012, where 21 cases were identified, of which 16 were unvaccinated, and over 3000 individuals were exposed.[11] Among the unvaccinated children, nine were age-eligible for vaccination, and of those nine, seven families had safety concerns about vaccines.

---

[10] Center for Disease Control and Prevention, "2013 Provisional Pertussis Surveillance Report," January 3, 2014, available at www.cdc.gov/mmwr/pdf/wk/mm6252md.pdf
[11] P. Gahr, A. S. DeVries, and G. Wallace et al., "An Outbreak of Measles in an Undervaccinated Community," *Pediatrics 134* (2014): e169-e175.

This decade, we are now witnessing a disastrous outbreak of measles, heaviest throughout the southwest U.S., particularly in West Texas, with over 1000 cases so far, three known deaths, and a hospitalization rate of up to 20%. Almost all are easily and undeniably prevented by a two-shot series of MMR. If Florida lifts their school mandate on vaccines, a visit to Disney World or other Florida parks may become riskier.

I know the epidemic firsthand because in 1988, I was the first to report two local counties measles outbreak with three known cases here thus far. We (our office and health departments) gave primary vaccinations and booster vaccinations to every appropriate child for the three local counties, and the outbreak died. Immediately. Gone. And then all single-dose patients received the requisite second dose at the appropriate time (3 months or more later). We have seen no measles cases in our area for nearly 4 decades. This will change shortly, I surmise, with the astonishing spread of child vaccine refusal.

Who Is Refusing?

In my rural general pediatric practice, about 75% of our parents agree with our philosophy on infant vaccines. About 15% are "fence sitters" who vacillate about vaccines and merely need some calm reassurance about their safety and robust protection. Around 7 to 8% of families will acquiesce to our stern warnings about the hazards of vaccine-preventable diseases or assertions that vaccines are critical for the health and safety of the child, and for the other unprotected patients. Some of these families may agree to my specific alternative schedule to the routine vaccine schedule, which comprises a rapid sequence of almost monthly injections during the first 15 months of life (see following article). The requirement for copayments at each nursing vaccine visit creates consternation in some families. The family will also need constant reminders that the vaccines must be given on time; also, none of the multivalent vaccines can be split, for economic, logistical, or manufacturing reasons. Some families later want to opt out of one or more specific vaccines despite their earlier agreement with you. This limit testing can be frustrating and daunting for the pediatrician.

But what should be done with the remaining 5% (up to 20% in some areas) of families who gospel-like believe the fabricated reports like those of Andrew Wakefield and his autism scare? And now RFK Jr.'s waffling opinion? These communicable diseases have become so rare that, in a certain sense, we pediatricians have become victims of our own immunization successes.

An impasse stands between the clinician's science-based pediatric infectious diseases training and expert medical recommendations, versus the family's science denialism resulting from a plethora of pseudoscience and misinformation (Google: the "Disinformation Dozen"). This produces a situation in which no one can win. The pediatrician is in an untenable position, having to decide whether to provide sub-standard medical care and risk malpractice suits if the child contracts the disease, or to sadly dismiss the family by "refusing the refusers" of infant vaccines. A concept we disdain.

Is the Refusal of the Vaccine Refusers a Reasonable Position?

The American Academy of Pediatrics (AAP) advocates a "wait and see" approach for these families, meaning that it is better to keep them in your practice and to continue your otherwise high standards of pediatric care. Some observers suggest that someday the family may come around and change their minds about immunizations; whether it is within 6 months, 2 years, or 6 years, it could happen. It could? But by then, most of **the protection needed from most of the vaccines will be mostly irrelevant for the child and the community.** This is a pointless vaccine stance. Will their vaccine "Russian roulette" decision have paid off? Some hold to the theory of the "soggy potato chip"—this delay is better than "no potato chip" at all. But it is not better, according to most experts.

A rate of pediatric practice dismissal for refusers was recently reported to be as high as 40%, while the national rate of families who refuse some or all infant vaccines in 2023 was reported as high as 35% in Oregon. However, pockets of counties in certain states may approach refusal rates higher than 40%. The most common reasons for refusal are "low vaccine safety and efficacy, low level of trust in the government, and low perceived susceptibility to and severity of vaccine-preventable diseases." (And non-vaxxers understand the concept of **herd immunity** quite well—your child's vaccination protects my child's not vaccinating up to a certain point.)

Exposing other compliant patients to communicable, preventable infectious diseases is not reasonable. For example, our office was seeing a 2-year-old child for his first visit with us. When we offered follow-up vaccination, we learned that no vaccines had ever been received. "We are just waiting a while and would like to come back later for them." After 3 more visits over the next year, and still no vaccinations were given due to a variety of excuses, we decided that the parents were never considering vaccination for their child, despite our lengthy discussions. So, we dismissed them from our practice in accordance with our office policy of 40 years' standing.

Two months later, the child contracted pertussis with significant morbidity and hospitalization. Furthermore, if he had been sitting in our main waiting room for the usual 5 to 15 minutes, coughing and hacking, exposing several sick and well newborns and infants, or some children immunosuppressed by chemotherapy or disease, one can imagine the potential dire consequences. Pertussis can damage the brain and even kill or hospitalize a significant number of infants annually, especially when only 0 to 2 doses of DTaP vaccinations have been received, which is typical for children younger than 6 months of age. Full vaccine protection of infants from pertussis typically occurs only weeks after the third dose of DTAP vaccine.

We believe it is our ethical duty to tell all of our families that we have tried to vaccinate all of the children being seen in our office to the fullest extent possible and according to the CDC vaccine schedule. We should be able to reassure all of our families that these highly contagious infectious disease hazards (measles, pertussis, pneumococcus, rotavirus, *Haemophilus influenzae* type b (HIB), etc.) have been optimally minimized in our offices by our diligent vaccine efforts. Clinicians should be able to honestly tell their families, "You will not be unnecessarily exposed in my office."

If this risk is not minimized, by contrast, and a practice accepts vaccine refusers, it should be their responsibility to fully disclose upfront to each visiting family that they may have in their office between 1 in 10 to 1 in 20 young children at any given time who rarely could be exposing other children to a devastating vaccine-preventable infectious disease. For instance, before the routine use of oral rotavirus vaccine, 1 in 15 children would end up in the emergency department with dehydration, and 1 in 75 were hospitalized. Over 100 children died annually. Pre-vaccine, rotavirus was a universal and horrific, specifically-<u>untreatable,</u> relentless, weeks-long vomiting/diarrhea infection (occurring 2-3 times in the first two years of life). Thus, with a notable rate of potential infectious vectors sitting in this office, should this "accepting" office consider preventively disallowing or sequestering newborn or immunodeficient children from their office?

Medico-Legal Risks of Keeping Non-Vaccinators

Few things are as devastating to a physician's career, self-image, and psyche as being the object of a medical negligence lawsuit. Nearly 30 to 50% of all pediatricians will be the target of a medical malpractice suit over their professional lives. Vaccine issues commonly play a major role. Most pediatricians will spend 4 to 5 (or 1/7) years of their professional lives dealing with the stressful vagaries of the adversarial and shaming tort system. Even worse, pediatricians on average have had the largest payment claims of all specialties—the mean payment exceeds $500,000. These awards could exceed the maximum coverage of many malpractice policies, placing the pediatrician at considerable personal financial peril.

Should a pediatrician be expected to blithely increase these odds of a harrowing malpractice suit by accepting non-vaccinators? Or even be mandated to do so??? Not in my book.

Many pediatricians have been sued for delayed or missed vaccines, or for failing to "fully inform" the vaccine-refusing family about all the consequences of a particular vaccine-preventable disease (HIB, pneumococcus, influenza), or for failing to offer the vaccine at a later visit. In a few cases, the physician had even obtained some form of parental acknowledgment regarding the hazards of not vaccinating, but they were sued anyway. I have personally defended two medicolegal cases for this very reason—a flu encephalitis case and a pneumococcal meningitis case–both irreparably brain-damaged. It was alleged that it was the doctor's fault; yet the parent refused or delayed the respective vaccine! Unbelievable!

Is Refusing the Refusers "Unprofessional"?

The AAP Committee on Bioethics has examined several questions in the arena of vaccination refusal, including the issue of professionalism, which is one of the most contentious. The option of refusing the refusers of infant vaccines has been chosen by nearly 40% of pediatric practitioners, and for this decision, some have been branded as "unprofessional." The following three areas of professionalism are relevant: disagreement about the goals of care, withdrawal from patient care, and integrity.

Parents and physicians may have conflicting goals of care that must be resolved. After the pediatrician explains the professional point of view regarding vaccines, provides much additional scientific literature and pamphlets, educates the family as much as possible, and allows for lengthy discussions in several office visits, the ultimate showdown comes—whether to start timely vaccinating the infant or not—usually by 3 or 4 months of age. At this point, the practitioner must decide whether or not to continue to provide parentally requested substandard medical care. And make no mistake: intentional infant non-vaccination or marked vaccination delay is simply substandard medical care.

Office Financial Costs of Keeping Non-Vaccinators

According to the CDC, for the non-vaccinator family, **each office visit requires a detailed discussion of each "refused" recommended vaccine** needed at the appropriate age. Thus, by 24 months, one will need to discuss and inform and present the CDC VIS forums for up to 14 different antigens at each of about 8 subsequent checkups. The amount of extra discussion time and declination signatures needed at each visit will add an additional 5 to 15 minutes per visit, depending on the pediatrician's fervor and litigation fears.[12] This represents **time that is lost** for other patients who have major psychiatric, behavioral, dietary, or disease problems that require extra time. The practice also forgoes administration fees and our additional overhead payments for at least 14 different vaccines in the first 2 years of life, which we must still store. One can calculate that subsequently, office receipts will be reduced by about 2 to 10%; many practices will suffer financially when retaining even a small percentage of refusers. And importantly, because of the major loss of available office visits, other compliant, willing families will not be afforded the opportunity to seek our expert pediatric advice or to get an appointment for acute illness care with our busy schedules.

Our office, which is a regional pediatric center, employs about 70 people, who are well-paid with benefits. Contrary to the salacious misinformation perpetuated by a famous plaintiff lawyer, vaccinations are not a major source of income for pediatricians!! The upfront costs, the hidden costs, and the nursing labor intensity costs typically make them only a break-even option for most practices. Insurance companies make it impossible to make much, if any, profit from them, especially with their 6-month or more payment delay of the escalating costs for any new vaccine that we are supposed to use. Meanwhile, we are underwriting the new higher cost. Several times, we have even required a bank loan to cover these new, higher costs.

---

[12] S. L. Block, "Taking a Pass on Alternative Immunization Schedules," *Pediatric Annals* 42 (2013): 399-406.

And again, because of the pediatrician's dedication to preventive care, we blithely continue this life-saving vaccine crusade and provide medical advancements. To besmirch our reputation over this is reprehensible and inflammatory.

Vaccine Costs: The Pediatrician's Scary Gamble

Let's get a handle on the disparities in costs and reimbursements for vaccines in an office setting. This is also partially dependent on the proportion of Medicaid/VFC versus private pay patients. First, all VFC/Medicaid vaccines are free; we pay nothing, and families pay nothing. That accounts for over 50% of vaccines in most peds offices. But, we still have all the ancillary costs (see below), and we typically lose money on this group!

Most pediatricians are administering 16 to 18 injections to each child in the first 2 years of life, and we are still not off the hook during pre-teen/teen years for an additional 3 to 7 expensive shots, which are typically covered by insurance. This topic is near and dear to every pediatrician practitioner.

The storing and buying costs in vaccines alone is the equivalent to nearly an entire 2 or 3 pediatricians' annual income in our refrigerators! To not get paid adequately for this critical, benevolent work makes this gamble for us look like we are either dilettante philanthropists or Las Vegas losers. And thus, it is the general office pediatrician who bears the almost entire brunt of this cost and gamble for society's children. No other specialty is involved to any extent like this. None.

Furthermore, one of the biggest vaccine costs in our offices is the hidden regular nursing and doctor teaching time. Then we must cover the salaries and work benefits needed to pay a shot nurse or two specifically because of the massive number of injections in a busy practice, which most peds groups (larger than 2) employ, I believe. For the patient half, who are commercially insured, we must then accept the long lagging lead time for any new vaccine—but we still pay, up front, hundreds of thousands of dollars. Sometimes, we must take out a bank loan to survive this hit. When we receive reimbursement, it is sometimes partial and sometimes full, and sometimes with a very small profit. We also depend on how quickly the insurers come on board and when federal ACIP mandates it (yes, the group in disarray!), often happening almost 4 to 6 months later. Thus, we must gamble on *post facto* receiving an adequate payment from cost-cutting insurers for 2 to 3 doses of an expensive new vaccine, such as rotavirus or HPV9 or Men ABCWY, for the first six months until payments start trickling in.

It is the most slippery slope economically for a pediatric practice. We often forgo some or any practice income during this transition phase for any typically new expensive vaccine.

The totally misinformed head health lawyer spreading disinformation about pediatricians generating massive vaccine income is disingenuous and irresponsible.

Resolving Conflicting Goals of Care

How much will the child "be put at significant risk of serious harm by following the wishes of the child and/or parent?" This is not known, but we do know, for instance, that a child who is under-vaccinated with the DTaP infant series is 19-fold to 28-fold more likely to become infected with the pertussis bacteria, which could cause death, brain damage, or respiratory failure. Resolving the conflict in favor of refusing to continue care for children whose parents persistently refuse vaccination may be most consistent with professionalism.[13]

Withdrawing from Further Patient Care

These are healthy children, so no abandonment occurs if dismissal proceeds correctly. As the AAP professionalism guidelines discuss, "If a physician...is unwilling to honor a family's refusal of intervention in a situation in which

---

[13] P. Offit, *Autism's False Prophets: Bad Science, Risky Medicine, and the Search for a Cure* (New York: Columbia University Press, 2008).

the family has chosen an established alternative, he or she should withdraw from the case and must provide reasonable assistance to the parent in making alternative arrangements for care."

The intervention at issue here is: routine and timely vaccination. Both parents and physicians acknowledge the fact that the alternative to vaccines is the parents' belief system (not science-based) that vaccines are not acceptable, yet they have still chosen to disregard the physician's vaccine recommendations. At some point, the philosophical differences between the two groups become irreconcilable, as one mainstay of the general pediatric practice is preventive medicine. The timely transfer of medical records to a willing provider is the pediatrician's final obligation.

Exhibiting Honesty and Integrity

Many pediatricians would consider continuing futile discussions with refusing families over years to be bordering on <u>disingenuous</u>, and not intellectually honest and straightforward. Nearly all pediatricians acknowledge that one of our professional goals must be "to provide the best patient care and social activism," and that "patient well-being should be the primary motivating factor in patient care, ahead of physicians' own interests and needs" (AAP). From the pediatrician's perspective, infant vaccines are the ultimate in "best patient care and social activism."[14] They are almost fully protecting the child from what were, in an earlier era, very common, devastating diseases. Infant vaccines also have a major impact on reducing disease among other non-vaccinated older and younger contacts by way of herd protection.[15]

Yet, what could be considered more optimal care or more altruistic care than fully vaccinating a child? To emphasize again: vaccine programs in

---

[14] D. S. Diekema, American Academy of Pediatrics Committee on Bioethics, "Responding to Parental Refusals of Immunization of Children," *Pediatrics* 115 (2005): 1428-1431.

[15] J. Gilmour, C. Harrison, L. Asadi, M. H. Cohen, and S. Vohra, "Childhood Immunization: When Physicians and Parents Disagree," *Pediatrics* 128, Supp. 4 (2011): S167-S174.

most offices are a loss-leader or a break-even financial proposition. Their administration is not clinician self-interest. [16] Rather, with vaccines, pediatricians want to provide only the best of established standards for all of the children under their care.[17] A visit to a pediatric intensive care unit, seeing a child on a ventilator, or brain-damaged, or dying from any of the vaccine-preventable diseases persuasively argues against accepting a parent's demand for the substandard pediatric care of non-vaccination.[18]

Emotional Costs of Dealing with Non-Vaccinators

As I grow older, my dislike for confrontational office visits increases. I need to keep a calm façade all day long for my young patients, to keep my blood pressure down, and to keep my catecholamine levels subdued. I lose too much sleep worrying about diagnosing and managing the multitude of other challenging and life-threatening problems in my office among vaccine-protected children, as you have read earlier in this book.

The problem is really accentuated when: Did I ask whether the febrile child was fully vaccinated or not? Is one dose of XYZ vaccine going to really protect against ABC disease? Was that rash really measles? Was that croup really epiglottitis? These are difficult diagnoses—often requiring a single emergency or multiple visits before the diagnosis is apparent, and meanwhile, the disease has spread to other unsuspecting victims.

For many vaccine-refusing families, when I must seek a rapid septic workup, spinal tap, intubation, bladder catheterization, chest X-ray, IM antibiotic, or a hospital admission for a moderately or very ill child, I might have difficulty convincing them that I need to act promptly. Vaccine

---

[16] E. A. Flanagan-Klygis, L. Sharp, and J. E. Frader, "Dismissing the Family Who Refuses Vaccines," *Archives Pediatric Adolescent Medicine* 159 (2005): 929-934

[17] S. Leib, P. Liberatos, and K. Edwards, "Pediatricians' Experience with and Response to Parental Vaccine Safety Concerns and Vaccine Refusals: A Survey of Connecticut Pediatricians," *Public Health Report* 126, Supp. 2 (2011): 13-23.

[18] M. E. Fallat, J. Glover, and the Committee on Bioethics, "Professionalism in Pediatrics: Statement of Principles," *Pediatrics* 120, no. 4 (2007): 895-897

refusal may be a marker for other major patient non-adherence issues. These families are often contentious, and if they have little trust in the heart and soul of my everyday pediatric practice (vaccines), I am afraid that they will not trust me in urgent life and death matters as well. Delays could doom a very sick child, as you have read here, and as every pediatrician is keenly aware, it would be emotionally traumatic to see a preventable catastrophe happen because of parental resistance and science denialism.

Classic Profound Autism: The "Real History"

Sadly, my group continues to disenroll any family who refuses most or all vaccines for their infant. The vaccine manufacturers, vaccine experts, even our own meticulous research office, and the previous science-based FDA have spent decades proving the overall safety and protectiveness of our current vaccine schedule, including the multi-component formulations. The vaccine science is sound; the seriously significant vaccine risks range from extremely rare to non-existent for vaccines. A return to the horrible pre-vaccine era is also unacceptable.

And reassuringly for the persistent vaccine skeptics, the **2025 International Society for Autism Research** has just published data confirming that the **rates of classic "profound to debilitating" autism have been stable from the years 2000 to 2016**. This obviously disabled subgroup of autistic children (with IQ <50) comprised 27% of all "autistic" children. In this study, **this autism category rate has actually dropped slightly over 16 years** from 1.5 per 1000 to 1.2 per 1000 children. Currently, this is the "classic autism" group that will unlikely move beyond a first- or second-grade school level, if that.

The reported increase in autism cases has actually only occurred in the more nebulous mild new cases or those with minimal disabilities, from 3.1 to 7.3 cases per 1000. This increase has been a result of the **major expansion of the autism criteria**, which now includes the "Asperger's" category since 2013, **which was actually a nonexistent category before then**. This milder version typically performs adequately academically and occupationally in the long term, but has social struggles in general. Often, they are considered eccentric, peculiarly behaved, with poor social skills, or with OCD, or anxiety, or stereotypical types of behaviors as well. But this group's outcome is most generally favorable.

(These reported data were based on health and school records only.)

A multitude of previous epidemiologic studies have substantiated that Tylenol (acetaminophen) does <u>not</u> cause autism when taken during pregnancy. Furthermore, expert medical societies, such as the World Health Organization, the American Academy of Pediatrics, and the American College of Obstetrics and Gynecology, have stated that taking Tylenol (acetaminophen) during pregnancy <u>is</u> safe. Mothers should not ever feel guilty for taking Tylenol during pregnancy in standard doses. As this issue has become a real quandary, please consult your obstetrician if you are pregnant. Standard doses of Tylenol are extremely safe in all other populations, except for those with liver issues or taking hepatotoxic drugs.

In a well-done study of over 2000 children, it was the maternal fever from an infection in the second trimester that was associated with a 2 times greater risk for documented autism. So Tylenol will actually look beneficial due to its fever reduction. As for autism links, aside from the overwhelming evidence for genetic influences, infectious causes (in my opinion) should be the next major research focus. Heck, we even have vaccines available or in advanced stages of development to prevent some of the most common febrile prenatal infections (RSV, flu, COVID-19, CMV, GBBS6, Zika).[19]

---

[19] Croen LA, et al, Infection and Fever in Pregnancy and Autism Spectrum Disorders: Findings from the Study to Explore Early Development. Autism Res. 2019 Oct;12(10):1551-1561

This illustrates the problem with alarmist "paper mill" data. *Retraction Watch* warns, "In 2021, around 100 studies mining The FDA Adverse Events Reporting System (FAERS), for drug safety signals were published. In 2024, that number was 600..."[20] "**By presenting mere statistical associations as 'safety signals', these publications can generate unjustified alarms** with considerable impact on healthcare provider practices and patient behaviors,"[21] says Charles Khouri, a pharmacologist at Grenoble Alpes University Hospital in France.

Folinic acid

On an optimistic speculative note, some unverified, **very** preliminary data suggest that the daily use of **high-dose folinic acid** (Leucovirin used for reversal of methotrexate inhibition) ($100 monthly) might somewhat improve meltdowns, along with a slight improvement in verbal and social skills in some children within this classic **profound autistic group.** This very limited data only applied: 1) if they do not have a known genetic basis (e.g., Fragile X, etc.), and 2) if they have an anti-folic acid antibody present (possibly present in the blood of 50 to 75% of these profound cases only). The theory is that this antibody blocks a key folic acid uptake in the brain, and folinic acid bypasses it. Studies of safety and effectiveness must be undertaken by the FDA to test whether this compound really works in these children before it becomes standard of care. Is this a knee-jerk approval from political pressure? Stay tuned. It does have some side effects.

Finally, <u>no-fault medico-legal protection</u> should be available for any clinician who is willing to provide care for any under-vaccinated or unvaccinated patient, if the patient subsequently contracts a vaccine-preventable disease! These clinicians are providing an invaluable service

---

[20] https://retractionwatch.com/2025/09/16/exclusive-journal-bans-drug-safety-database-papers-as-they-flood-the-literature/?utm_source=chatgpt.com

[21] Khouri C, Fusaroli M, Salvo F, Raschi E. Transparency and robustness of safety signals. BMJ. 2022 Nov 3;379:o2588. doi: 10.1136/bmj.o2588. PMID: 36328354.

with notable liability risk. This would also eliminate one of the many disincentives for dismissal of the vaccine-refusing family.

See the article below for an alternative vaccine schedule that often appeases those demanding to delay vaccines.

The Vicar of Vicarious Vaccine-Preventable Diseases

(Adapted from Block SL, The Vicar of Vicarious Vaccine-Preventable Diseases, *Pediatric Annals 43(6)*, June 2014)

On this spring day early in your career, you have seen your fourth patient younger than age 24 months with a fever of 103.5°F for the past day or so, including your own granddaughter, who was being examined by your partner. Each child was without other symptoms except for being cranky, anorexic, non-toxic appearing, and totally unappreciative of any physician examination.

In the past, before our life-saving vaccines were available, many of these children would likely have been the unwelcome recipients of a chest X-ray, venipuncture for both a complete blood count and possibly a blood culture to ascertain whether they had become occultly infected with either *Haemophilus influenzae B* or pneumococcus in the bloodstream. You may have also obtained a catheterized urine sample if you stumbled upon a leukocytosis in your female patient or if the patient had persistent fevers. A critical dose of IM ceftriaxone would be typical, too. Lumbar punctures (spinal taps) were also commonplace.

In today's world, during the first few days of these symptoms, you can usually cavalierly administer calm reassurances and instructions for ibuprofen/acetaminophen for most of these children, with one notable exception—the unvaccinated or undervaccinated toddler. Why? The terrifying specter of vaccine-preventable diseases (VPDs) may be resurrecting.

As a young or middle-aged pediatrician, you will not be old enough to have experienced firsthand the morbidity and mortality of these VPDs for which we now have effective and safe vaccines. Thus, you may approach the vaccine schedule with an inkling of trepidation and with some "empathy" for the stressed and worried mother who has read somewhere or been told by some "mommy blog" or by an outspoken celebrity or by a notorious trial lawyer that vaccines are unnecessary and perhaps unsafe. After all, the child will likely cry when the injections are administered, and who wants to see their baby cry, even if your intentions are good? You might even think it may be satisfactory to avoid the "entire mess" along with the time-consuming "messy" discussion about routine infant vaccines. Your patient's parents have been scared out of any scientific logic.

You are a busy professional. You know you can wait out these non-vaccinators (possibly for years), and you seem to even have the equivocating approval of your own medical society. Somehow, you apparently have forgotten your infectious disease training, in which you learned that **these communicable diseases mostly occur in and are most devastating for infants and very young children.** You think that you can be lackadaisical about vaccines and the oft-forgotten monster of VPDs, but this infectious nightmare is lurking, as the following examples show.

Your Vicarious Vicar's Experience with VPDs

I personally do not need to be reminded why these infant and preschool vaccines are critically important for infants and children. I have seen the malevolent monster of these infections up close and personal, and it is a scary picture. I have lived the pre-vaccine nightmare scenarios while fully awake, and, unfortunately, most of the details are indelibly etched in my memory. This resulted in far too many sleepless nights worrying.

I therefore think it is important for my somewhat forgetful or younger colleagues to vicariously experience the sheer terror of some of the worst days of my life as a private practitioner, as told in this book. Heaven forbid that you become complacent about the microscopic pathogenic barbarians that are still circulating and occasionally banging at your doors.

During the course of a 40+-year career in pediatrics in a rural area, I have probably saved at least one to two children/teens per month (perhaps close to 500 patients) from all sorts of obvious and not-so-obvious catastrophes and illnesses. These would include meningitis, septicemia, epiglottitis, Rocky Mountain spotted fever, tularemia, cancers, asthma, prematurity, antifreeze ingestion (anion gap), suicide, depression, schizophrenia, and so on.

Thus, parents may think they can count on us pediatricians to always be able to save their children from these devastating VPDs if the illness should ever strike their child. That is a very dangerous gamble with any child. The mother who said she was not scared of pertussis has not seen the several pertussis-induced brain-damaged infants or deaths that I saw three decades ago, despite all the marvelous medical technical skills of our pediatric intensive care units. She is also gambling with the lives of other infants and toddlers who are unwittingly exposed to her own highly contagious, unprotected vectors (i.e., her children). It is not just about you. "We do so depend on the kindness of strangers!" (Blanche DuBois in *A Streetcar Named Desire*)

Cases of VPD

The specifics in each of the following cases have been changed for privacy reasons.

Case 1

As a recent graduate of the top-notch Wake Forest University pediatric training program, I had been enjoying my autonomous private pediatric practice for a few years here in rural Kentucky. The busy practice consisted of two pediatricians (James Hedrick, MD) at the time, and seeing 30 to 35 patients per doctor during a 9-hour day was the norm during the winter.

One dank and frigid February afternoon, my office received a phone call from the emergency department (ER). These time-consuming disruptions were not uncommon back then. At that time, there was no in-house ER doctor covering the small, 35-bed hospital.

The highly experienced and trustworthy ER nurse seemed frantic and said there was no time for the patient to come over to the office, which was only about a block away. The patient, a 2-year-old White boy, had a fever of 104°F and seemed lethargic. Which one of you was going to traipse over there? By default, seniority won out. My partner stayed in the office. I was designated for the septic workup.

I quickly run over (young and without bad knees then) to the ER only to encounter the dreaded predicament: a lethargic, pink, and minimally moving male toddler.

My rapid but complete physical examination revealed one of the pediatrician's greatest professional fears—a lethargic, highly febrile but stable child who had a few bruises on his trunk. Petechiae and/or ecchymoses in a febrile child are ominous. However, his vital signs were stable with only moderate tachycardia and a normal blood pressure; his neck was slightly stiff. It was time for the "full court press"—better known as the complete septic workup.

In my training during the heyday of pneumococcal and HIB disease (like this patient), old-time (and hopefully still for the "New Age") pediatricians were generally taught that if the diagnosis of meningitis seriously enters your differential diagnosis, then one best act on this hunch and perform a spinal tap. In my 3-year residency stint, I would have probably performed at least 30 or more spinal taps, and for a few years, about one per 2 months in private practice since then. Spinal taps were a trained automatic reflex performed on infants who looked very ill from infection, who had a full fontanelle, or likely with meningismus (neck stiffness). The complex procedure is relatively easy to perform in young children and infants, and success is actually highly dependent on my experience and the person holding the patient. A child had to be in shock or critically unstable or too combative before one would consider delaying this procedure. In fact, the tiny amount of spinal fluid drawn off by the procedure may be theoretically brain- and life-saving in purulent meningitis cases under CSF pressure.

Thus, within minutes, I had the obligatory blood culture, complete blood count (later chest radiograph), and a less traumatic bagged urinalysis/urine culture. These were nearly always performed prior to the prompt requisite infusion of broad-spectrum antibiotics, lest one obscure the important potential bacterial growth. Thus, intravenous access was also critically needed for both the IV antibiotics and fluid resuscitation. This itself is a highly technical and challenging skill infrequently practiced by our current pediatric trainees.

Then, the stable, alert but lethargic child was rolled on his side, restrained, and positioned as usual for a spinal tap while he received blow-by oxygen. At L1-L2, I hit the ½ cm "sweet spot" and felt the tiny pop. Three milliliters of clear, colorless fluid were obtained without difficulty. The needle was withdrawn. The intravenous line was started, and the ampicillin and ceftriaxone infusions were initiated. Resuscitative doses of IV fluids were being administered.

And similar to the Israeli experience of a 4% HIB fatality rate despite optimal care and for unknown reasons, a half-hour later, while waiting for the ambulance to arrive and take off, the previously stable and monitored patient abruptly developed apnea. He went into asystole before we were able to load him onto the ambulance. He could not be resuscitated despite all our heroic medicines and life-support efforts. HIB septic shock can just be that deadly. Pre-HIB vax, I saw way too many deaths already in my training. One will always be affected by and never forget this type of tragedy. A gut-wrenching and horrific discussion with the family was the next step. Severe VPD bacterial infections, like HIB, are totally unpredictable. He had no chance. God bless his innocent soul. His funeral was heartbreaking.

Case 2

Sound asleep at 3 a.m. on an icy January night, the local ER physician called you with some bad news: "I think your 2-year-old Black patient with 102°F fever may have epiglottitis." This was a true medical emergency. When you arrived, the patient was struggling to breathe, was drooling, and maintained a forward-lurching tripod sitting position. He had a distinctly different non-croup stridor. His lateral neck X-ray showed a positive thumb sign (swelling) of the epiglottis.

The tertiary care hospital intensive care unit (ICU) was 45 minutes away. The emergency medical technicians, who were an additional 20 minutes away, would not be able to handle an obstructed airway on the road. The urgency was palpable. He was struggling to breathe and was now experiencing mild desaturation spells, manifested by slight cyanosis of the lips and dropping oximetry readings. In his unstable condition, transporting him by ambulance could be lethal. In fact, any upsetting disturbance of the child could trigger complete obstruction of the airway and death.

The local friendly excellent general surgeon, Dr. Mickey Anderson, was called in for a potential backup tracheotomy in case the intubation went awry. Children with epiglottitis are among the most difficult intubation procedures to perform due to the obscured landmarks and marked swelling of the epiglottis portal for your endotracheal (ET) tube. The experienced nurse anesthetist provided some blow-by inhaled low-dose nitric oxide (if you remember correctly, during all the commotion).

Under immense pressure, you chose a 3.5-mm French ET tube, the size normally used in a smaller full-term infant. Maintaining any fair-sized airway was paramount the first few hours. As you suspected, when the laryngoscope was inserted and the tongue was lifted, the cherry-red epiglottis was swollen. The laryngeal opening was partially obscured as he inspired. (Your heart almost expired at that moment.)

All those newborn and child intubations during your pediatric training at the local teaching hospital were about to pay off. With the straight laryngoscope and an inserted ET tube stylette, you were able to firmly force the ET tube with a sorta pop past the tight, swollen epiglottis. With the airway stabilized, you could now perform blood cultures and deliver intravenous antibiotics and IV fluids. The stress of performing these other invasive procedures before the airway was stabilized could have triggered an airway collapse and a nightmarish medical emergency like the one you were trying to avoid by keeping the boy off the road. Even the lateral neck radiograph in the ER could have been perilous.

As expected, VPD HIB was recovered from the blood culture a few days later. He did well and survived without any sequelae. Yes, we can save most of these deathly ill children, but not all.

Case 3

About a decade into your practice, a healthy-looking 10-year-old Hispanic boy from Elizabethtown was seen in the office in the past week with a relatively mild case of chickenpox for 48 hours. He was alert, febrile to 101°F, drinking well, but itching furiously. His family was reassured about the self-limited nature of varicella and no Zovirax was prescribed. He was sent home in good condition. They were told to administer diphenhydramine and acetaminophen, and to use oatmeal baths daily for his itching and hygiene in an attempt to prevent the increasingly common secondary Group A strep necrotizing fasciitis, being increasingly witnessed in the past decade.

He was apparently doing well for several days, but you heard over the weekend that he had been seen in the ER and then admitted to the hospital for altered mental status. You knew what that meant. You find out that he is now comatose and on a ventilator. An intracranial pressure monitor has been inserted into his skull.

You found out that his initial liver function tests were 10- to 20-fold above the normal range, his prothrombin time was twice normal, and his serum ammonia was markedly elevated, too.

At your earlier office visit, you had warned the family not to administer any aspirin to him. Earlier reports in the 1980s had noted some occasional association of Reye's syndrome with aspirin use during either influenza or varicella infections. But were other sources of salicylate still available to the unsuspecting family? Yes.

After a week-long battle with his Reye's syndrome, the patient succumbed to his unrelenting high brain pressure. During his hospitalization, the family asked you questions as to why he became afflicted by this deadly condition. He had taken no aspirin. However, he had developed some vomiting during his early illness that they treated with the adult version of Pepto-Bismol (Procter & Gamble, Cincinnati, OH), otherwise known as bismuth salicylate. (You may have uncovered the first ever case among several local Reye's syndrome cases theoretically precipitated by ingestion of bismuth salicylate during a bout of varicella.)

Although he did not use any of the following substances, you also suspected that Reye's syndrome could also possibly be triggered by topical applications of wintergreen or salicylate liniments for muscle aches.

An additional lesson to be learned here is that any type of salicylate compound should be avoided during an unknown febrile illness or during known chickenpox or influenza-like illnesses. Yes, we can save most of these deathly ill children, but not all. If only the mandatory chickenpox vaccine were available back then. I am so thankful that later, our research group was at least able to help develop this life-saving chickenpox vaccine for future generations.

Case 4

In a not-so-hypothetical medico-legal situation, a 4-year-old child from an urban area in Kentucky is confined to a wheelchair; he cannot speak, cannot feed himself, and has spastic hemiplegia (cerebral palsy). His disability is due to pneumococcal meningitis that he developed at age 9 weeks.

One of the major medico-legal complaints from the plaintiffs was the lack of administration of the first dose of the then just-approved pneumococcal conjugate vaccine (PCV7). But the parent had cancelled a well visit at age 8 weeks and had subsequently rescheduled the visit at age 10 weeks, which was 2 days after the boy developed meningitis. The office schedule was busy, and this was your "earliest available" appointment.

Is the defendant physician responsible for the unfortunate delay? Will this parent's allegations be similar to any family who chooses to delay infant vaccines and whose child subsequently develops a VPD?

The other critical legal unknowns are as follows: Would one dose of PCV7 have made any difference in preventing invasive disease? Would you not need to know the serotype of the pneumococcal strain (7 of 90 possible serotypes in PCV7), which was not assessed, to make any plausible case of this? If the wrong non-vaccine serotype caused the infection, then the vaccine would have had absolutely no protection. Would high rates of community vaccination have provided herd protection–perhaps here too?

CONCLUSION

I do not fully profess to be saintly, or an actual vicarious vicar of VPDs and their afflictions; for this, read your pediatric infectious disease textbooks. But I have personally felt the sting of death and devastation from VPDs, which can almost always be prevented by the minute "sting" of some particularly impeccably studied safe shots.

As stated previously, we can save most children who become infected with many VPDs, but not all of them.

Pediatricians must also realize that continuing to provide care for children whose parents are willfully either keeping them non-vaccinated or in a state of delayed vaccinations is fraught with multiple problems. These include the following:

- A presumptive medico-legal sanctioning of substandard pediatric care
- A child who continues to be at significant risk for a devastating VPD, especially when population vaccine levels drop a little too low, like measles and pertussis currently.
- Becoming enmeshed in a deadly gamble for your patient, and the terrible personal anxiety about the course and outcome if one of your patients should become afflicted with a VPD. The haunting "if only..." question.
- A profound and very expensive change in the way you approach these patient encounters for fevers, rashes, and bad coughs, both on the phone, in the office, and in lab test ordering.
- Eventual likelihood of medico-legal conundrums and disparaging smearing lawsuits.

With the increasing rates of non-vaccination and undervaccination in your practice, these are examples of the many potential VPD infections and possible legal crossroads that many pediatricians will likely face in their careers. Remember that in a peds career, the odds of being dragged into court as a defendant are already somewhere between 30% and 50%. That means at least 30,000 to 50,000 of the nearly 100,000 currently practicing pediatricians will have to spend about 5 years of their active 35 career years in a state of shock, high anxiety, depression, insomnia, and self-doubt. Despite the **unavoidable** bad outcome for the patient in most legal cases, your personal and professional integrity will still be completely lambasted. "Jackpot justice" is terrifying.

✸ Vaccine-Preventable Diseases: The Measles Epidemic

I stopped our area's first and only measles epidemic.

In the spring of 1988, a 4-year-old girl presented with a whole-body red bumpy rash, high fevers, a clear runny nose, red conjunctivitis (not draining), red throat, a bad cough, and obviously feeling terrible. What really differentiated her from every other rash-afflicted child was the two white dots on her inner buccal mucosa (inside her cheek). This finding was nearly diagnostic for measles and is called Koplik's spots. So, the constellation of fever/rash with "3 Cs and a K" (cough, coryza, conjunctivitis, and Koplik's) indicated to me that this young lady was infected with measles, despite no recently reported cases and having received an on-time, earlier single dose of the measles vaccine.

The measles vaccine had been available since 1975 and was known to be very effective as a single dose. However, some breakthrough measles cases had been reported, but at this time, not enough for the CDC to warrant routine booster shots after the first dose. Subsequently, we found out later that a single dose of measles or MMR (measles, mumps, rubella) vaccine was only 90% effective. The entire pediatric population would need booster immunization rates of 95% to achieve full herd immunity or herd protection for the entire unvaccinated population, many of whom either refused the vaccine or were too old or too sick to get it routinely for school. The second dose would raise her patient protection to 97%.

Upon further questioning of the mother, who had just recently delivered another baby, it appeared her obstetrician was concerned that she might have the measles as well (very few obstetricians have observed a case of measles in their careers). So, his entire waiting room was exposed, thus requiring all of them to receive post-exposure prophylaxis shots.

This is vital to know because measles is one of the most contagious viruses ever. It can lead to blindness, serious illness, and hospitalization for dehydration (about 15 to 20%), brain damage (1/500), and even death (1/500). (83 deaths occurred on the small island of Samoa in 2020, possibly due to advice from a lawyer to health officials there that the measles vaccine was not beneficial.) And over 1/3 of patients lose their entire immune memory, thus predisposing the patient to other innumerable serious infectious diseases for a few years to come.

So, I contacted the state health department in Frankfort. I felt as if they thought, since I lived in the bourbon whiskey capital of the world, Bardstown, KY, that maybe I imbibed too much. I explained that I was a board-certified pediatrician and knew what I was doing. On the other line, crickets chirping.

Then, three days later, another case rolled into my office with nearly identical findings on history and examination. This sicker child had not received any measles vaccine. I became more adamant about my diagnostic skills. I contacted the health department chief and reiterated my conviction that I was seeing the beginning stages of a measles outbreak. Well, two days later, our office nurses and the state health department mobilized the entire area's three-county health department staff and nurses to enter every school and daycare. They would vaccinate every child who received one dose with a second dose of the MMR vaccine over a 3-day period. They would administer an initial dose of MMR to all those unvaccinated. And if the child was younger than 12 months old who was exposed, an initial dose of MMR was likewise administered, knowing they would have to receive a 2nd dose after 12 months old.

This was essential to squelch the brewing measles epidemic. Because two doses of the measles vaccine would provide over 97% protection to the population, thus achieving herd protection for all children and minimizing any breakthrough cases. Even if a breakthrough case should occur, it would be milder, less severe, and much less contagious.

Thus, with my input, the 1980s epidemic of measles in our three counties was aborted. Also, routine vaccination with a second dose of MMR was implemented later that year by the CDC for all school-age children, preferably at age 4 years, but as early as 3 months after the first dose. Take heed, all U.S. sites with measles outbreaks.

(Post-exposure prophylaxis with either a dose of MMR or a shot of immunoglobulin, depending on timing, is also a key to prevention.)

This is how you stop the otherwise likely carnage of measles. Herbals, cod liver oil, and vitamin A for exposures are a fool's errand.

💥 An Acceptable Alternative Immunization Schedule

By contrast, for the vaccine-hesitant family, I have devised a potentially workable compromise—the "Block almost timely/tenable alternative to Sears schedule" (BATTASS)—which can work within Dr. Sears' principles (but only the second edition of the Sears' *Vaccine Book,* as the first edition is not suitable*).*

Case: 'The Anxious Family'

Today, you are seeing for the first time this 5-day-old full-term healthy infant girl who was born by spontaneous vaginal delivery to a 31-year-old healthy G3P2 mother. You are excited that the mother has picked your practice for her daughter's pediatric care. As you review her history, you uncover that the child has not received the hepatitis B vaccine at birth. You inquire whether there is any particular reason for not vaccinating her infant.

The mother calmly explains to you that she has "read up" (she has done "her research") (on the internet, on the blogs, and the op-eds on TikTok!) on the hazards of the infant hepatitis B vaccine and has declined any hepatitis B vaccination based on the guidelines proposed by Dr. Sears, one of the nation's leading proponents on alternative vaccine schedules. She says that, as he explains in the second edition of his book, infants are getting too many shots at one time, which may overload their immune systems, and that many injectable vaccines contain too much aluminum, a "known toxin" (debunked below) when injected in large amounts in certain susceptible populations (none of which is true).

'Dangers' of Newborn Hepatitis B Vaccine? C'mon, Really???

In his book, Sears unequivocally and vocally states that the hepatitis B vaccine is actually unnecessary until the teen years, but feels it should still be given to preschoolers.[22] You can actually almost accept this assertion that when the hepatitis B vaccination is not received at birth, and parents who have no risk factors, along with a maternal negative hepatitis B screen, hepatitis B infection would be almost unheard of until the teen years. Almost.

Dennis Murray, MD, pediatric infectious disease specialist of Medical College of Georgia, [in personal communication] warns that he has seen cases of postnatally acquired hepatitis B in young children. At this age, it is associated with a nearly 50% chance of chronic active hepatitis B, often with later cirrhosis or liver cancer.[23] Sears also worries that the hepatitis B vaccine at birth may precipitate some cases of fever, irritability, and poor feeding, which in turn may trigger a hospitalization for a newborn septic workup. He cites a 1999 inpatient retrospective study, which showed a twofold increase in rare newborn hospitalizations by 5 days of life after implementation of a birth HBV dose. Statistical fluke? Or, cause and effect? My conclusion is the former.

Other than with maternal fever, chorioamnionitis, or flu, I have never seen this early-life fever adverse event personally in our practice over the last 4 decades while dealing with a cohort of over 40,000 births. In addition, Niu and colleagues reported that the VAERS data from 1991 to 1994, after 12 million doses of birth dose HBV vaccine, revealed only 13 potential cases of

---

[22] Dyer, BJ. Do you fire parents who refuse to vaccinate their children? *Infectious Diseases in Children*. February 2009.

[23] Gilmour J, Harrison C, Asadi L, Cohen MH, Vohra S. Childhood immunization: when physicians and parents disagree. *Pediatrics*. 2011;128(Suppl 4):S167-S174. doi: 10.1542/peds.2010-2720E

newborn fever and hospitalization. Admittedly, VAERS is underreported, but this tiny number is most reassuring.

Not without some risk, this immediate HBV newborn decision to decline, however, is now irretrievable for this newborn. Before 1991, about 18,000 cases of hepatitis B were reported in young children, mostly acquired from a mother/family member with unknown status. So you move on to see how many other immunization compromises may be needed to appease this family.

Immediately, you have become skeptical, wary, and somewhat defensive about how you should optimally approach the issue of the remainder of routine vaccines for this family's infant. Having recently dealt with many families with similar "belief systems," you recollect that the markedly delayed and separate vaccine antigen tactics proposed in the first edition of Dr. Sears' book had driven an insurmountable wedge between your staunchly pro-CDC and pro-ACIP "timely" schedule, and the parents' "pick 'em" and "choose 'em" terribly delayed schedules. Have you reached an impasse?[24] Or can you blithely accept a willy-nilly, unorthodox, and untested approach to the vaccine schedule from a set of parents who really do not fully comprehend all the rigorous testing that goes into vaccine development, safety, and schedules? They also have no actual idea about the devastation that these vaccines prevent. By contrast, you know this or have seen this way too many times.

In the interest of connecting with your patient, you decide to take a dip into this murky literary pseudoscience pond. During your reading of Sears' book, you learn quickly that Dr. Sears claims to be "pro-vaccine" as he clearly alleges several times. Most of his discussions about infant vaccine side effects and efficacy are actually fairly well-researched, but very over-exaggerated. Most of his warnings about side effects are no more "scary" than reading the actual CDC Vaccine Information Sheet (VIS), which each

---

[24] Sears R. *The Vaccine Book. Making the Right Decision for Your Child.* 2nd ed. New York: Little, Brown, 2011.

parent is supposed to read anyway. He clearly explains the rationales and benefits of each vaccine as well. This is not true about his ideas for older children. To sum up his approach, in order to gain cooperation from vaccine-doubters, "We need to offer schedules that acknowledge their concerns but don't compromise disease protection."

Well, here I go, Dr. Sears.

He also tries to maintain some balance between the vaccine clinical trial data and the post-marketing vaccine-negative publications. He does warn the reader about potential self-interests of both respective groups, although I cannot fathom how a group like the well-respected and blatantly impartial PAST iterations of the FDA, the CDC, or the ACIP can be portrayed as having any self-interest here. They did not in the past. (In 2025, it is a mess.) For instance, if the FDA uncovered any irregularities in vaccine manufacturing processes, any major negative "scientific" clinical trial data about a new vaccine, or any off-label advertising of a vaccine, they will shut down vaccine manufacturing, prevent vaccine licensure, or heavily fine the accused company, respectively. This would occur no matter how vital and life-saving the vaccine usually is—think HIB vaccine shortages.

Sears acknowledges that many of the negative vaccine articles he quotes were non-scientific, and he notes that many of these negative authors were involved with their own competing "complementary" unapproved products for personal financial gain. Similar to many of the newly appointed ACIP committee members.

The Near Impossibility of Bias in Current Clinical Trials

Dr. Sears, along with other non-medical officials, however, does not seem to fully understand the true "science" behind the clinical trial process of double-blinding, randomization, and comparator or placebo-controlled vaccine trials. Placebo-controlled trials can only be performed on previously unapproved vaccines as well. No reasonable parent is going to forego the standard of care when performing a comparison trial to advance an established vaccine with an improved version of the vaccine.

All clinical trials and protocols for vaccine approval must be conducted strictly under the most stringent FDA guidelines. With all current investigative trials during the last 25 years or so conducted in this fashion, there just is no way to bias or taint the data—you, the investigator, never see the data until it is totally locked into the main computer and then later analyzed by the coldly calculating computer. You are just recording patient diaries, physical examinations, and adverse events into case books—totally blinded to the treatment arm or outcome.

In addition, the company's own internal and external auditors constantly monitor the entire data set as it pours in from the office, also in a totally blinded fashion. And the (external) FDA itself audits a large portion of the trial data for fraud, irregularities, and good research compliance—audits that I have personally experienced and survived unscathed from multiple times over the course of my prodigious research career.

Whether any discovered problems are due to intentional or human error, sanctions, fines, or data exclusion (meaning all that work for no pay at all) by the FDA additionally ensures that you do your job as a scientist correctly. Unlike Andrew Wakefield, MD of "MMR and fabricated autism" infamy, you, as an investigator, are not even remotely thinking about veering from the protocol, inappropriate patient enrollment, or data manipulation. You have no way of doing so, regardless. In addition, the overall sample size of patients enrolled must be sufficient enough to show statistical significance or at least non-inferiority via effectiveness or patient-obtained blood antibody levels.

Dr. Sears, via his followers coming into each of your offices, also has trouble grasping the implications of the vaccine adverse event reporting system **(VAERS)** relative to true background rates and "noise" always simultaneously occurring with any reported vaccine adverse effects. Nearly a third to one-half of national VAERS reports originate from plaintiffs' lawyers trying to drum up litigation. When it comes to the adverse effects of vaccines, these "temporal" or anecdotal associations **rarely ever** translate into "causal" associations, once they are independently evaluated. Smoke screens? For example, just because the child was riding in a car seat and dies from SIDS later that night, it does not translate as the association: the car seat caused SIDS. The rate of naturally occurring "background noise" versus actual vaccine adverse effects must always be considered in reliable, accurate science. Not because Aunt Fran heard her cousin had a COVID-19 reaction of blood clots 4 months later, which is sadly "reportable."

The Unproven Aluminum Toxicity Contention

Aluminum adjuvants are critical to the high immunogenicity, durability, and reduced number of doses for many of our vaccines. Because the aluminum content of vaccines during each visit is such an important point of contention for Dr. Sears, let's examine the amounts in those aluminum-containing vaccines. Aluminum toxicity has mostly been reported in two populations: premature infants and dialysis patients. The toxicity is due to chronic, very large exposures and is characterized by dementia, memory loss, fatigue, depression, and learning impairments. However, Keith and colleagues calculated that a standard immunization dose of aluminum is eliminated within 1 to 3 days!

Also, injection total doses of 850 mcg or 1,225 mcg of aluminum via vaccine(s), respectively, did not cause any changes to normal plasma concentrations in either adults or premature infants. In another study of aluminum adjuvants, up to 60% and 70% of aluminum in adult vaccines was excreted in the urine by 1 week and 5 weeks, respectively. Thus, vaccine-injected aluminum is so rapidly excreted that it produces minimal, if any, elevations in serum aluminum concentrations, and only for a few days, and definitely not near any toxic range, from the total possible 2000 to 3000 mcg injected over a 6-month period. Thus, it accumulates little more than the **infant's 6-month oral total (38,000 mcg-117,000 mcg)**

intake of daily regular dietary aluminum via formula, with a 1% absorption rate.

Aluminum Content Within Specific Infant Vaccines Containing Aluminum	
Vaccine	**Aluminum Content (mcg)**
HIB (PedVax HIB Only)	225
PVC13	125
DTaP	170 to ≤ 625
Hepatitis B	250
Hepatitis A	250
Pentacel	330
Pediarix	≤ 850
Vaxells	319

Table 5. Aluminum content within specific infant vaccines containing aluminum
Note: Aluminum content may vary slightly by manufacturer formulation. The value for
Vaxelis (DTaP-IPV-Hib-HepB) is based on published manufacturer data:
approximately **319 mcg** of aluminum as aluminum hydroxide.

And just recently published in the *Annals of Internal Medicine* (August 2025), a population study of over 1 million young children in Denmark 1997-2018 observed no increased rate for the diagnosis of **classic autism** or even other neuropsychiatric or autoimmune disorders in children who had received routine, somewhat higher doses of adjuvanted aluminum from the new enhanced vaccines in the improving immunization schedule. Once again demonstrating no increasing rates of classic profound autism (it had actually decreased) despite slightly higher doses of aluminum in vaccines. For some reason, Heads of Human Health Services wanted this article retracted and buried. Real science does not work that way.

The Block Almost Timely and Tenable Alternative to Sears Schedule (BATTASS)

Age	AlternativeAge (months)	"Main" Vaccine	Concomitant Vaccines
4 Weeks	1 Month	Hepatitis B vaccine*	
6 weeks	2 Months	Pentacel	RV5 or RV1
10 weeks	3 Months	PVC13	
14 weeks	4 Months	Pentacel	RV5 or RV1
18 weeks	5 Months	PCV13	
22 weeks	6 Months	Pentacel	RV5
26 weeks	7 Months	PCV13	
9 months/ 10months		Injectable flu vaccine (preservative-free)+	Hepatitis B vaccine
12 months		MMR	PCV13
13 months		(Hepatitis A vaccine)+	
15 months		Pentacel	Varicella

*Hepatitis B is administered at 1 month for those infants enrolling in day care, although no hepatitis B vaccine is supposed to be administered in the first 2 years to accommodate Dr. Sears' usual schedule.

+The intranasal vaccine is only FDA approved after age 24 months, and definitely should NOT be given as early as age 9 months, as stated by Dr. Sears, due to increased risk of hospitalization under 12 months.

+First dose of Hepatitis A vaccine can be given as late as 24 months, and still "almost" be within the ACIP guidelines, unless an outbreak occurs.

Table 6. The Block Almost Timely and Tenable Alternative to Sears Schedule (BATTAS)
*Vaxelis could replace 1st dose of Pentacel and Hep B and Pentacel at 4 and 6 months and Hep B at 9 months

Sears' Vaccination Restrictions

Dr. Sears has espoused the following restrictions on alternative infant vaccinations.

- Give only one aluminum-containing vaccine at a time;
- Receive no more than 2 vaccines at a time;
- Delay shots for "milder" diseases or non-infant diseases, specifically hepatitis A and hepatitis B shots, respectively. Hepatitis A vaccine may be given at 12 and 21 months. For daycare requirements, hepatitis B vaccine (HBV) may be given at 1 month (birth dose is still much preferred), with a second dose at 3 months and a third dose at 9 months. (Sears still otherwise recommends hepatitis B as a preschool vaccine);
- Give only one live-virus combo or single vaccine at a time;
- Receipt of MMR at 12 months is adequate for him, but Sears prefers giving patients separate monovalent components, which he acknowledges is not going to happen! They do not exist anymore! The varicella vaccine is typically given at 12 to 15 months. If they are dosed in separate months, each vaccine needs to be given at least 3 months apart. Per the CDC, the MMR vaccine is currently recommended to be administered separately from the varicella vaccine for the first dose anyway. So the risk is minimal for merely another 3 months delay. With the impending measles epidemics, just give the MMR first, and it is still compatible with the ACIP schedule. **However, the MMRV combo is still FDA-approved at 12 months and older.**

He also discusses 3 different possible delayed first vaccines scheduled at 6 months, 12 months, or 24 months, for those parents who insist upon it. Yet, these would never be palatable for most pediatric practices.

Almost timely and tenable? If parents are adamant and balk at the irrational and totally disproven association of MMR with autism (see the recent report by the autism society)[25], then reverse the order. But only if there is NO measles epidemic ongoing!!!—Give MMR at 15 months instead, and varicella at 12 months. This is still within the ACIP guidelines, but it does allow the child to have an extra 3 months unprotected from measles and mumps. Note, if a child does not show signs of "moderate to significant" classic autism by 15 months, then they are extremely unlikely to ever spontaneously develop this category of the profound classic autism disorder. Remember, mumps infection can cause sterility and encephalitis.

Issues With Sears's Adolescent Schedule

But, I have several major issues with his adolescent schedule, for example, adherence to and the scheduling of the several shots, and the use of only a single dose MCV4 at age 16 years old—by then it's just too late for many, as I have personally experienced. I suggest that he watch our video on the National Public Broadcasting Network's program: "Healthy Bodies/Healthy Minds" [26] regarding the prevention of meningococcal disease in preteens as well.

Finally, his discussion of the HPV4/9 vaccine is too biased and will lead to tragic outcomes. It is fraught with errors and background "noise" (claims of unproven: pregnancy issues, severe reactions, autoimmune disorders, and fictional serotype replacement issues). And he creates a dangerous mindset medicolegally for you. It particularly downplays the terrible consequences of severe female and male HPV disease (over 330,000 surgeries for high-grade CIN 2/3, etc.) and cancers (over 40,000 cervical, vaginal, vulvar, rectal, and oral), over 90% of which will be preventable with the HPV9 vaccine. His book seems to be advocating the failed and dubious "just say no" to sex policy for teens. This is unlikely to work in real life for

---

[25] https://autismsociety.org/national-disability-groups-unite-to-protect-lives-and-dispel-vaccine-myths-in-the-autism-community/?

[26] Healthy Body Healthy Mind. To catch a killer: Preventing meningococcal disease {DVD}National Public Broadcasting Network; 2012. Available at: www.itvisus.com/programs/hbhm/episode_2204.asp. Accessed Sept. 23, 2013

HPV, as has been reported in college freshman students. The staggering fact is that up to 25% of college-age who were initially virgins will become infected with preventable high-risk types of HPV within 3 years. Perhaps, we all need to investigate the HPV vaccine better by catching up on the huge available data sets showing the extreme safety and efficacy of HPV9 in true scientific studies (many of which I am also an author on – look it up).

Alternative Infant Vaccine Schedule Using Pediarix When Pentacel Is Unavailable (Not Preferred by Dr.Sears' Schedule Due to High Aluminum Content in Pediarix (850 mcg)

Age	AlternativeAge (months)	"Main" Vaccine	Concomitant Vaccines
4 Weeks	1 Month	Hepatitis B vaccine*	
6 weeks	2 Months	Pediatrix	
10 weeks	3 Months	PVC13	HIB vaccine/RV5 or RV1
14 weeks	4 Months	Pedicatrix	RV5 or RV1
18 weeks	5 Months	PCV13	HIB vaccine/RV5 or RV1
22 weeks	6 Months	Pediatrix	RV5
26 weeks	7 Months	PCV13	HIB vaccine/RV5 or RV1
9 months/ 10months		Flu vaccine (preservative-free)+	Hepatitis B vaccine
12 months		MMR	PCV13
13 months		(Hepatitis A vaccine)+	
15 months		HIB vaccine	Varicella
18 months		DTaP	IPV

*Hepatitis B is administered at I month for those infants enrolling in day care, although no hepatitis B vaccine is supposed to be administered in the first 2 years to accommodate Dr. Sears' usual schedule.

+The intranasal vaccine is only FDA approved after age 24 months, and definitely should NOT be given as early as age 9 months, as stated by Dr. Sears, due to increased risk of hospitalization under 12 months.

+First dose of Hepatitis A vaccine can be given as late as 24 months, and still "almost" be within the ACIP guidelines, unless an outbreak occurs.

Table 7. Alternative Infant Vaccine Schedule Using Pediarix When Pentacel Is Unavailable (Not Preferred by Dr. Sears' Schedule Due to High Aluminum Content in Pediarix (850 mcg))

✸ Block Almost Timely and Tenable Alternative to Sears Schedule (BATTASS)

Or The Pediatrician's Alternative to Sears Schedule (PASS) for Infants (See above table 7.) This is the first published complete and acceptable "alternative" schedule.

The key to my compromise with the Sears schedule and my new BATTASS schedule is his allowing the use of Pentacel (Sanofi Pasteur) in his second edition.[27] Sears states, "Pentacel is an OK choice, and it easily fits into an alternative vaccine schedule." It has a much lower aluminum content than does Pediarix (GlaxoSmithKline)—330 mcg versus 850 mcg, which he does not advocate except when Pentacel is not available.[28] (Not that it matters really.) The good news for us "traditionalists" is that, despite his multiple simultaneous antigen concerns, the two extra antigens in each of these vaccines do not preclude their beneficial utility for him. The much lower dose of aluminum in Pentacel is actually lower than giving the single-component vaccines simultaneously. Thus, he gives a waiver to Pentacel, which is almost perfect for us and you. And the recent data from Denmark shows that vaccine aluminum is not a culprit in any way!

CAVEATS TO THE USE OF BATTASS

Adherence

When using BATTASS, parents must be willing to adhere to and be totally accepting of the clinician's vaccine timing. For those practitioners who are more compulsive about ACIP recommendations, you can ask parents to come in for vaccines on the 4-week interval schedule instead. Thus, they

---

[27] Diekema DS; American Academy of Pediatrics Committee on Bioethics. Responding to parental refusals of immunization of children. *Pediatrics*. 2005;115(5):1428-1431

[28] Omer SB, Salmon DA, Orenstein WA, de- Hart MP, Halsey N. Vaccine refusal, mandatory immunization, and the risks of vaccine-preventable diseases. *N Engl J Med*. 2009;360(19):1981-1988. doi: 10.1056/ NEJMsa0806477.

will be finished with the primary series by 6 months as well. The vaccines at 12 to 15 months old in BATTASS are relatively the same as ACIP, except for the separation of MMR from varicella by 3 months, yet still fall within ACIP guidelines. Each physician will have to decide when to pull the plug on families who procrastinate too long for their comfort.

Costs

Parents must be willing to accept the extra visits and the additional slightly higher charge incurred for first vaccine administration at the 3-, 5-, and 7-month visits as opposed to the reduced charge for simultaneous 2 to 3 vaccines at one visit. Many clinicians have a separate additional nurse visit charge for shots not occurring during a checkup. (Use CPT code 90471 [first shot] and CPT 90472 [additional shots]). Further "spacing out" of visits would not be acceptable.

Availability of Pentacel

Pentacel must be in full supply to make your and their acceptable transition to BATTASS fully work. Using Pediarix could create significant friction for the family who still does not believe in low-dose aluminum safety. Pentacel reduces the number of shots by two for each of four visits—a real time/cost saver for our nursing staff. Some offices may complain about the three to four possible extra visits and extra time in the room for vaccines. I sympathize. But it does not seem too much different than giving a child one or two weekly allergy shots apart from any office visit.

Hepatitis A and Hepatitis B Vaccines

Hopefully, we can convince many of the delayers of the birth dose of the hepatitis B vaccine to receive the first dose at 1 month and the second dose by 9 months of age, and the third dose after 15 months. The daycare attendance policy requiring the hepatitis B vaccine may be compelling for over half of the families. The delay of the hepatitis A vaccine is an issue we will just have to possibly compromise with until the child is older, perhaps by 23 to 24 months, almost compliant with ACIP guidelines. For the missed birth-dose hepatitis B vaccine, you will need to have the family sign and acknowledge the AAP vaccine refusal form either at birth or within the first weeks of life.

Vaxellis

It just became available in 2021, and some offices can replace two other injections for hepatitis B. It consists of the Pentacel formulation with an added Hepatitis B component built in, and it uses 3 doses instead for the first 6 months of life.

CONCLUSION

In 2005 and 2009, the AAP Bioethics Committee said that "continued [vaccine] refusal" after adequate discussion (between physician and parent) should be respected unless the child is put at significant risk of serious harm. In our quest each day to "do no harm," I think we can do better than becoming a willing partner to needless severe or catastrophic illness and deaths because of untenable vaccine hesitation and refusal. It is distasteful being placed in this position, which is in defiance of everything pediatrics stands for.

However, when adopting a Physicians' Alternative to the Sears Schedule (PASS), we are acknowledging both that we have found a way to compromise within limits and that we still insist upon providing the best possible care for our patients, families, and the community. By using my BATTASS schedule, it should allow you now to finally work with the numerous families who follow a frequently invoked, previously untenable "belief system."

✳️ Playing Newborn Intracranial Roulette: Parental Refusal of Vitamin K Injection

(Adapted from Block SL, Playing Newborn Intracranial Roulette: Parental Refusal of Vitamin K Injection, *Pediatric Annals 43(2)*, February 2014)

Hemorrhagic disease of the newborn, also referred to as vitamin K deficiency bleeding (VKDB), is a totally preventable, potentially deadly condition that most of us pediatricians don't routinely give much thought to.

However, internet bloggers have once again apparently made pediatricians unwitting victims of our success with the standard use of intramuscular (IM) vitamin K prophylaxis in every newborn since 1961. That is more than 50 years of routine use in every newborn nursery, adding up to nearly 200 million doses in the United States alone. And for newborns, vitamin K delivered intramuscularly has shown almost no known adverse effects except possibly a total of seven dermatologic reactions.[29] The only reported serious adverse effect I could find in the literature happened not in the United States, but in a newborn in Turkey.[30] This was a single case of potentially severe anaphylaxis reaction from a dose given at birth. This is the only English-language report in any of the reputable medical literature that I could find, despite administration of probably more than a billion newborn IM doses. If this one-in-a-billion occurrence should ever happen again, then what better place for it to happen than in the presence of a trained physician and at least two nurses?

I think that because the internet bloggers and parents posting in chat rooms may not have seen severe VKDB themselves, they have assumed cavalierly that severe VKDB must no longer exist. They are dead wrong, and they are

---

[29] Munz M. Four babies hemorrhage after parents refuse vitamin K shot, a practice on the. St. Louis Post-Dispatch December 8, 2013.

[30] Centers for Disease Control and Prevention (CDC). Notes from the field: late vitamin K deficiency bleeding in infants whose parents declined vitamin K prophylaxis-Tennessee, 2013. *MMWR Morb Mortal Wkly Rep.* 2013;62(45):901-902.

gambling with some infants' brains and lives in a dangerous game of intracranial roulette. No matter how much they want it to be true, VKDB is not a myth concocted by the medical establishment, which is a falsehood these bloggers try to perpetuate.

History Is Doomed to Repeat Itself

For those young scientists and naive parents who claim that VKBD is a myth, I say not so fast. For example, we need only to look at four babies in Tennessee whose mothers unfortunately declined vitamin K to see that the threat of devastating VKDB still lurks, as reported in the November 15, 2013, issue of *Morbidity and Mortality Weekly Report*. Three of these babies had potentially life-threatening blood clots evacuated from their cranium and will likely suffer from some form of permanent neurological damage.

And why did this happen? Let's explore how something so tragic and preventable could still happen in these days of modern medicine. It must be remembered that VKDB is not caused by a lack of available medical care, but instead caused by a conscious parental misinformed decision to refuse customary known optimal care.

"Doctor, we know better. We've done our research."

One of my older partners recently stormed into the office, notably upset about his current trip to our newborn nursery. The parents of a 12-hour-old newborn had just informed him that they were declining all "extraneous" medical interventions for their newborn boy. They desired that no "unnatural" substances be given to their newborn, and that their baby not be "unnecessarily disturbed or poked." This included A) two state-mandated therapies: newborn metabolic blood screening and prophylactic eye ointment; and B) two highly recommended prophylactic therapies: hepatitis B vaccination and, for the first time in our experience, vitamin K1 injection.

My partner was totally flabbergasted by the hour-long discussion it required to explain the conventional pediatrician's point of view about the importance of these potentially morbidity-sparing and mortality-saving interventions, only to casually hear the following rebuttals about his recommendations:

"We have read on the internet." We want only the "natural way." "God does not want us to perform any unnecessary procedures." "These newborn shots will cause permanent psychological and emotional damage." "Vitamin K has been associated with cancer."

These last two objections were a first for our practice, and thus inspired us to perform further research into the recent voicing of these objections. With 17 keystrokes in an internet search engine, we had our answer. The very first "hit" with a single search on Google under "newborn vitamin K" led us immediately to one source of such inspirations of medical paranoia about routine newborn care: Joseph Mercola, DO, and his website (http://www.mercola.com). Part of the vaccine "disinformation dozen."

Why is there such pervasive parental anxiety about an **"act of commission"** or doing something preventively, no matter how bad the disease that this "something" prevents and how well-known the safety of this "something" is documented? This is diametrically opposed to an **"act of omission,"** or merely passively letting Mother Nature wreak her own havoc by doing nothing. Then, if the rare bad thing actually happens to our child, then it would not be our fault, even though established medical advances, such as a vitamin K injection, could have prevented it.

Have we as a society become so distrustful of our medical scientific methods and of our pediatricians that we would rather trust the unsubstantiated, unscientific innuendos and claims of a single person or group of naysayers and science denialists? Perhaps next they will do their "research" on simple jobs like airplane pilots and architects? I think that most pediatricians would welcome an open-minded question from the parents and a chance to explain the science and to provide credible internet sites, rather than dooming a baby to potentially devastating, substandard care.

Newborn Intracranial Roulette

Without standard IM (or even oral) supplemental vitamin K during the immediate newborn period, the totally healthy infant is at notable risk for significant hemorrhaging during three specific time periods:

1. **Early-onset hemorrhagic disease** (within the first 24 hours), which is usually associated with cephalohematoma, gastrointestinal bleeding, or intracranial bleeding, such as subarachnoid bleeding that we have all seen. The last two prolonging hospitalization by many days.

2. **"Classic" hemorrhagic disease** (days 2 to 7), which occurs with a staggering incidence (reportedly as high as 0.25% to 1.7%) during the first week of life. This bleeding tends to be milder and more often from the umbilicus, gastrointestinal, circumcision, and at puncture sites.

3. **"Late" hemorrhagic disease** (2 weeks to 6 months), which occurs with an incidence ranging from 4.4 to 7.2 per 100,000 live births from ages 2 to 12 weeks, based on reports from Europe and Asia. However, an even more alarming statistic is that late VKDB can develop in 1 in 15,000 to 1 in 20,000 infants who are exclusively breast-fed. Infants who do not receive IM vitamin K at birth are estimated to have an 81-times greater risk for late VKDB than those who receive the shot. And 50% of infants with late VKDB present with intracranial hemorrhage, with a 20% mortality.

Overall, the typical sites of VKDB or hemorrhaging include intracranial (usually late disease), subarachnoid bleeding and extracranial cephalohematoma (both of which all pediatricians have seen, usually early disease), gastrointestinal (usually classic disease), epistaxis, intrathoracic, circumcision, and skin. More subtle, milder bleeds and infant failure to thrive may herald the more catastrophic events.

Risk Factors for VKDB

Note that late VKDB mostly occurs in healthy breast-fed infants. Who are the parents most likely to decline the birth dose of vitamin K? The breastfeeding mother, whose infant will now remain highly deficient in vitamin K for a month or longer.

How Commonly Do Parents Decline Vitamin K?

From January to October 2013, in three Nashville-area hospitals, an alarming 3.4% of 3,080 newborns did not receive vitamin K by the time of discharge. Even more disturbing, 28% of 218 neonates from Tennessee "birthing centers," run primarily by midwives, did not receive a birth dose of vitamin K. A similar rate of refusal has been reported at a birthing center in Missouri.

Some experts think that the rates of VKDB are grossly under-reported because it is always assumed that any young infant with gastrointestinal bleeding, or with a subdural or other brain bleed, who enters an emergency department or intensive care unit has received the birth dose of vitamin K. According to these recent data, we could be totally wrong.

I cannot begin to estimate the notable number of exclusively breastfeeding, otherwise healthy young babies with some significant hematochezia (blood in the stool) who were seen in our practice during the past few years. Like many pediatricians, our practice had always just assumed that they had an atypical "cow's milk allergy" from milk proteins being transferred through the breast milk. We have usually switched the breastfeeding infant to one of the casein hydrolysate formulas (e.g., Alimentum), and then noted remarkable amelioration of blood in the stool in the next few days to weeks. Perhaps recently, many of these infants had not received the birth dose of vitamin K or they were hyper-metabolizers, and their ingestion of the larger concentration of daily oral vitamin K manufactured into the formula was the cure instead.[31]

---

[31] American Academy of Pediatrics. Vitamin K Ad Hoc Task Force: Controversies concerning vitamin K and the newborn. *Pediatrics*. 1993;91(5):1001-1003.

Are there any valid concerns with vitamin K injection for the newborn? Let's explore the alleged issues with vitamin K injection of the newborn.

Parental Reports to the U.S. Centers for Disease Control and Prevention

According to the CDC's report in 2013, three reasons were attributed to vitamin K refusal by parents. The first was the belief that IM vitamin K doubles the risk for leukemia. This idea was first touted by Golding et al in a case-control study from Great Britain. For multiple reasons, including lack of plausibility and reproducibility, this theory has since been totally debunked. Even the website of Dr. Mercola has acknowledged this as pure mythology. And as for triggering leukemia, why would an IM injection be much different than oral ingestion of either small daily doses or weekly small boluses of vitamin K? Each method achieves some improved levels in the bloodstream.

The second reason was that parents felt the injection was unnecessary. Thus, they allege that they were not made fully aware of the possibility of late VKDB by our "experts" or by our website.

Mercola.com: "The Potential Dark Side of the Routine Vitamin K Shot"

Dr. Mercola, a mass marketer of multiple diverse, controversial, and unproven homeopathic products, does acknowledge the lack of any link between IM vitamin K and leukemia! He also acknowledges that vitamin K is essential to prevent VKDB.

However, www.mercola.com has three additional complaints about IM vitamin K. He argues that the multiple oral doses are better than a single IM dose, that a single shot will cause psycho-emotional problems in the newborn and may "jeopardize breastfeeding," and that an IM injection within the hospital may create a site for infection. None of these claims is based on scientific data.

Studies show that there are more, albeit rare, breakthrough cases of VKDB with the oral doses than with the single IM dose.

He obviously dislikes the notion of any shots for the newborn. I agree that the avoidance of pain in any child or newborn is an admirable goal. But preventing all tears in a baby is just not practical, even for their routine care that is required. As anyone who works or lives with babies knows, babies will cry, and they will often even act like babies! No matter how gently anyone tries, crying often also accompanies the doctor's newborn examination or care while trying to check their eyes' red reflex, hip dislocation, femoral pulses, posterior pharynx, temperature, or even when diapering, bathing, and unclothing them. Are babies really that fragile?

Yet, in our hospital, we actually do quite well without fussing or tears with the vitamin K injection during the "kangaroo care" time period. Sometimes, we even give the injection using the calming effects of the feeding itself to prevent any crying. To say that one or two shots or heel sticks will cause permanent psycho-emotional trauma is perhaps ludicrous. No, it is ludicrous! This objection is not based on any credible science. Again, we are not talking about weeks or days of necessary heel sticks every 2 hours for glucose, blood gas, or bilirubin in a sick infant, which truly is a pain-management problem.

As for iatrogenic site infection being caused by a routinely and correctly done single IM injection into a newborn, no data support this allegation, either in the literature or in my daily practice of 43 years. Perhaps he is referring to an unrelated iatrogenic intravenous catheter site infection? To call an IM injection of morbidity-sparing or life-saving medications or immunizations "damaging" is inflammatory and has no merit.

CONCLUSION

We must now be ever-vigilant about whether each of our patients younger than 6 months has received vitamin K in some form at birth or beyond, **especially if the child is breastfeeding.** For any infant who presents to your office, emergency department, or intensive care unit with any bleeding problems, the parents must now be interrogated as to whether supplemental vitamin K was administered IM or orally during the newborn period. The 3% to 25% chance of not receiving vitamin K is terrifying. I would personally not perform a circumcision in a breastfeeding boy during the first 6 months of life who has not received IM vitamin K. (Think: possible additional not-yet-identified rare liver or intestinal problems in the newborn, or even more common medication adherence issues. Also, have you ever witnessed the rare terrifying "free-bleeding" circumcision site?) The optimal dose of IM vitamin K in premature infants is still debated, and some have recommended using a lower dose of 0.2 mg IM.

Back to our newborn case: We were finally able to convince the baby's family that it was in the best interest of their child's future health to at least proceed with the metabolic screening and prophylactic eye ointment. Sadly, we were unable to convince them to give their child the hepatitis B shot or the newborn vitamin K by injection or orally.

I hope that their spin of the intracranial roulette wheel is a lucky one. They will be seeking their care outside of our practice due to their total infant vaccine refusal.

I continue to be amazed at how a single person or group without a medical or any postgraduate degree, or an internet site, or with a megaphone can spout incredulous speculation(s). They can totally undermine the standard of care and recommendations of an entire legion of medical experts who used massive, credible scientific data. Such is the power of the internet today, of the famous non-medical town criers, and Google's known "disinformation dozen."

✴ Importance of the Newborn Checkup

Simple Checklist for the Full-Term Healthy Newborn Visit

(Adapted from Block SL. *Pediatric Annals* 2012; 41(7):270-274. July)

When I am in the nursery discussing routine newborn care with postpartum mothers, I run through a list of pertinent advice that I have developed over the years. The clinician may find the entire article of my essential tips helpful to use or distribute in their own practice, like I do.

Tips for Moms/Dads of Newborns: 'Back' to Sleep/Preventing Crib Death

A newborn should sleep on his back only; no side or prone sleeping. Never let your baby sleep in your bed, especially during the first 4 months of life when the risk for sudden infant death syndrome (SIDS) is many-fold higher. We have seen three **"crib deaths"** from this in our practice. Cosleeping with an older infant/child is also fraught with other repercussions, such as poor sleep for all, and in my clinical experience, inevitable marital discord. Additionally, as early as 2 weeks, co-sleeping babies are at significant risk for falling out of your bed at night (particularly if you get up to use the bathroom, even for just a few minutes) and fracturing a major long bone or skull, just the kind of event for which child protective services have been known to remove babies from households. Also, creating the baby "pillow fortress" is too risky, as I recently explained to my daughters, both of whom were new mothers. One older baby even sustained a **deadly subdural hematoma** falling off the bed! Likewise, I would advise to **never** leave a baby alone high up on a changing table, bed, sofa, highchair, etc., at any age.

To help condition your baby, try to lay her down while she's still partially awake. Over a few months, **this will help her learn that being held is not essential to fall asleep. It is still acceptable to pick her up after a few minutes of crying during the first few months. As she ages,** rocking the baby completely to sleep will usually become a nightly ritual that is traumatic to break. Sleep comes much easier for all if the baby eventually learns to "self-soothe" at night after the first few months. Lots of in-bed hand patting and soothing talk will make the transition easier.

Your baby's crib mattress should be somewhat firm with a minimal touch of cushioning. Avoid blankets and pillows inside the bassinet or crib, as these may increase the risk for crib death. Typically, the room temperature for a sleeping baby should be less than 77°F. Another way to gauge it is that the room should be comfortable enough for a parent wearing lightweight clothing.

Pacifiers

Although controversial, these can actually be a soothing tool, as most babies want more non-nutritive sucking than the typical 14 to 20 minutes they get per feeding. Pacifiers sure make life easier if you have a temperamental baby (personal experience). **Early pacifier use may reduce the risk for SIDS and has been shown to improve rates of breastfeeding.**

Breastfeeding

Breastfeeding is the best for your baby, but pace yourself—too often, too soon can create unnecessary discomfort. This is like long-distance running. By gradually increasing the feeding duration during the first week, then somewhat more during the next few weeks, your breasts will have a better chance to acclimate to the increasing vigorousness of nursing a robust baby. Bottle-fed babies only eat 1 to 1.5 ounces per feeding over the first few days. Similarly, a breastfed baby only eats about 1/2 to 3/4 of an ounce per breast per feeding for the first few days. Thus, both the bottle-fed and breast-fed baby only require small volumes of milk per feeding for the first 3 to 4 days of life. **Note: breastfeeding will also provide a major reduction in the mother's lifetime risk for breast cancer.**

During the first 3 or so days of your baby's life, the milk you are producing is called "colostrum." The "pins and needles" feeling of the breast "letdown reflex" usually occurs after 3 to 5 days old. Not every mother experiences it, but if you do, it is a very reassuring sign that your milk production will likely be adequate.

After 4 or 5 days, your full milk supply comes in. At each feeding, about 80% of the milk you produce in the first 5 minutes is the "foremilk," which is lower in calories than the nutrient- and fat-enriched "hindmilk" that is delivered in the next 4 to 5 minutes. Thus, initially allowing your baby to continually nurse for more than 10 minutes on a single breast during the first week is probably unnecessary, since you will not actually produce any additional milk for the baby. But it might cause you unnecessary nipple pain. To avoid this most common reason for breastfeeding discontinuation, try to limit nursing during the first week to feeding intervals of 2.5 to 4 hours for 8 to 10 minutes on each breast. After using both breasts, you can also return to the first breast to suckle on if the pacifier is not sufficient.

Be aware that during the first 24 hours of life, all babies are so sleepy that they may eat very poorly. This common pattern can be extremely stressful, especially for the first-time mother. The mother may think that her breasts are producing inadequately. However, after 24 hours, the baby will typically become much more alert and eat more. So, be patient with the breastfeeding process during the first two days of life.

During the first few weeks, it may also help tremendously to read books about breastfeeding or to talk with any close relatives or friends who have successfully breastfed.

Try to avoid baby bottles until the second week of life at the earliest. Otherwise, your baby may refuse to breastfeed due to the slower flow of your milk and "nipple confusion."

Breast Care for Nursing Mothers

Some experts suggest that breast pain caused by nursing may be alleviated by applying warm, wet tea bags (due to tea's tannic acid) to the nipples. Some women may also find nipple pain relief by using soft silicone nipple shields. Also, try frequently changing the angle at which you hold your child while he nurses.

Routinely apply medical-grade lanolin cream or emollients to your nipples after every feeding. Do not routinely use soap to clean the nipples; just rinse them with warm water. For sore, cracked nipples, or really tender breasts, consult your expert. Ensure that the baby is properly latched onto the areola, and that the baby's suction is removed by your finger, before latching off.

The breastfed baby needs extra daily vitamin D (preferably with the much more palatable "Just D" formulation available at most drug stores or Amazon.com) after the first week. Administer 1 cc daily while you are mostly breastfeeding. A recent report has documented that breastfeeding mothers may safely ingest some caffeine while nursing, so feel free to enjoy a daily coffee or tea.

Bottle Feeding

Boiling or sterilizing bottles for formula feeding is likely unnecessary; wash your baby's bottles the same way you would your dinner dishes. Mixing tap water with powder or concentrate formula is acceptable. But if you instead choose to use bottled water products for mixing formula, I encourage you to be sure to specifically purchase the "nursery water" formulations, which have some tiny fluoride supplementation. Introduction of an extra few ounces of water alone after the first week is fine. Be aware of the need to change nipple sizes as the infant grows, as the size of the nipple controls the amount of formula your baby receives with each feeding. Avoid bottles with an internal device that slows feeding. (See article on bottles.)

Growth Spurts

Nearly all full-term infants will experience a week-long **growth spurt** at about 2, 6, and 12 weeks of life. This can be alarming because it will seem as though your baby's appetite is almost insatiable, with frequent demands for feedings every hour or so, for nearly a full week. The baby is experiencing a temporary increased need for more calories to grow. No need to start cereal yet.

Bowel Movements and Urination

The baby usually has one or two stools per day in the first 2 days. After that, the infant typically will produce three to eight stools per day, with the breast-fed infant likely having at least one bowel movement per every feeding. This frequency is usually a good indicator of adequate milk intake for the bottle-fed or breast-fed infant. The appearance of healthy stools may range from soft, seedy, to watery; they may be any color—even green—but not red or bloody. If that happens, time to call the pediatrician. By 1 week, more than six wet diapers daily is typical.

Hard balls of stool or bowel movements less frequently than every 48 hours probably indicate constipation. In that case, contact your pediatrician.

Scalp Care

The small "soft spot" on the top of the head, called the "fontanel," is where the bony plates of the baby's head remain open to allow the large amount of brain growth during the first years of life. This is a normal feature. The fontanel usually closes after about 9 to 18 months. Do not be afraid to scrub this area gently with baby shampoo along with the rest of the scalp several times weekly.

If your baby's scalp is scaly or he has developed orange plaques of "cradle cap," I suggest shampooing the scalp daily with baby shampoo, but twice weekly, substituting a dandruff shampoo that contains selenium sulfide.

Umbilical Cord Care

About two to three times daily, use a cotton swab to apply rubbing alcohol under and between the cord and the skin until the cord falls off. This will occur somewhere between 2 and 10 weeks. Do not give your baby a full immersion bath until the cord falls off. These measures will usually prevent the wet, putrid cord smell.

The Single Umbilical Artery: Mythology

I have seen many reports on the internet lately about the single umbilical artery (SUA) scare, which is supposedly related to an increased risk of kidney abnormalities after birth. Two older reports from over 45,000 infants observed that there was no increased risk for kidney abnormalities in children who have a 2-blood-vessel cord (or SUA). Thus, this post-natal or prenatal observation does not need a post-natal kidney ultrasound. The risk is the same as if there were no SUA observed; it is about 1%, just like in the general population. Spare yourselves the worry and cost of any further kidney testing. They did have a slightly increased risk for inguinal hernia, but this will be obvious as the child ages, for the most part, and there is no screening procedure for this condition anyway.

Genitalia

Boys

If your male infant is circumcised, apply petroleum jelly to the wound after every diaper change. If uncircumcised, leave it alone; do not try to forcibly retract the foreskin. Circumcision is mostly a personal, social, or religious choice, although much data support its benefits in reducing early urinary tract infections and in later life, some sexually transmitted infections such as HPV, HIV, syphilis, and possibly others. About one-quarter of circumcised infants will develop some form of mild scar tissue or adhesion at the head of the penis; this is easily removed, but only by your pediatrician when your baby is at least 2 months old.

Girls

A thick, white vaginal discharge is common for several months after birth. Gently wipe it off using a tissue, cotton ball, or soft, damp washcloth. Rarely, a moderate amount of brief, spontaneous vaginal bleeding can occur during the first 2 weeks of life; this is temporary, normal, and due to the maternal passage of hormones across the placenta. Be sure to clean between labial folds after each stool.

Fingernails

Filing your baby's fingernails with an emery board every few days is the preferred way to trim your baby's nails. If you use nail clippers, it's easy to accidentally clip the skin on the fingertips. (The wife yelled at me for this one.) Chewing your baby's nails off with your teeth can transmit staph or herpes infections.

Skin Care

In the first month of life, most babies peel and molt skin, just like snakes. Apply lotion specifically to the trouble spots—usually wrists and ankles— several times daily. Daily application of emollients or skin creams may reduce atopic dermatitis in eczema-prone children. However, avoid the use of "calming creams" or any products containing tea tree oil or lavender because of their possible connection to the development of gynecomastia (breast lumps).

Skin Marks

Frequently, children have coincidental, innocuous skin spots, such as flat nevi, flammeus nevus ("stork bite"), dark Mongolian spots, hemangiomas, milia rubra, etc. The duration and benign nature of these findings can be explained to you by your pediatrician.

Jaundice

In the uterus, the baby produces extra red blood cells to carry oxygen. After birth, the breakdown of these extra red blood cells may cause an excessive orange skin discoloration. Occasionally, this breakdown can lead to bilirubin (jaundice level) that is too high, requiring treatment with special lights. Some doctors think that exposing the baby to indirect sunlight (never direct sunlight!) from a window may occasionally help reduce the levels of jaundice. A heel stick on the day of discharge from the hospital is commonly performed to determine the blood bilirubin level. Call your pediatrician if your baby starts to look like a little bronzed sun-god in the first few weeks.

Preventing Infections

Crowds are best avoided during the first 2 months of your baby's life. A newborn with a fever is a parent's—and pediatrician's—nightmare. Contact your pediatrician immediately if your newborn develops a fever of 100.5°F or higher.

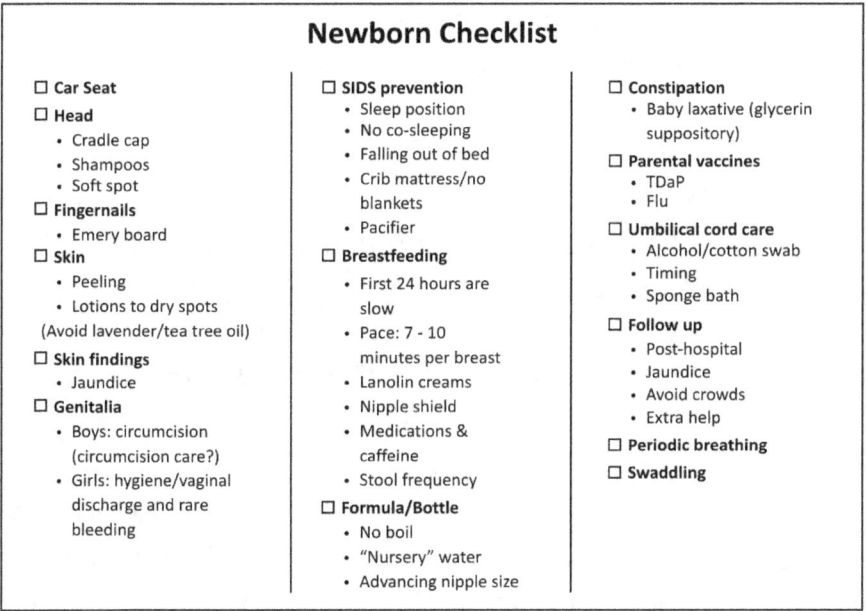

Newborn Checklist

☐ **Car Seat**
☐ **Head**
  • Cradle cap
  • Shampoos
  • Soft spot
☐ **Fingernails**
  • Emery board
☐ **Skin**
  • Peeling
  • Lotions to dry spots
  (Avoid lavender/tea tree oil)
☐ **Skin findings**
  • Jaundice
☐ **Genitalia**
  • Boys: circumcision
    (circumcision care?)
  • Girls: hygiene/vaginal
    discharge and rare
    bleeding

☐ **SIDS prevention**
  • Sleep position
  • No co-sleeping
  • Falling out of bed
  • Crib mattress/no
    blankets
  • Pacifier
☐ **Breastfeeding**
  • First 24 hours are
    slow
  • Pace: 7 - 10
    minutes per breast
  • Lanolin creams
  • Nipple shield
  • Medications &
    caffeine
  • Stool frequency
☐ **Formula/Bottle**
  • No boil
  • "Nursery" water
  • Advancing nipple size

☐ **Constipation**
  • Baby laxative (glycerin
    suppository)
☐ **Parental vaccines**
  • TDaP
  • Flu
☐ **Umbilical cord care**
  • Alcohol/cotton swab
  • Timing
  • Sponge bath
☐ **Follow up**
  • Post-hospital
  • Jaundice
  • Avoid crowds
  • Extra help
☐ **Periodic breathing**
☐ **Swaddling**

Source: Stan L. Block, MD, FAAP. Used with permission

Table 8. Newborn Checklist

Parental Vaccines

Both parents should be vaccinated with annual flu vaccines during the season, and with TDaP (especially the mother after 20 weeks of gestation but before delivery to best protect the baby). Maternal RSV vaccine in pregnancy is also recently recommended now. If not given then, give the baby the RSV vaccine for the right season.

Cabin Fever

If allowed by your obstetrician, taking short walks several times a week postpartum can help alleviate the stress of round-the-clock caring for a newborn.

Especially for first-time mothers, having a grandmother stay with you in the first weeks of a newborn's life is usually an excellent way to ensure you can take a break when you need one and receive the advice and help of a seasoned mother. Having the baby's father to share most newborn care, e.g., changing diapers, holding the baby, also gives you a break and the father a chance to bond.

Newborn Tests

A vital heel-stick metabolic testing is performed on all newborns. Your pediatrician will call you with the results within about 10 days. This test can be life-saving. A pulse oximeter via a probe is usually performed at 24 to 48 hours of life to screen for some serious lung and heart diseases.

Periodic Breathing

In the first months of life, nearly all babies will have periods when they actually stop breathing for nearly 5 to 10 seconds. The baby will then progress into a pattern of more rapid breathing for 30 or so seconds. This breathing cycle often repeats itself and is totally normal. However, a baby who stops breathing for more than 20 seconds or develops any persistent blue color of the lips is cause for alarm. You should contact your doctor or emergency services immediately.

Spitting Up

Nearly all babies spit up or regurgitate some feedings. Even vomiting an entire feeding once a day is common. Contact your pediatrician if the problem seems excessive or the baby seems constantly fussy.

Swaddling

Many temperamental babies respond to swaddling, or tight blanket wrapping, of the upper body. However, do not swaddle the legs, as this may be associated with hip dislocation.

CHAPTER 8

More Pediatric Enigmas

Blue Tumor of the Spine

My Faulty Memory?

Three decades ago, the mother of a pleasant 3 1/2-year-old girl from Bloomfield, KY, was in the office on a quiet summer day, where we discussed her growth and development. She was doing quite well with her verbal skills and motor milestones. Her weight and height had been on the appropriate growth curve, and her temper tantrums were to be expected— and ignored. Then she reminded me of the following: "Do you remember when you missed it?"

I asked, "Sorry. What are you talking about?"

She said, "Yeah, about 3 years ago, when you saw my baby, she had a small, slightly blue lump on her back."

When I saw her earlier as a little 4-month-old baby for that routine well checkup, I performed my usual complete and thorough physical examination. I discussed her growth with her mother, noting that her percentiles were appropriate. Her motor milestones were reasonable for a 4-month-old infant. I also noticed that she had an unusual small blue lump, about 2 cm wide and protuberant by maybe half a centimeter, in the middle of her spine around lumbar spine L1 and L2. It had a strange, unusual, slight blue discoloration (Figure 38). It wasn't a hemangioma (a collection of blood vessels), nor was it a solid mass. It could have possibly been a covered myelomeningocele (spinal cord defect). It was somewhat movable but seemed to be adherent to the spine. No other lymph nodes or lumps were felt anywhere else on the child's body. Her abdomen was normal with a normal-sized spleen and liver.

I informed the mother that I wasn't certain what the lesion was, but because it was directly over the spine, I was certain that the child needed to have an MRI (magnetic resonance imaging) of the blue lump soon. All sorts of possibilities emerged from the differential diagnosis of what this could be, from myelomeningocele to tumors. I recommended that she get the MRI done as soon as possible.

However, she decided to wait. Some people are skeptics. The possibility was sounded. She returned to the office for a six-month check-up, examination, and immunizations. At that point, when the lump was pointed out to one of the doctors, he told her that the lump was nothing to be concerned about. Her thorough examination was still otherwise totally normal.

She subsequently returned to the office at age 7 months when her mother found multiple lumps and lymph nodes in her groin—many about 2 to 3 centimeters scattered throughout her inguinal area. Apparently, her liver was now enlarged as well. She was subsequently referred to the hematology oncology group at the tertiary care hospital. Upon further examination of the spinal lump with an MRI and multiple other screening tests, they initially determined she had what was termed "a blue tumor" and needed a biopsy done immediately. The biopsy revealed a neuroblastoma, as did the biopsies of her lymph glands in her inguinal area. Although we see a few cases of neuroblastoma every decade, it is a very rare, aggressive, potentially deadly cancer of the nerve cells, initially found mostly as an abdominal mass in children.

Subsequently, she was treated with radiation and chemotherapy over a period of several months. Fortunately, the tumor was lower grade and still in its early stages and had not invaded above the diaphragm, which greatly improved her prognosis. After she finished all her chemotherapy and radiation therapy, she was considered to be in remission, and happily, there were no further signs of the tumor a few years later when I saw her.

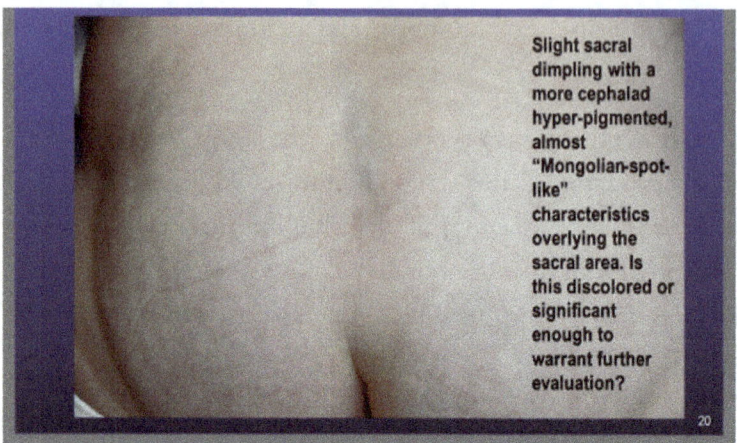

Slight sacral dimpling with a more cephalad hyper-pigmented, almost "Mongolian-spot-like" characteristics overlying the sacral area. Is this discolored or significant enough to warrant further evaluation?

20

Figure 38. Sacral Dimpling with Cephalad Hyper-Pigmentation. A 4-month-old White female with a midline "blue lump." What is this?
Source: Dr. Block

So, at this 3 1/2-year-old visit with her, her mother finally remembered that I had actually urged and recommended, at 4 months old, that she obtain an MRI of the midline spinal blue lump.

It's really amazing how the initial discussions of potentially bad diseases are often jumbled and misconstrued in parents' memories. It is easy to deny a problem, which we are all guilty of. I even went back to my original note, written at the 4-month-old check-up, where I wrote that I had asked that she get her an MRI. I had to be certain that my memory wasn't confused, which does happen. Oh well. The mental and emotional stress of a potential or actual cancer diagnosis in your child is beyond brutal. As Shakespeare reminds us: "**All's well that ends well.**" Thank goodness. My diagnostic skill was not appreciated here.

Earlier diagnosis is usually better.

The innocuous hematocrit?

I sadly had just read the obituary of this lovely, vibrant 20-year-old, Deborah, from Shepherdsville who died in a motor vehicle accident last year, and it jogged my memory.

She had been a patient of ours since birth. She had received her routine checkups and was thriving quite well. She came in for her routine preschool kindergarten checkup at age 4 years old, where I performed a complete examination that was normal, except for two benign-looking, tiny spider hemangiomas on her torso. The family history was also unremarkable at that point. However, when I received the report that her routine finger-stick blood test for hemoglobin was elevated at 15.2 (normal is 11–12), I became quite alarmed. It is exceedingly rare to see a prepubescent child with polycythemia (high red blood count). Thus, I decided to do further evaluation for apparent polycythemia. Could the tiny spider hemangiomas have any relationship?

Testing included venipuncture with a complete blood count (which confirmed the prior elevated hemoglobin), serum chemistry with liver functions, chest X-ray (for chronic hypoxia), EKG (for heart defects), and renal ultrasound (for kidney tumors and failure). I also rechecked the pulse oximeter, which was still significantly low at 92%. Normally, a child's oximeter should read above 94%. So, with all the non-hemoglobin initial lab testing being within normal limits, I pursued a more invasive arterial blood gas, which showed a PO2 of 50% (normal >94%). At this point, I speculated that she had an arteriovenous shunt somewhere in her body. A high volume of venous blood was pathologically mixing with the arterial blood in some blood vessels' aberrant connection.

In light of the two spider hemangiomas, the first three tests I ordered were CT scans of her chest, abdomen, and brain. The abdominal/liver and brain tissue and blood vessels were normal, but the chest CT scan showed two small arteriovenous malformations (AVMs) in the lung tissue. This defect consisted of a vein and an artery that had erroneously congenitally connected to each other directly as blood vessels, rather than connecting at the normal tiny capillary level. This was also putting a major strain on her leftside heart (like my own PDA).

In the 2000s, no simple surgical intervention for an arteriovenous malformation (AVM) was available, except from an interventional radiologist procedure at an Ivy League university. She was thus referred there across the country, where they were able to insert a small coil into the AVMs to ablate them. Her hemoglobin subsequently returned to normal over the ensuing several months.

Further discussion with the family revealed that she had experienced some heavier-than-usual nosebleeds. And so had her mother and grandfather as well. Add the fact that she had a few "spider angiomas" on her skin. These are typically innocuous findings, but in the face of either frequent nosebleeds, "free bleeding," bruising, heavy menstrual periods, or skin AVMs, I determined that she had familial Rendu-Weber-Osler syndrome, causing her AVM malformations. It is apparently highly variable in its autosomal dominant pattern and presentation, although giving it a 50/50 chance of being inherited (runs in families).

All this was uncovered due to a simple finger prick uncovering a seemingly innocuous laboratory abnormality during a routine checkup. Untreated, over time, this AVM would have triggered complete heart failure in her. The devil's in the details.

God bless my poor young friend and her later demise.

Case: A Long Leg

Checkup Incidental Findings

Again, Artificial intelligence will NEVER replace the skilled pediatrician!

"Yes, Bart is now doing well," the newly minted grandmother of this 2-year-old boy told me.

People often wonder why we perform so many seemingly mundane and "meaningless" maneuvers and observations during our routine checkups at any age. Amazingly, there are hundreds of subconscious observations going on in every pediatrician's mind during an exam.

This is again one of the many reasons why!

Two years ago, the pleasant young Hispanic working mother from Elizabethtown brought her 12-month-old infant boy, Bart, for a checkup and immunizations on a hot summer day. "Yes, if you don't mind, **please take all the clothes off the baby**," I said. We discussed the baby's progress with motor milestones, solid food consumption and meat intake, teeth brushing, and growth parameters. Then I proceeded to fully examine the child. All was normal until I arrived at the last component: examining the spine (see above case), the genitalia, and the legs. (We examine all boys' genitalia at each checkup through the first 6 years of life, hunting for that important occasional undescended or high-riding testicle, and for hernia.)

Also, usually, we examine all infants for hip dislocations, and as part of that hip assessment, we look for leg length discrepancies until 6 months old. I happened to notice that his right leg was distinctly longer than his left leg at this visit. The foot seemed larger, too. After several maneuvers, I confirmed the finding. Then I noticed his right arm seemed to be subtly larger in volume and in length. "OMG." I then measured them with a tape measure. It was real.

When one entire side of the body is larger than the other, we term that "hemihypertrophy." In continuation of my good pediatric training, I remembered that hemihypertrophy is sometimes associated with an initially asymptomatic tumor: Wilms tumor, a non-hereditable bad cancer of the kidneys, which is almost always uncovered as an incidental abdominal mass. Not here... I ordered an ultrasound of his kidney, which revealed a 4 cm tumor on the kidneys, consistent with Wilms tumor. I called her the next day to refer him to a regional pediatric cancer center.

Wilms can be associated with a more obvious syndrome of Beckwith-Wiedemann syndrome (very large tongue and liver) and aniridia (no or defective iris) and undescended testis, none of which this child had. Five to seven percent of cases have bilateral tumors. Most children present with a large abdominal mass on exam. The primary competing diagnosis is neuroblastoma, a cancer of the kidneys, as previously described above. Wilms is also the most common malignancy in childhood.

Fortunately, this was caught in stage 1 development, which has an excellent prognosis. He was treated with surgical removal of the tumor along with chemotherapy. He did very well and is now a healthy, thriving youngster. Earlier is better.

Hemihypertrophy, Hmmm. You better bring your "A" game to rural Kentucky.

A Visit to CVS Drug Store

"Hi Sara, how are you feeling after your last visit with me?" I asked the friendly 16 y.o. female clerk while I was searching for some acne cream. It's a tricky confidentiality business to discuss anything about a patient's care outside the examination room, but I wanted to seem friendly, not arrogant toward her. She muttered some short pleasantry in response and excused herself.

Sara, a long-term patient from Boston, KY, was in the office earlier that month for her routine follow-up of her oral contraceptive pills, prescribed to her for heavy periods and pregnancy prevention in 2010.

I insist routinely to have my female patients who are on contraception return for follow-up at 6-month intervals—for compliance, physical, and mental health screening issues. It's unbelievable what I uncover anew within this short interval with a few simple queries. I also always perform a cursory but relevant physical examination too (mouth, neck, thyroid, lungs, abdomen, skin). On the last portion of her exam that day, I palpated her abdomen and could not find anything soft in either lower quadrant. As I poked and prodded, she seemed to be in the early second trimester of pregnancy, with a firm "uterus" covering up to her umbilicus (belly button). "You didn't tell me your periods were gone and that you were pregnant," I proclaimed, seeming somewhat badgering. She flat-out denied that she was pregnant and insisted that her periods were totally normal. How could that be?

Incredulous at her denial (I have heard this similar denial many times before in this office–immaculate conception not likely.) I asked, "Would you mind if I get a urine pregnancy test?" I thought she was obviously pregnant. But could this be a scary hydatidiform molar conception? But then this mass was enormous.

The pregnancy test was negative. Totally perplexed, I informed her that we needed to perform an ultrasound of her pelvis promptly. This abdominal mass was actually a 20 cm solid ovarian cyst. Commonly, any ovarian cyst over 8 cm is considered to be most likely cancerous. Terrified, I promptly referred her to our local gynecologist, who felt that this was still a benign cyst. However, it was too large and too vascular to be removed anywhere but at the major medical center. She may need blood transfusions.

Upon surgical removal, the cyst was benign, no transfusions were needed, and she recovered rapidly to good health postoperatively. She returned to work at the pharmacy fairly quickly and began taking her oral contraceptive pills again.

She was still not pregnant several months later, with continued normal menstrual cycles. I quietly bought my acne cream and headed back to the parking lot. Another saved soul.

Currant Jelly Stools!! (Not a "Smucker's Jam" Problem)

A few years ago, a mother brought her two-month-old African American baby girl to the office because she had moderate diarrhea, major abdominal pains, a low-grade fever, along with poor feeding and poor fluid intake. On examination, she appeared ill and pale, with signs of moderately severe dehydration. Her doughy skin had lost elasticity due to a lack of fluid in her system. She had no signs of tears and showed dry mucus membranes in her mouth. She was tachycardic and had a mild fever of 100.5°F.

During her office visit, she defecated a stool that appeared as "currant jelly," a dark, gelatinous, blood-mixed stool. This type of stool most likely indicated intussusception—a condition where the terminal ileum intestine folds into itself at the cecum or large intestine opening, leading to intermittent bowel blockage and compromised blood supply. It telescopes in and out intermittently for several minutes. In the previous twenty-four hours, the baby had displayed major intermittent crying episodes lasting ten to fifteen minutes, followed by calm periods of about thirty minutes. This intermittent severe crying pattern is another key symptom pointing to intussusception.

The rare condition can begin after viral infections and mesenteric lymphadenitis (swollen lymph nodes in the intestine), but it can also develop due to an intestinal node from lymphoma or leukemia. I immediately hospitalized her, started her on IV fluids with a fluid bolus for hydration, and continued these fluids for rehydration. On admission, her BUN was elevated, although her electrolytes and creatinine were still normal. Initially, her white blood cell count reached 23,000, with 10% band forms detected.

A simple upright abdominal X-ray revealed a classic presentation: right lower quadrant air-fluid levels in the large intestine. I had seen this finding two times before. The presence of these air-fluid levels on an upright abdominal X-ray can strongly suggest the diagnosis even before performing a barium enema or CT scan. Novice practitioners need to be aware of this radiologic clue when this constellation of symptoms is observed.

A second surgical opinion was immediately obtained from my local talented general surgeon, Mickey Anderson, MD. The team considered the standard non-operative treatment with a barium enema for intussusception.

However, due to the severity of her symptoms and the distinct possibility of an already infarcted (or dead) bowel, the surgeon opted for surgical intervention.

Fortunately, open abdominal exploration confirmed small bowel intussusception into the cecum, which had not yet reached the stage of bowel necrosis. The surgeon successfully reduced the telescoped bowel manually. Enlarged lymph nodes on the cecum were identified as the "lead point" for the intussusception. Lymph node biopsies were performed (particularly for lymphoma).

However, postoperatively, the situation became even more concerning. The child's white blood cell count continued rising daily until it reached 45,000, with 35% band forms. Her fevers were now spiking to 103°F. This could not be explained by a post-surgical response alone. It suggested a secondary or even a primary bacterial infection was ongoing—likely related to her diarrhea. Her repeat chest X-ray remained normal.

When bad diarrhea is accompanied by severe leukocytosis, especially a high band count, this often indicates a Salmonella or Shigella bacterial infection of the bowel. The stool culture was already underway, so I added ceftriaxone and gentamicin to cover for these other, more resistant gram-negative infections. Within 24 hours, the culture grew Salmonella bacteria. Our patient had a severe Salmonella infection—not typhoid fever. While Salmonella rarely triggers intussusception, it clearly contributed to her case this time.

She remained hospitalized for a full seven days. Her intussusception, although removed, her symptoms did not resolve like typical cases due to her persistent bloody diarrhea and fevers that lasted for over three days postoperatively. But that problem was due to her concomitant now uncovered Salmonella infection. The eventual decrease in her white blood count was reassuring after changing the antibiotic therapy as above. Pathology reports on the lymph nodes showed reactive lymphadenitis without evidence of lymphoma or other malignant conditions.

This medical scenario demonstrated once again that Occam's razor—the idea that the simplest explanation is usually the correct one—often fails in real-world pediatric diagnosis. Intussusception alone did not fully explain her symptoms. The persistent diarrhea, high white count, fevers, and delayed recovery pointed to an additional infection. Pediatricians must remain vigilant in complex cases.

Guardian Angels

Case 1

The following case of mine was part of a nationally televised program from National Public Radio entitled: "Catching a killer: preventing meningococcal disease." Healthy Body, Healthy Mind. "The best doctors in the world are making house calls."[32]

The Story

The winsome, taciturn young lady brought her daughter in for her annual checkup and to discuss some of her school issues. The mother's presence almost brought on an attack of acute PTSD in me.

"Hi Tanya, how are the kids today?"

"How is your new job treating you?"

"Any changes in your household?"

She replies that all is well with her and her new husband.

"Dr. Block, do you remember when?" she asks me.

How could I forget that day?

---

[32] Healthy Body Healthy Mind. "Catching a killer: preventing meningococcal disease. The best doctors in the world are making house calls. National Public Broadcasting Network: the TV series and DVD. 2012. Episode 2204.

That Day

I had received an urgent phone call from the local ER on Sunday morning about my 17 y.o. patient who came to the ER complaining that this was "the sickest she had ever been." The first few hours of her illness started as a seemingly bad cold and rapidly escalated to her "feeling on fire, could not move, severe joint pains, lightheadedness." These symptoms were so bad that her dad had to carry her into the ER room. The mother was terrified and said she felt like her daughter was on her "deathbed."

Her vital signs: pulse, blood pressure, oximeter and respirations were all within normal range, but her fever was 102°F. She had a mildly elevated white blood count of 16000, and her serum chemistries were normal. The ER doctor was somewhat concerned, enough so that he performed a lumbar puncture, which revealed a normal, clear spinal fluid. When I talked directly with the ER doctor on the phone after her evaluation, he reported her as being somewhat hysterical and histrionic, and he was going to send her home subsequently. I told him that I had known Tanya since she was a toddler, and she never struck me as being overexcited. In fact, she was always so stoic, docile and introverted. "Please stay in the room until I can get a look at her shortly." So out goes my own plan for church service this Sunday morning. I was obligated to another important Christian service— a sick teenager.

When I arrived, I noted that, as the ER doctor reported, she was in no distress, not in shock, and appeared reasonably well, based on my thorough physical examination. But my *spine tingling* struck me hard. She was sick.

However...

"Ms. Bray, have you ever noticed those 4 dark red spots on her back?" (The critical importance of examining almost every square inch of her body and skin, when a patient is really sick, despite being a teenager.) "I think so," she replied. They appeared to be tiny cherry angiomas, which are occasionally seen normally in menstruating females. "Are you sure?" I interrogated her. Affirmative still.

Well, anyway, *I will go upstairs to the newborn nursery and visit with my most recent baby delivered last night, but I want to examine Tanya again.* Repeated serial exams and assessments are often the pediatrician's best friend when trying to decipher acuity of illness.

After my pleasant nursery visit upstairs, when I returned to the ER room, I lifted up her gown in the back, and voila! 8 dark red spots were now present. Now, that had to be more than coincidence. In the meantime, her sed rate results, testing for general inflammation, were quite elevated at 45 mm.

I told Tanya and her mother that I felt it was imperative that I admit her to the hospital for IV antibiotics and further observation with IV fluids and hourly vital signs. I explained that I thought Tanya likely had a very early infection with either meningococcus or a rickettsial infection with Rocky Mountain spotted fever or Ehrlichiosis. A patient in Louisville recently died from Ehrlichiosis in April 2025. These infections can often be deadly, but both can be cured with the appropriate and timely IV antibiotics and lots of IV fluids to prevent the impending shock syndrome. I was not sure as to which infection, but I was starting both IV ceftriaxone and IV doxycycline for her. Blood cultures were already drawn, and although she had an elevated white blood count with some immature bands, her platelets and sodium were normal as well, making the Rickettsial and RMSF diagnosis much less likely.

After getting her admitted and IV antibiotics initiated, I went to her room to check on her status after about an hour. Her aunt had arrived. Chaos. She was a nurse, and she demanded that Tanya be transferred immediately to the children's hospital. I asked the quiet mom if she agreed, but she deferred. I have learned over the years that it is pointless to argue with "almost knowledgeable" medical relatives. The misconception applies here: "If the child dies at the local hospital, it is presumably the doctor's fault; if the child dies at the Mecca (tertiary care hospital), it is thought to be God's fault."

So, I transferred her by ambulance to the children's hospital along with all of my notes and findings and impressions. She is still febrile, stable, and conscious, so I do not need to accompany her on this trip. The transfer is uneventful. And they continue with the same antibiotics and high-dose IV fluids.

The next morning, I called the hospital to the pediatric infectious disease specialist, Dr. Jerry Rabolais, who is a long-time medical friend of mine. "Jerry, how is Tanya doing?" "She is great, and we are going to send her home this morning." I fell off my chair. Excuse me? Did you not see the 8 petechiae on the skin on her back? "Dr. Block, no one here saw anything like that," he explained.

OMG; the antibiotics had worked that fast in this very early septic infection, I guess. I said, "Jerry, humor this old fool, but would you mind keeping her there a few more days, and wait to see what her blood and spinal fluid cultures grow in the next two days?" I said, "I swear on my mother's varicose veins that she really did have a few petechiae yesterday. They just disappeared that fast? Have you ever seen anything like this before in all your years of experience?"

Nope.

Since Jerry knew me well and knew that I was one of those savvy country docs, he agreed to do so. In the next 24 hours, the blood culture grew a type C meningococcus bacteria, which was sensitive to ceftriaxone. The spinal fluid culture was negative, too. She was now also feeling much better and afebrile. They discharged her after another five days of antibiotics. I surmise that if given only 24 hours of antibiotics, they would not likely have completed saving her from devastation. Note that, with meningococcemia, 1/8 of teens will die, 1/4 will lose a limb or two, and ¼ will suffer some type of neurologic sequela. This is the deadliest, rapid-onset bacteria we see.

Although she went home after 5 full days of IV antibiotics, she subsequently missed almost 2 months of school due to chronic malaise and fatigue afterwards, almost like a chronic arthritis or chronic fatigue type of patient. We also had to arrange for immediate antibiotic prophylaxis for her family and all her close contacts—a lot of exposed people when one is dealing with a social teenage girl.

As Tanya's mom explained in the video, "He saved our angel; if it weren't for him, she would not be alive today." Yes, I was very fortunate to have a guardian angel looking over both of our shoulders that eventful day.

(I was proud to be a part of the incredible expert team of infectious disease specialists on this insightful video—Dr. Pichichero (U. of Rochester, NY), Dr. Krilov (Winthrop Medical School), and Dr. Judelson (Erie County Health Dept), and then they added this rube (me) as part of the team of "world's best doctors" video.[33] Who knew?

Case 2

Making the Case for Adolescent Vaccines: Sepsis

Around 11 p.m. on one spring night in the middle of my pediatric career, before we had coverage by ER doctors well-trained in pediatric medicine, I received a frantic phone call from the ER nurse: "Dr. Block, your 14-year-old Black patient from High Grove, is here in the ER, thrashing, incoherent, and out of control. We need your help." Sounds like a PCP (phencyclidine) or meth overdose patient, eh?

Earlier in the evening, this previously healthy youngster had abruptly developed a low-grade fever and a severe headache just after supper while he was home alone, according to his father. When he called his dad at work,

---

[33] "Catching a killer: preventing meningococcal disease." Healthy Body Healthy Mind. "The best doctors in the world are making house calls." National Public Broadcasting Network: the TV series and DVD. 2012. Episode 2204.

he thought nothing of it, as the boy had a history of frequent headaches. This time, however, it would be different—unbeknownst to him. Both of his parents were working the second shift. His condition later worsened to the point where he collapsed on the floor at home, barely conscious. Through some actual miracle, he fell near the home phone, which had fallen on the floor next to him. Totally confused and semi-conscious, he somehow managed to dial his dad's phone number, but his conversation was completely unintelligible, according to the father. The father rushed home to find him on the floor, thrashing around and crying out gibberish. He was able to lift him into his car and drive him to the local emergency room about 10 minutes away.

This began one of the multitude of long, stressful, capricious nights in my career.

I crawled off my couch, said goodbye to my lovely wife, and told her not to wait up for me. This might be a long night. As I sped to the hospital, about 1 mile away from my quiet, dark house, I contemplated what the problem could be. I really had no idea—perhaps drugs, overdose, or a psychotic break?

When I arrived on the hospital grounds, I jumped out of the car and raced to the emergency room door, where all the commotion was coming from. Beds and hospital tools were rattling, some on the floor. As I came upon the chaos, a strong, muscular, stocky young Black male was yelling at the demons he was seeing. He was too strong for the nurses to restrain him, but his father was able to calm him down enough for the nurses to at least obtain his vital signs: Temperature 102°F, tachycardic, blood pressure 150/90. He was obtunded and irrationally muttering.

I calmly introduced myself and was able to perform a very cursory exam with his father holding his arms for me. Thankfully, his dad was a larger, athletic man himself. While he was lying down, I noticed that his neck was stiff, and I could hardly bend it. He had what we term "nuchal rigidity," which nearly always signifies a deadly condition known as meningitis, especially with the presence of a fever and an abnormal high or low white blood cell count. In sicker children and teens, it is usually bacterial in origin, often caused by the pathogen known as *meningococcus*, and rarely caused by *pneumococcus*. (*Haemophilus influenzae* type B was a very common cause in children under 4 years old before the 1990s, until we developed the routine Hib vaccine for infants.) There are also cases of viral meningitis, which are much less severe, but these typically occur in younger children infected with enterovirus. Rarely, herpes simplex virus, West Nile virus, etc., may cause a meningoencephalitic pattern. And by contrast, we almost never see fungal or tuberculosis meningitis in our area.

Yes, bacterial meningitis can devastate a healthy patient, transforming them from normal to deathly ill in just a few hours, as it did here.

Normally, we would perform a spinal tap or lumbar puncture to draw off spinal fluid for testing and cultures whenever we suspect meningitis. But that would never happen tonight with this robustly combative young man. This procedure, unlike in babies, requires much cooperation from the older patient to insert a needle into a specific area in the lower back, similar to a spinal or epidural anesthetic procedure in a laboring mother.

Nonetheless, if he survives the next 48 hours, this young man will still require immediate and repeated courses of IV antibiotics, ICU-level monitoring, and probably a later spinal tap (once he was more stable and cooperative). He would also need a rapid ambulance trip, 40 miles down the road to my excellent intensive care doctors at the tertiary care hospital. Getting him there could be quite precarious, as with meningitis, he could: 1) stop breathing, 2) herniate his brain stem down his rigid bony foramen magnum opening into the spine, or 3) develop septic shock and asystole. My job now became the life-saving backup for this youngster.

Before we left in the ambulance, it dawned on me that I knew this youngster from his playing football at one of the local high schools. Also, his kind mother had done some domestic work for my household for a few years, but had since moved on to factory work on the second shift, where she currently was tonight. Now, I had an even more major vested interest here, not that it mattered.

I quickly explained the likely diagnosis to her over the phone and how precarious his life was at that moment. I was sorry to relay the bad news, but assured her we would do everything we could to save him. I was transporting him to the tertiary care hospital as we spoke.

As I always did, I hopped into the back of the ambulance after we had established IV access and administered IV ceftriaxone. I had immediate access to the Ambu bag and oxygen for ventilation (though he vigorously yanked off any mask or nasal cannula), IV lorazepam for sedation, laryngoscope and several sizes of ET tubes for shock or apnea, and IV mannitol and dexamethasone for brain herniation in case his pupils became "blown" with non-reactive dilation. On the way downtown, to Louisville, I had to physically restrain him myself several times when he attempted to yank out his IV catheter or jump off the gurney. A small dose of lorazepam calmed him somewhat—minimally, actually. The bumpy, shaky ambulance ride in the back was quite unsettling. I even had the ambulance stop once and pull off the interstate halfway during the trip when he appeared to stop breathing for several seconds. I was preparing to intubate him, but Interstate 65 was still in desperate need of resurfacing. Suddenly, his respirations and oximeter returned to normal, and his heart monitor stabilized as well. (I could never intubate a patient in a moving, shaking ambulance.)

Finally, the exit sign for the hospital ER was in sight. Perspiring, I took a cleansing breath and acknowledged that we had both survived the trip so far. We pulled up to the bay, unloaded the gurney, and I continued to move him inside while he continued to flail as much as he could. I proudly walked beside his gurney past the ER, into the elevator, and into the ICU, where I finally relinquished my death grip on his arms to prevent him from rolling off. The ICU had already received the nursing report that this teen likely had meningitis and was quite unstable.

The staff knew what I had gone through. His next 24 to 48 hours in the hospital, with IV fluids, antibiotics, and critical-level monitoring, would determine whether he would recover without long-term issues or suffer limb loss, cognitive damage, or be wheeled down to the morgue. He would receive the best care here.

Between me, his guardian angel at home that night, and the ICU staff, he totally recovered from his meningitis. Once his belligerence and mental status had cleared in 24 hours, they were able to obtain a spinal tap. His spinal fluid showed a pus-like distinct pattern for bacterial meningitis, but the fluid was culture negative—meaning he had already cleared the bacteria from his spinal fluid, likely from the prior antibiotics. A good sign, actually. However, his blood culture from our ER and later from the ICU both grew a vaccine strain of *meningococcus*. After seven days of IV ceftriaxone, he was discharged home without any residual sequela. Unfortunately, historically, even in the best-case scenario, the death rate is 15%, and neurologic damage and limb amputation rates are about 15% to 25%.

To think, I've had the terrifying misfortune of diagnosing and initially managing 10 cases of this deadly meningococcus sepsis or meningitis in my career here. Most pediatricians may witness only one case in their entire career. The sudden death and bad outcomes caused by this bacteria have often contributed to many doctors' early retirements due to guilt and the adversarial "jackpot justice" of the medicolegal system. But I can fortunately report that each of my cases had survived without any sequela. Skill or luck? I don't care. Most likely, I have a guardian angel too.

The two peak age incidences of this meningococcal sepsis or meningitis (split 50/50 for each type of presentation in most meningococcal series) are 1) under 12 months old and 2) 14 to 18 years old. Most of the cases I have cared for were middle school or early high school age. The best news is that we now have vaccines covering over 80% of the serotypes causing this infection. But it is only given routinely at age 11-12 years, with a booster dose at age 16. So, there is no routine baby coverage so far, and this is an age population dominated by the B serotype as well, a vaccine which has only recently been developed for older children and teens.

To add complexity to this issue, about half of the cases are caused by C, W, and Y strains, which are included in the older quadrivalent meningococcal vaccine (A, C, W, Y combo), as part of the routine vaccine schedule for over a decade. A separate and newer combo meningococcal vaccine contains the B strain, which is suggested but not recommended at the same age intervals.

The good news is that we now have a pentavalent (five serotypes: A, B, C, W, Y) vaccine that was just FDA-approved. Our Bardstown research center was instrumental in developing all three of these formulations. In fact, I am the first author on the first paper reporting the efficacy and safety of this newest pentavalent version over a decade ago. This B strain is one incredibly complex family of bacteria, which I learned while sitting through numerous advisory board meetings on the formulation of this life-saving vaccine (See later paper on this). We hope that the two-shot pentavalent series for teens will provide durable protection for many years, as expected, but this is still unknown.

The cost-effectiveness question is whether the pentavalent version could next become part of the infant or childhood vaccine series, with so few cases now being reported. We must acknowledge that overall, only 600 to 1000 deadly meningococcal disease cases are reported annually in the U.S., down from about 3000 cases in the past decade. This huge drop in cases is attributed to 1)the good uptake of the quadrivalent vaccine (especially in epidemic settings), and recently, 2) the reduced rates of blood cultures being obtained in febrile children, 3) along with the widespread use of ceftriaxone without drawing blood cultures in febrile children, which has blunted uncovering breakthrough cases. We take our victories where we can in the fight against deadly diseases.

The Persistently Itchy Child

Six years ago, our facility was contacted during the spring season by a mother from Lebanon, KY, who was concerned about her four-year-old son's intense, body-wide itchiness. The phone nurse assumed he had a typical case of eczema or dyshidrosis—dry skin is an extremely common cause of itching. Thus, we advised her to use lotions and a nighttime Benadryl in combination with a morning dose of cetirizine. She was instructed to bring the child to the office for assessment if his symptoms did not improve.

The child later visited an allergist who added a higher dose of antihistamines to the treatment but failed to perform an extensive physical evaluation. The boy took additional doses of Benadryl while continuing to use antihistamines. About nine months into his chronic itching condition, she made an urgent phone call late on Friday afternoon to report that he was still itching severely, had stopped eating, felt sick for one week, and now had a pale complexion.

When the phone nurse asked me about this patient, I immediately requested that she rush him to the office because of the persistent nature of his condition. I would even wait for her after our office had closed. The first noticeable finding during the examination was his jaundiced eyeballs. He had no fever. His whole body appeared to be jaundiced as well. He also had an enlarged liver, three centimeters below his rib cage, and a spleen enlarged four centimeters below the ribs. All the patient's lymph nodes appeared normal. The rest of the examination was normal.

That night, I referred him to the local hospital to perform stat blood tests because I wanted to rule out several life-threatening, hidden medical conditions (although mild jaundice of Gilbert's disease is common (bilirubin <2.0)). Otherwise, any significant jaundice after the newborn age is usually serious. The blood tests revealed a bilirubin level of 4.5 along with elevated liver enzymes (ALT and AST), which exceeded normal levels by six to seven times. His pancreatic enzymes of amylase and lipase levels were also mildly elevated. I advised the mother that her son needed a prompt medical referral to a hematology-oncology specialist. The specialist performed a liver biopsy procedure the next day. The diagnosis: Hodgkin's lymphoma.

In this case, the lymphatic and liver involvement of the disease created bile duct blockage that resulted in the chronic itching and jaundice, and elevated pancreatic enzyme levels of amylase and lipase. After starting immediate treatment followed by months of chemotherapy, his disease entered remission. Years later, he is still in good health and accompanies his mother to my office; the disease has never returned.

This situation emphasizes that it is critical to perform a careful physical evaluation of any child with persistent or unusual symptoms. The lengthy nine-month delay before diagnosis, while symptoms persisted, might have produced a considerably worse medical outcome. We got lucky here, but he had not visited our or other offices during this interval.

Fever and Cough, Plus Tea-Colored Urine

On a busy winter Saturday morning twelve years ago, while the office was experiencing an intense flu wave, the 10-year-old boy from Rineyville, KY, was sitting uncomfortably and sweating in his office chair. The patient had experienced regular fevers for several days, along with a productive cough and poor appetite. His complexion seemed pale. He also reported that the color of his urine had recently changed to tea-colored.

A careful examination revealed normal ears, nose, throat, and neck. Lung breath sounds revealed wet crackles throughout his lungs, indicative of pneumonia. He exhibited distant heart sounds but no heart murmur. His abdomen was soft with diffuse mild tenderness; his skin was pale-looking, most likely indicating severe anemia.

His chest X-ray revealed bilateral fluffy infiltrates, or pneumonia. The white blood cell count was moderately elevated at 20,000, consisting mainly of neutrophils and immature bands. His hemoglobin was mildly reduced at 9, along with slightly reduced platelets at 100,000. The kidney tests showed early kidney failure with a BUN of 25 mg/L and creatinine of 2.5 mg/L.

Furthermore, his urinalysis demonstrated the presence of 4+ red blood cells, along with numerous red cell casts and occasional white blood cell casts. You must perform (an old school) microscopic urine analysis to observe these "cast" findings, which always indicate acute glomerulonephritis. Unfortunately, most offices will have to send a urine sample to a reference or hospital lab to get this test. This importantly signifies kidney inflammation—not infection. Thus, this very ill youngster appeared to have an extremely uncommon autoimmune disease (his bloodstream immune cells attacking his own kidneys and likely his lungs), causing both his pneumonia and kidney disease—not a bacterial infection!

According to my clinical best guess, **Goodpasture Syndrome** appeared to be the most probable diagnosis, as it represents an autoimmune disease that abruptly damages both kidneys and lungs. (See, I paid attention during medical school.) Although exceedingly rare—and I had never seen a case of it—the most feasible diagnosis for this patient was Goodpasture's Syndrome, even though other autoimmune kidney diseases like Wegener's granulomatosis and systemic lupus erythematosus remained possible alternatives.

I instantly referred him for care by a nephrologist, not an infectious disease specialist, at a tertiary care center located 60 miles from our office. Their hospital staff scoffed at my written presumptive diagnosis, as I expected. But they started high-dose corticosteroids and peritoneal dialysis immediately. After a few weeks, he had an arm shunt placed and then renal dialysis initiated regularly.

The kidney biopsy was performed a day into the hospitalization.

And guess what? Perhaps the "rube" old country doctor knows a little bit. The biopsy revealed linear immunofluorescence antibodies detected along the glomerular basement membrane, establishing the Goodpasture Syndrome diagnosis (known as one type of a specific "rapidly progressive glomerulonephritis" (real bad kidney inflammation), which is caused by only a very few rare kidney disorders).

The boy received long-term dialysis treatment before receiving a kidney transplant after the sixth month. He visited my office years later as a father of two children, who was now thriving after his transplant procedure. He reminded me of that stressful, chaotic Saturday years ago. Oh yeah, I remember you! The ominous illness findings!

Once again, the sound of beating hooves is not always a cattle stampede, but rather sometimes a zebra stomping in rural Kentucky. Better bring your "A" game to practice pediatrics in the rural areas. Uncovering a complex diagnosis earlier more frequently leads to a safer, better prognosis. This was a severely ill young man in acute renal failure, closing in on acute respiratory failure as well. High-dose steroids and immunosuppressants, not antibiotics, were acutely life-saving.

Visual Spots In a 3-Year-Old

An otherwise healthy three-year-old Hispanic child from Springfield, KY, visited the clinic with symptoms of headaches, poor appetite, and some malaise. A previous examination by a partner physician one week earlier had shown no abnormal physical findings—including the absence of lymphadenopathy and a normal throat, neck, chest, and heart findings. The mother had also reported that the child was experiencing visual disturbances described as seeing "stars."

When headaches persist beyond one week, are atypical, or are associated with any other neurological findings, the cardinal rule for the practitioner is to perform an eye (fundoscopic) examination (per Dr. Robert Bauman at U of KY, pediatric neurologist). This is one of the most challenging procedures to perform in younger children, particularly since they are usually uncooperative. That's why we tend to avoid it in practice—but as you will read here, it is often of utmost importance in determining which further diagnostic tests are needed—or not.

I observed a normal eye structure, fundus, and optic nerve in the left eye, while the right eye showed a complete whiteout—no red reflex! This indicated a dangerous underlying medical issue.

This was a case of **retinoblastoma**—a deadly malignant tumor that can be fatal when it spreads outside the orbit. <u>Retinoblastoma is rarely diagnosed after age one year, and unheard of at age 3.</u> (But, not in my practice over the decades!) Within hours of my phone call to the referral ophthalmologist, superb Dr. Douglas—who knows my penchant for bizarre cases—the diagnosis was confirmed in his office. The child was then promptly referred to a pediatric ophthalmology cancer center that night, where they employed a novel intra-retinal radioactive isotope therapy to destroy the tumor. Because of early detection, they were able to use this method instead of resorting to enucleation (removal of the eye), which was the prior standard of care. No other chemotherapy was needed.

Happily, the child even demonstrated some recovery of sight in the affected eye by six months after treatment.

The genetic basis of retinoblastoma is strong, as the disease passes down through families in an autosomal dominant pattern (a 50/50 chance). We stressed to the mother the importance of genetic counseling and continuous eye monitoring of future offspring of anyone in the family. Early detection testing for any potential future children of the patient herself would again be critical.

Retinoblastoma is seen in only about 1 in 250,000 children annually. Do cases occur in rural Kentucky, and at an older age of 3 years—who knew? Examine the eyes! Save a life.

The Headache in a 6-Year-Old!

A six-year-old boy experienced prolonged, severe headaches for the last five days. He was also seeing flashing stars. He had already consulted with two other doctors before coming to see me. Mom had known me for over a decade with her older, complicated children. Again, this case highlights the necessity of performing a fundoscopic examination in cases of unusual headaches. Unfortunately, I was unable to perform the eye exam successfully, but my gut instinct told me that something was off. This was not a typical headache. Overreacting or not?

So, I ordered a head CT or MRI scan, because the findings made my spine tingle with trepidation. But we could only get the MRI scan 4 days later. Still, I opted for the more definitive MRI scan, because I just knew something was OFF, and the CT scan is not nearly as sensitive for smaller brain lesions.

The children's hospital performed the MRI, which showed equivocal results that could indicate either an older brain bleed or possibly a tumor. A spinal tap was then performed, which revealed atypical cells—possibly early cancer cells. He was sent home the next day but returned to my office shortly that afternoon, still complaining of bad headaches. When the mother told me more about the scan and spinal tap findings, I told her she didn't need me anymore—she immediately needed the cancer center's expertise. He was too sick, and the situation too dangerous, for him to be at home.

A repeat MRI with different contrast and a lumbar puncture with more positive cell findings the following day confirmed the diagnosis: **medulloblastoma**, a brain cancer located in the brainstem. Because of its location, it was inoperable. Although very small and early, survival rates in such cases are often poor. The family chose aggressive chemotherapy and radiation therapy.

Amazingly, the child's treatment resulted in complete remission of the cancer after several months, and he has remained cancer-free for years. Recently, the patient returned to my office at age 15 for a check-up, nine years since his initial diagnosis. (Figure 39)

Early diagnosis, combined with intense, novel medical intervention, have saved his life. Although low yield in most cases, **early fundoscopic examination cannot be emphasized enough for atypical headaches.** When it comes to cancer or serious infections, earlier is better.

Well I'm so excited to finally announce that Joe Charles is 10, yes I said 10 years CANCER FREE!! What a journey he has been on. We are blessed and so grateful for all your prayers and support. Dr. Stanley Block will forever be our hero along with the other amazing medical staff along the way; James Brown Cancer Center and Norton Children's Hospital staff to name a few.

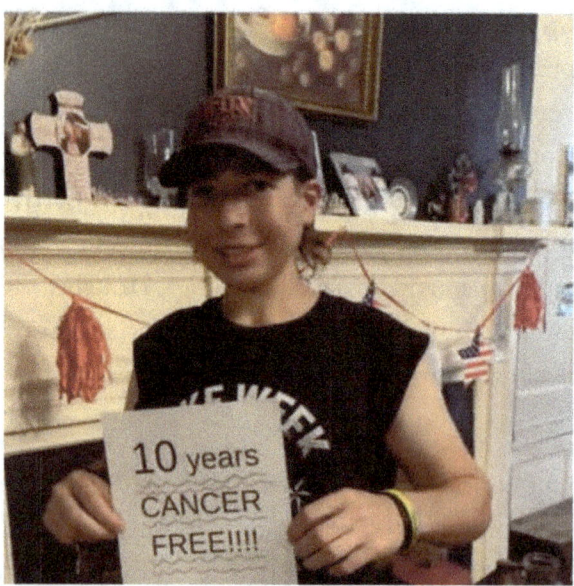

Figure 39. 10 Years Cancer Free. Quote from his mother.
Source: Kentucky Standard Tri Weekly Newspaper

Hysterical Young Adult Female or Major Problems?

Twenty-five years ago, an otherwise healthy 20-year-old biracial female from Cox Creek, KY, had persistent headaches for three weeks. She was pleasant, with an insightful and loquacious demeanor. In high school, she had been diagnosed with inattentive ADHD, which resulted in poor academic performance. Treatment with Concerta led to improved grades until she began dabbling in substance abuse, primarily marijuana—another known inhibitor of academic achievement.

She had a long history of chronic migraine-like headaches. Her association with a troubled boyfriend led to more frequent marijuana use, which further worsened her short-term memory, concentration, and grades. Due to the high risk of stimulant abuse, her medication was switched to atomoxetine, but this alternative proved less effective. During her early teenage years, she had several tumultuous arguments with her mother, resulting in months-long periods of estrangement.

Despite these challenges, she managed to gain admission into PT school after high school, thanks to her determination and intellectual capabilities. However, early academic struggles placed her on academic probation. Her emotional state continued to decline, exacerbated by her boyfriend's abusive behavior.

Reinstating stimulant therapy for her ADHD, along with a significant reduction in marijuana use, helped her markedly improve both academically and personally.

During her visit for the three-week headache complaint, she revealed that the headaches caused morning vomiting (a red flag!). At-home testing confirmed she was not pregnant. Her physical examination showed no abnormalities with generic assessments, but a detailed neurological evaluation uncovered a few more major red flags.

She had 4+ hyperactive deep tendon reflexes (DTRs) in both patellar tendons—her leg extension was so rapid it nearly goosed me—along with neurological "recruitment" of other abductor tendons in the contralateral leg simultaneously, an incredibly rare finding in a healthy adult or child. This strongly suggested that the problem originated in the brain, not the spinal nerves. There couldn't be this many findings???

Several other subtle but significant neurological tests were also abnormal, worthy of a *Dr. House* TV episode:

- **Positive Babinski reflex**: toes moved upward with plantar foot stroking
- **Positive Romberg test**: she easily lost her standing balance with eyes shut
- **Poor coordination**: she really struggled to hop on one foot
- **DTR recruitment** of 4+ quadriceps reflex to the contralateral leg–really unusual.
- **And the *coup de grâce***: fundoscopic exam revealed loss of spontaneous venous pulsations in the optic nerve—the earliest detectable sign of intracranial hypertension

An MRI was immediately performed the next day, and it revealed an 8 mm pituitary tumor located in the brain's pituitary fossa. Though often considered benign and non-cancerous, these can still lead to several neurological complications, particularly intracranial hypertension, blindness and severe debilitating headaches. Given her worsening balance and cognitive dysfunction, I believed this tumor needed to be removed as the root cause.

However, over a month or so, multiple regional specialists—including neurosurgeons and neuroradiologists—recommended against surgery because the tumor was smaller than 10 mm and did not meet the standard threshold for removal.

Her resourceful mother, dissatisfied with the available treatment options, sought outside help at Mayo Clinic. There, a specialist in pineal and pituitary tumors decided to operate. The tumor had almost grown to 10 mm. Despite the mortifying aftermath of shaved hair and a skull scar, the surgery was a success. All of the patient's symptoms—headaches, balance issues, and cognitive problems—vanished completely within weeks.

With her neurological health restored, she went on to graduate from PT school with honors and found employment at a nearby hospital. She left the abusive relationship and eventually met a new partner who brought genuine love and support into her life—and to her children. Another amazing recovery story for an earlier "lost cause." I love my job some days.

Always listen to the patient—and the mother

Persistent headaches, especially when accompanied by unexplained cognitive and motor disturbances, demand a fundoscopic exam, a comprehensive neurological exam and usually head scans. Patient advocacy and continued support may very well be life-saving. Persistence is critical, often in the stodgy medical system.

Burger King Memories—The Medical Whopper!

On my way back home from visiting my own kind elderly mother in Louisville last year, I happened to stop at the local Burger King restaurant in Elizabethtown, KY, halfway home to Bardstown. I placed my Whopper burger order uneventfully on the intercom. As I pulled up to the cashier, the smiling, friendly, garrulous Hispanic young teenager said; *I recognize you! You're Dr. Block. Do you remember me?*

OMG, how could I ever forget you? Yes, Brian, I remember you. I almost lost sphincter control when you were in the office that time. How are you doing? I inquired.

I am working part-time here, and I am starting my business degree at the local community college.

That is great progress. And how is your sweet elderly grandmother?

We exchange further pleasantries. I quickly rehash the medical nightmare that we shared. I pay him, and then I start my drive home. All this was following the Whopper of a story. All this information was exchanged while in the drive-through window at Burger King!! Thank goodness for credit card expediency.

Here is his story.

His office visit was on a warm spring day, when he presented as a robust Hispanic 16-year-old with moderate abdominal pain, along with several days of low-grade fever up to 102°F, and some occasional vomiting. He also said that his pain was mostly in the right lower quadrant (appendix area) and somewhat in the epigastric area, too. He had been coughing somewhat. The ibuprofen was helping a little bit. His grandmother was present, but she was quiet and had given him instructions. He had just seen my partner 3 days earlier, and he presumed that he had viral gastroenteritis. His white blood count was only slightly elevated then, and his fever was also down.

He was a star receiver on the high school football team, known for his speed and athleticism. He was a good student. He was always very polite and deferential in the office. He was living with his grandmother, who had obtained sole custody of him a few years ago, due to some major parental issues. But he was adapting wonderfully to his grandmother's love, sternness, and rules.

With his elderly grandmother in the room, on my physical examination, he was talkative, smiling, in no distress, and seemed only mildly uncomfortable. He was mildly tachycardic, the oximeter was normal, and his blood pressure was slightly low—typical of super athletes. He showed some moderate discomfort with his abdominal examination, more so in the RLQ. I was still worried about his appendix, especially when his white blood count had risen to about 16,000 this day. I explained to both parties that I was still a bit worried about his appendix possibly being inflamed, thus I ordered a CT scan of his abdomen with contrast dye at the nearby hospital. The appendix is not always located in the right lower side. I told him and his grandmother to go home and wait for the results, as he looked that good.

About 90 minutes later, I received the urgent phone call from the radiologist. That was never good news, typically.

He informed me that Brian did not have appendicitis, but...

On a lower cross-section of the chest on a CT scan, he observed that he had a large pericardial effusion. He estimated it as about 750 cc of fluid—when there should be no fluid present.

Brian was home, so I called him and his grandmother, instructing them to rush to the office for a repeat evaluation (which was unchanged from earlier) immediately. I would explain the problem as soon as they arrived. His vital signs were still stable, and he was still loquacious. I then called the ambulance to take him down to the children's hospital ER immediately. I gave them my chart notes and results to take with them. I then called one of the ER attending doctors, thoroughly explaining the reason for transfer. They were prepped.

Well, that conversation went nowhere.

Two hours later that afternoon, after they had left the office, worried, I decided to call the ER to check on Brian's status. They connected me to the resident trainee doctor. He calmly stated they were sending Brian home, and that he looked that good (I know that, too), and they could find no reason for concern.

I don't fluster very often at the office in my station. But this one got me.

I requested the resident go out to the parking lot right now and retrieve the patient. Now, I was in a state of panic. I explained that the boy had an estimated 750 cc acute pericardial effusion on the CT scan report that I had sent. For unknown reasons. And that if he did not consult the cardiologist and have him promptly remove that fluid and put a drain in, Brian was at risk for sudden death, despite his benign clinical appearance. All this was conveyed in one breath. The pericardial fluid would very shortly constrict the blood flow out of the heart so much that the heart pump would not be able to compensate for the restriction. The surrounding heart sack could only expand so much, then it would be a ball game over.

After some sedation with ketamine, the on-call cardiologist had removed 800 cc of pericardial fluid from his sack and placed a drain—within 1 hour of the phone call! He was recovering nicely after the surgery, I found out shortly. The most likely pericardial culprits were lymphoma and the fungal infection of histoplasmosis. Thus, they selected the latter diagnosis to empirically treat with IV antibiotics for several weeks while waiting on his cultures and blood titers, which later confirmed the diagnosis. Histoplasmosis is endemic (native to) in the Ohio Valley, and over 90% of people here will become infected, but almost never this severely. Most infections are like a bad cough and a common URI. Shockingly, he never displayed any of the classic signs of massive pericardial effusion either. All of us were fooled by his continued affable demeanor and lack of cardiac findings despite his deadly disease. Super male athletes are often the most challenging to diagnose.

By contrast, I have made the diagnosis of **pericarditis** (inflammation of the heart sack) in otherwise healthy patients at least 3 times in my career. When carefully listened to, they each had an obvious scratchy-sounding **friction rub** over the lower cardiac area, which was very patient-positional and increased notably on inspiration—I surmise when the heart was pushed upward closer onto the chest wall. They were all viral-induced and likely related to the current epidemic of enterovirus or flu in the community. Recovery was uneventful with only doses of ibuprofen. This milder condition is also commonly reported recently with COVID-19 infection, too, and extremely rarely an even milder version after the COVID-19 vaccine, especially in young adult males.

Scarily, sometimes it is better to be lucky than good. Suspicions, thorough testing and team effort pay off. It takes a village in pediatrics, too. I called the radiologist and personally thanked him effusively for his due diligence, as he likely helped to save this young man's life.

Commonplace syncope in an adolescent female

When passing out is not just simple orthostatic (postural) hypotension.

I was ready to board the airplane to Dallas, Texas, for a pediatric conference where I was presenting the latest data from my office on ear infections. My cell phone began chirping. It was Ms Jones. Her 18 y.o. daughter, Lucy, was hyperventilating and lightheaded. Lucy thought that she was dying. She had been terribly worried about her heart and was sure she was having some sort of serious heart pain, albeit the chest pain was totally in the wrong spot anatomically. She had not been sleeping for days. It was all becoming too much for her to handle, she explained. The last month of weekly counseling was not helping at all. Was she just a hysterical teenage girl, or did she really have a reason for concern?

I knew better.

Because of the lack of any progress, Mom was begging me to start her on daily Ativan because she was totally distraught and unable to function—Except when she was given a few Ativan pills from the emergency department during one of her earlier panic attacks. I had never prescribed chronic benzodiazepines before, because of concerns of drug addiction. Could this be the exception?

The story: I had been taking care of the brunette, long-haired, pleasant, and taciturn Lucy for years. When she was 12 years old, she presented to the office on a sunny autumn day with complaints of fainting spells a few times in the last week. Hot weather? Dehydration? One must realize that 42% of all teenagers experience fainting or syncope spells, mostly from orthostatic /positional hypotension (low blood pressure) in their teen years. It is especially common in teen girls during flu season and in hot weather due to mild dehydration. It can also occur frequently in teenage girls during an emotional spell when exacerbated by heavy periods and anemia.

But we must always listen carefully to the patient and obtain a precise medical history. This story was different. In most benign postural fainting spells, the patient rarely ever sustains an obvious injury or contusion. As I looked at Sally, I noticed that her nose was very bruised, and perhaps she had a hint of a black eye.

Were you unconscious? Do you remember fainting? Do you remember falling flat on your face? Did you get lightheaded?

YES. NO. NO and NO.

Not my run-of-the-mill patient fainting spell, I thought.

So, I ordered a CBC (for anemia), chest radiograph, and an ECG (hunting for SVT, atrial flutter, WPW, long QT, etc.) in the office. These tests were normal. Still. This history did make my pediatric sixth sense tingle...and bristle. Without any obvious source for fainting, I asked her to start taking an iron pill daily, along with a women's multivitamin (increasing iron levels and B vitamin levels have notably been shown to reduce benign orthostatic hypotension spells).

Return to the office promptly if any more fainting spells occur.

Well, the next week she had another, of this more severe type of fainting spell. So, I called up and referred her directly to my brilliant cardiac electrophysiologist, Dr. Johnsrude. I explained that I had no hard evidence, but I suspected something more nefarious was happening here.

During her visit there, he likewise could find nothing wrong on her physical exam, ECG or echocardiogram either. So, he tentatively proceeded to obtain a treadmill test on her the next day, just to be thorough, and because he knew that I was worried.

Interestingly, he almost had a metaphorical heart attack when she developed a long run of ventricular tachycardia on her ECG after about a lengthier-than-usual 20 minutes of treadmill testing. (Ventricular tachycardia is a deadly arrhythmia originating in the main pumping chamber or ventricle, which renders it useless, and can cause death if not treated or not spontaneously resolved within minutes.) Long QT syndrome is one of the major silent causes of this V. tachycardia in otherwise healthy adolescents.

An amazing number of families in our area have uncovered the same phenomenon over the years. However, in 2015, she most likely was in that newly frequently discovered category of 20% of patients with **Long QT syndrome** who had a normal routine ECG. Typical ECG positive Long QT syndrome was in itself very rare, and was usually obvious on ECG. Or she could have been a case of exercise-induced ventricular tachycardia, as just recently reported in an Italian series of otherwise healthy patients who developed sudden exercise-induced catecholamine ventricular arrhythmias. Management was the same, regardless: beta blockers orally and a subcutaneous cardiac defibrillator inserted surgically.

So, I told the cardiologist the following story, and he proceeded to obtain the very expensive and very novel blood test for a normal ECG-long QT, which insurance did not cover the ~$5000 cost at that time. Only the University of Pittsburgh was routinely performing the blood test then. I knew this because a doctor friend of mine in the Northeast just had his young, healthy teenage son die from this syndrome while riding a rollercoaster with his dad. They found this genetic marker was everywhere in his family's maternal side. It appeared to be autosomal dominant inheritance, like other long QT syndromes—50/50 chance genetically.

Thus, she was started on daily (forever) beta blockers, and quickly placed on the schedule for an implanted cardiac defibrillator—to shock her back into normal cardiac rhythm if she ever went into the lethal ventricular tachycardia again. And she was given an extensive list of drugs to avoid, which could trigger the arrhythmia.

Back to the phone call. My plane was about ready to take off. Apparently, she had received defibrillator shocks to her heart at least twice in the last few months, which worked. But she was now terrified to perform any daily activities. She was clearly agoraphobic, too. Fear of sudden death will do that to any person.

Thus, I phoned in a short-term prescription for Ativan daily (my first case ever) from the airport, and we would just have to take our chances with a low-grade addiction. I asked her to call the cardiologist to get his approval as well (which he did), because there was no other simpler alternative for her crisis and terror.

Although I had attempted for months to place her on an oral contraceptive, it became really interesting when she showed up pregnant a few years later. Because of the total novelty of this form of the disorder, we had no good evidence as to how her heart would tolerate pregnancy. Fortunately, pregnancy did not trigger any more spells, but her child, over the years, tested positive on his blood test as well. Leading me, as I take care of her future children now, to some harrowing treatment nightmares when they developed recurrent wheezing, as bronchodilators can be an easy trigger for v. tachycardia in long QT. Some of her siblings had also tested positive. The cascade of discovery of this lethal disorder has been astounding in this family.

Thus, a whole lot of lives in our area have probably been spared the ravages of sudden death from a previously "unknown" cause. We are always learning as physicians.

Diagnosing Serious Rash Illnesses Without Seeing the Rash: X-ray Vision of Superman?

Case 1 Telemedicine before telemedicine was an option

On a sunny spring Sunday, while I was enjoying the NCAA basketball tournament game between my two favorite teams, the phone call rang in. I turned down the volume (my late wife always politely complained that the TV was too loud). Ms. Perfidy from Springfield introduced herself on the phone as the mother of the 2-year-old child I had almost exclusively seen in the office. She was so thankful that I answered the phone call, as she did not want to speak with the answering service. *I only trust you, Dr. Block. Thank goodness I caught you...* (Each of my partners has their own cadre of very allegiant parents as well.) I had helped her daughter through numerous episodes of severe acute otitis media and an occasional pneumonia with great success, fortunately. But this time was unique.

In 1995, I had known this family for a decade and had great rapport with them. We had crossed paths socially off and on at school functions as well. I could sense the mother's intuition in her voice that this was something ominous. Her concern was oozing through the phone line. After answering 30 to 50 phone calls on any weekend on call day for decades, you just know. And I knew that the mother was a very courteous, caring, highly rational, appreciative parent. That made my course of action even easier.

Sarah has been running an unrelenting high fever up to 103°F for 4.5 days. She has been really cranky. She has this peculiar rash all over her body—not hives—more like smaller bumps. It is even distributed on her hands and feet. Her neck glands appear a bit swollen, her eyeballs are reddened, and strangely, her tongue looks red too. She has no cough or earache or sore throat. Her neck is not stiff, I checked. The Tylenol does not seem to be helping. She is drinking fairly, with an adequate urine output. No history of tick bites or strep throat exposure. What should I do now?

Dr. Block: No one will be in the office until tomorrow, and I hate to make her wait a while to figure out her potential illness. But I think fairly certainly she has a peculiar bad illness which requires early intervention to avoid major problems later. Your history tells me she meets almost every criteria. Would you do me a favor and take her to the local hospital laboratory for some stat blood work and a strep test? I will call them with the orders shortly. This may be one of those rare cases where I can make a diagnosis by her lab values alone.

Could this be RMSF, scarlet fever, systemic lupus, enterovirus hand, foot, and mouth, or other diagnosis?

I think it is the "other" diagnosis. It is an extremely rare pediatric-only illness.

Two hours later, my suspicions were confirmed. Her white blood count was normal, but her band count was only slightly elevated. Her sed rate (86) was markedly elevated, as was her platelet count (750,000). Her chemistries and liver functions were all normal. Her strep test was negative. I was fairly certain that she had **Kawasaki syndrome**, an unusual, autoimmune, treacherous disease which is also known as **muco-cutaneous lymph node syndrome**. She fit all the criteria by history—over 5 days of high fever, inflammation of the eyes, tongue and generalized rash and big lymph nodes, and by extraordinary laboratory findings—2 inflammatory markers like high sed rate and a very high platelet count with a normal white blood count.

I told the mother to gather up her lab report findings and take some overnight clothing, to drive Sarah to the children's hospital emergency room in Louisville, and to tell them to consider admitting her for Kawasaki's syndrome.

She was promptly admitted to the hospital for a week. She fortunately had a normal echocardiogram, which was searching for the ominous coronary artery aneurysms and aortic abnormalities, in order to prevent its predilection for these most unusual secondary inflammatory complications of Kawasaki syndrome. She was then immediately started on IV immunoglobulin and months of oral aspirin therapy. The cardiologist was integrally involved upon admission. She responded superbly to these interventions and did not develop any cardiac sequela. She remained healthy over the ensuing years of my follow-up in the office. She was also mandated to obtain the chickenpox and annual influenza vaccines, while being on aspirin for a while (to prevent the most common triggers of Reye's syndrome).

Case 2. No rash—so is it just strep throat?

Thirty-eight years ago, the 18-month-old Black child presented on a cool October morning with severe irritability and inconsolability, a high fever to 103.5, and a very dry-looking mouth, bordering on dehydration. We were in the midst of our usual autumn strep throat epidemic. Yet, if I did not know for certain that she had no nuchal rigidity and that she definitely had a totally supple neck, I would have sworn that she had meningitis. She was that irritable.

But my physical examination revealed no focal or obvious findings of a major bacterial illness. But she refused to walk. And she did have several healing old chickenpox-like lesions scattered over her body, which looked innocuous at this point. But these were the clues to this deadly disease process I would soon uncover in her.

Her joints had full range of motion, so that eliminated the not uncommon pre-vaccine, horrible septic joint possibility. But I still noticed that I could only barely touch her left calf muscle without her objecting vociferously. It appeared to be mildly swollen when I compared it with the right side, and it was not reddened at all. Something was really amiss.

My pediatric sixth sense was screaming at me. One of the axioms in pediatric diagnosis is that if you think the child may have meningitis, no matter the findings, you pursue a spinal tap looking for it. Meningitis can sometimes be subtle in its early phases, as every experienced older pediatrician is aware.

But I just knew that she DID NOT have meningitis. So what was her illness? First, I obtained a fingerstick white blood count—which was extremely elevated at $35,000/mL^3$.

Then I knew. I next obtained a rapid antigen test for group A strep on her throat, despite the lack of redness or throat complaints. This test was positive.

She was in a deadly crisis.

Even though her calf did not show any obvious findings, she had developed one of the other most feared complications in young pediatric patients. She most likely had early **necrotizing fasciitis,** I surmised, and needed an emergency operation to surgically filet open up her leg muscles in her lower calf—or she could either lose her leg or develop overwhelming lethal bloodstream sepsis from Group A strep. Normally, the body can contain the Group A strep bacteria to the throat or superficial skin (impetigo). But for some unknown reason, particularly after a chickenpox infection, the Group A strep had notoriously recently become known in the 1980s (as I had read then) to rarely invade the lower leg muscles, producing this horrific muscle and fascial infection. (Keeping up with the accurate CDC and medical literature is so important in pediatrics.) She was not vaccinated for chickenpox at this time.

(Note well: with the recent high rates of unvaccinated children, this severe strep illness had better again appear in the physicians' differential diagnosis of a febrile irritable child. Group A strep is not preventable, but the essential antecedent chickenpox illness would be. Likewise, in addition, examination for the septic extremity joints of the vaccine-preventable deadly Hib bacteria now needs to return to your diagnostic radar. I have observed multiple cases of devastating septic arthritis in my early career.)

She was subsequently hospitalized. And after an immediate Doppler ultrasound of the legs, it confirmed my suspicions—necrotizing fasciitis. Our superb surgeons then took her directly to the operating room to decompress the deadly compartmental pressure by making a foot-long open incision of the calf muscles, which would remain open for weeks. Per the advice of our pediatric infectious disease colleagues and myself, she also received, along with IV ceftriaxone, the obligatory IV clindamycin antibiotic, which was crucial to shut down the strep exotoxin production by the bacterial ribosomes. This was causing all the tissue destruction. Administering this antibiotic concomitantly was often a life-saving measure as well, since the death of the strep bacteria from ceftriaxone, if given alone, accelerates the additional release of the destructive strep exotoxin. Who said pediatrics was easy?

She recovered well after a week of both IV antibiotics. Her leg was intact. The permanent surgical scar on her leg was a small price to pay to save her leg and her life.

My guardian angel's sixth sense was to be thankful for.

What Disability?

We provide care to mostly generally healthy children and teenagers. Our population is about 90% White, 8% Black, and 2% other ethnicities. About 50% of the patients are insured by Medicaid, a low-paying but reliable federal/state insurance for low-income children under 19 and pregnant mothers up to 1 year postpartum. If a child has Medicaid and while staying in college, they will continue to be covered as well after age 18. Medicaid also covers indigent nursing home patients. The rules of coverage for adults with low income are obtuse to me.

As such, I also have many disabled and chronically ill patients that I and my excellent partners provide routine and acute medical care for.

My patient, Katy, requests to only see me in the office for her illnesses. She is 16 years old and is basically healthy, but she has no legs, no femur, and no tibia beneath her pelvis. She was born with **caudal regression syndrome**, i.e., no legs for unknown reasons.

She is quiet but always smiles when I see her. I clown around a bit with her and directly engage her about her own medical and academic issues, and she enjoys the attention and the "normal" treatment. She is amazingly quite self-sufficient except for the obvious mobility problem. But she can hop out of her wheelchair readily and deftly into a regular chair or onto the exam table. She is quite bright and responds well to the questions I ask her. She is now in puberty, and this has created some problems for her with her menstruation. I try to make her life easier, so I prescribe the 90-day version of oral contraceptive pills, which she appreciates. Today, she also has a mild cough and respiratory infection—all viral related, I am sure.

She does well socially with her peers at school. I am not sure about any dating aspects of her life. That will be a new hurdle for her.

She was just another special patient of mine who had adapted incredibly to her handicap.

I should be so brave.

Straighten Up, Dr. Block

Jennifer is a pleasant 15-year-old White female from New Hope, KY, who is sitting on the exam table with her respiratory ventilator chugging away. Sometimes she will ambu-hand-bag herself with some difficulty during the exam, as it tires her out to do so. Speaking is a struggle, too. She whispers mostly–less air needed for the lungs. She sits in a forward-leaning tripod position on the table. She likewise prefers to see me for her doctor... She "gets mad" at our nurses when she discovers that I am not in the office during some of her visits. She likes to tease me. This forces her mom to sorta lie in order to coax her to come in sometimes. She does have a temper, and she will show it.

I remember during the first few weeks of her life when I noted that she was severely hypotonic with a floppy neck and poor body tone, and she had struggled to feed. She required a surgically inserted gastric tube to feed her within a few weeks of life. Next was a necessary tracheostomy tube to be able to ventilate her because her chest muscle tone would fatigue quickly, including those muscles used for breathing. From her referral doctors, her muscle biopsies and tests revealed my suspicions were correct, that she had **Werdnig-Hoffman**, or spinal muscular atrophy type 1—a non-progressive, lifelong severe neuro-muscular weakness. Despite her need for constant caregiver help with every daily living aspect of her life, she went to school daily, and most of her classmates have accepted her unconditionally. Her special education teachers were amazing—what they will learn to do for their disabled students—complex ventilator care in her case.

During her puberty years, she really never grew much and weighed about 45 pounds and was barely 3 feet tall. And ironically, she had a few of the typical teen meltdowns at home, but she generally was happy.

I smile and joke around during her visits, and she often scolds me for my unkempt hair, my off-kilter buttoning, or my lack of ironed pants. "Tighten your belt, Dr. Block." She can hardly sit up alone and has extreme generalized weakness. She always goes on a ventilator during sleep or quiet times at home. On her examination, she is quite bright and insightful and has some atypical facial features due to her weakened condition. But she has the sweetest disposition unless she is very ill.

Her lungs always sounded congested and full of fluid and bronchitis sounds. Half of one of her lungs has been removed as well from chronic infection. This and her severe spinal scoliosis also always throw me off during my lung exam. She has a G-tube in her stomach and a "trach" in her neck, which she has to suction with tubing during the visit if she has a respiratory infection. Routine stuff for her. I really have learned to overtreat with antibiotics during many illness visits due to the very fragile nature of her physiology. She can get hospitalized quite easily for severe lung infections.

Unfortunately, the newest early-treatment monoclonal injections proven to ameliorate spinal muscular atrophy weakness were not available to her at the time of her diagnosis. I have seen firsthand how effective this therapy is if the new treatment regimen is started early in life. They can grow up to just look like clumsy kids as they age. Wow. My grandson's coach has a daughter with this treated affliction. She is incredible to watch her mobility and to semi-run around the gym retrieving basketballs.

And to think that some current U.S. health leaders want to restrict pediatric research funding by the National Institute of Health, which was instrumental in the development of this life-saving drug. (Who speaks for the children?)

After the visit, again, I am always impressed by the resilience of all these special needs children. And the mothers! They are surefire saints who should all be canonized by our new pope. What dedication and sacrifice for their children. This is a lifetime commitment by them.

Mother's Gut instinct: Apnea.

It was 1 a.m. on Friday, 5 years ago, and I had just dozed off into a nice, deep sleep when the phone buzzed. This Autumn day in the office was typically busy with respiratory illnesses, RSV, and fevers. It was a long day, and I was beat. I was glad I was going to have the weekend off-call to recover. I had just returned home from the football game, where I was busy on the sideline as team doctor. There were many collision injuries that I had to attend to.

Then a family friend called. "Dr. Block, this is Abby, the mother of Burton B., your 15-year-old patient. He went out tonight to a party, and since he has been home for the last hour, I can barely arouse him. I tried pinching him and shaking him, but he still will not wake up. He smells of alcohol, too. He is breathing, but it seems really slow. I am very worried about him. I do not want to take him to the ER. What should I do?"

I asked her: "*Does he respond to any stimulation at all*? (Not really.) *Does he seem to be breathing ok, or is it really slow breaths, like less than 15 times a minute?* (Almost.) *Is his pulse beating regularly?* (Yes.)"

She said, "This is the deepest sleep state that I have ever seen him in. I know he has been drunk before, but never like this."

My brain was beginning to wake up, and I realized that he may be in too deep a stupor from his alcohol intake tonight, such that he may become apneic.

I tell Abby, "*I think that you need to rush him up to the ER right now, and get him assessed and monitored. I will come up there shortly as well. He may be in a coma within minutes, so get going promptly.*"

On her drive up to the ER, which is 5 minutes away, I recall that this upper-middle-class family with 4 teen sons is quite active in the community. The boys are all extremely smart, very athletic, academic achievers, and well-mannered. They are always pleasant to talk with. The parents are quite loving and command their boys' respect. But like a lot of good larger families, one particular child seems to be like the proverbial "black sheep."

That would be Burton.

I was correct. This was a life-or-death situation.

As I arrived at the ER, the highly capable ER doctor had already assessed Burton, found him to be intermittently apneic with oxygen desaturations in the 70% at times, and he subsequently intubated him without problems. His blood alcohol was in the 290 range. His intoxication was possibly cross-affected by some other recreational drugs, like marijuana.

The ventilator was humming along smoothly, and he seemed much too relaxed in the bed. He did not arouse with any stimulation now. I obtained further history from Abby. He had been having a bad year at school, and he dropped off the football team. His grades were now marginal, despite his incredible intellect. Apparently, he recently broke up with his girlfriend. He was at a friend's party earlier that evening. His mother had just called his friends a few minutes ago. She found out that he most likely had polished off an entire "fifth" of vodka at the party. The friends had brought him home early, as they had become worried about his sleepiness, too.

I now fully examined this robust, healthy-looking young man who almost died in his sleep that night. This was our office's 3rd toxic alcohol case in a teenage boy in the last year. The teens just do not respect the possibility of a deadly alcohol overdose for a multitude of naïve reasons.

So, I let him sleep it off overnight while on a ventilator in the intensive care unit. By 6 a.m., he was awake and restless, and he suddenly jerked out his ET tube, to the nurses' chagrin and appall. Breathing on his own now, he was hoarsely asking for breakfast. That was quick.

I arrived at 7 a.m., re-examined him, and re-interviewed him.

He was ready to be discharged home, and I discussed the need for follow-up in the office on Monday to screen for all possible precipitating factors.

He was physically fully recovered from his naïve overdose. Emotionally, I was not so sure.

His mother and I discussed his past medical history in more detail. She reminded me that he was the baby who had an apneic spell as a 2-month-old infant. So, history repeats itself in strange ways. He wound up on a ventilator at that time as well.

He was one of our early **pertussis** infection babies from a few decades ago.

At 2 months of age, she recounted how he had suffered from a bad cold for about a week with a congested cough and heavy, runny nose needing constant suctioning. And how his cough had graduated to a more severe, almost croupy-sounding cough, a similar cough which her other sons had experienced as toddlers. But this cough was just a bit different. When she put him in the cradle that evening, he seemed fine. As she checked on him an hour later (call it mother's instinct), he appeared to have turned blue (cyanotic) in the lips and face. She shook him vigorously, and after several harrowing seconds, he woke up, began crying, and then produced that unmistakable 60-second inspiratory whoop of a cough. He then finally turned pink in the face. She rushed him to the hospital about 5 minutes away, where he was placed on a cardiac/oximeter monitor along with 4 liters of nasal oxygen. I promptly admitted him to the hospital floor, performed the usual septic workup for bacteria, started IV ceftriaxone and azithromycin (for pertussis), and obtained additional pertussis PCR testing. He was also placed in respiratory isolation. But his severe whooping cough spasms soon started again with a spell of major oxygen desaturation and near apnea again.

I then transferred him by ambulance to our sophisticated high-level ICU within the children's hospital. They decided to intubate him and place him on a ventilator within a few hours of arrival.

He was removed from the ventilator and IV antibiotics after about a week. He still had a severe cough and difficulties feeding for several days. He also had multiple episodes of post-tussive vomiting, which were quite debilitating as well. He required over a month before he started gaining weight adequately again. The stress on the family was nearly unbearable as they watched their baby boy's unrelenting coughing spasms.

In 2025, our office saw 3 non-lethal pertussis cases among partially vaccinated older infants. In the state of Kentucky alone this year, over 500 cases have been documented so far, with 3 deaths in unvaccinated younger infants. Nearly all severe cases in the USA have occurred in unvaccinated children.

Children, typically younger than 12 months and who are unvaccinated, die from pertussis due to one of three ways: 1) apnea (stopped breathing), 2) seizures/encephalopathy (brain damage), 3) severe pneumonia—usually as a secondary bacterial complication with shock and likely heart damage.

Pertussis deaths and severe cases can almost always be prevented with the timely current "acellular" pertussis vaccines in the 2-, 4-, 6-, and 12/15-month combo-DTaP infant series. Since community herd immunity is much less assured with the high number of families refusing the infant DTaP vaccine, maternal TDaP during the 3rd trimester has become an infant lifesaver for mothers who choose to get vaccinated then. Also, it usually requires the 3rd dose of DTaP at 6 months to achieve nearly complete protection from pertussis, so that vaccine timeliness is vital. Do not delay these critical vaccines, as with the other infant vaccines.

The newer "acellular" pertussis vaccine, compared with the older "whole cell" vaccine, has practically eliminated the more significant adverse effects previously seen with the older vaccine decades ago. The earlier office phone calls arising from reactions to infant pertussis vaccines have nearly disappeared.

Our teenager in the story has since required a few spells in drug rehab. He is still trying to put his life together, but his alcohol and new drug addiction have become major obstacles to his achievable success. He has been given myriad opportunities. Becoming a father has not helped either. We can only pray.

CHAPTER 9

My Family

The Medical Student

(Adapted from: Block SL, The medical student in *Infectious Diseases in Children*, October 2008)

As a fourth-year medical student, one is expected to apply to multiple programs for residency, whether it be surgery, pediatrics, or internal medicine, etc. However, upon examining and visiting various programs across the U.S., I decided that the pediatric residency at Wake Forest would be ideal for me. They seemed to have a very talented, intelligent, and approachable faculty. The program was very outpatient, general pediatric-focused, not merely a feeder system for academic subspecialties. I was especially enamored with the chief of the program, Dr. Jimmy Simon, who seemed to be quite the taskmaster but also one of the premier teaching pediatricians in the U.S. His very erudite and friendly pediatric residents seemed well above average in terms of their knowledge base and skill sets. And with their sense of humor! Now, we are talking on my level!

In medical school, I truly enjoyed my family medicine and obstetrics rotations as well. But I chose pediatrics. One of the kindest and smartest pediatricians I ever met, Dr. H. David Wilson, renowned for his work in pediatric infectious diseases at the University of Kentucky, told me that I would be foolish to use my skills anywhere else but in pediatrics. My fondness and acumen for helping children—newborns, adolescents, and everything in between—won me over. One could also sense the innate dedication and love most mothers have for "nearly all" of their own children...now my "little" patients—although some were 6 feet 6 inches tall. This was a team I could easily join.

But why did I say "nearly all…"? Sadly, in my career, I have seen a few too many mothers who were also abusive to their child, or who became a "Munchausen by proxy," or who were sociopaths, drug addicts or neglectful with their progeny. Ugh.

I was completely hooked on a pediatric career during a rewarding 1.5 months on my third-year medical school pediatric rotation. I had to perform a spinal tap on a 4-month-old, mildly obtunded and very irritable infant with *Haemophilus influenzae* type B meningitis, while also inserting his IV catheter as he screamed and cried. Some painful procedures are necessary to save the baby's life. And I was getting really good at these pediatric skills, too.

(Yes, this is the same bacteria now routinely included in the infant vaccine series (thank god), as this bacteria used to wreak havoc on the lives of young infants and children, often killing them or brain-damaging them. **In the pre-vaccine era, it incredibly afflicted 1 in 200 young children and babies!!** Awfully common numbers. Awful disease.)

Now, almost unheard of for decades, in the year 2025, a previously healthy vaccinated young boy died from overwhelming sepsis due to the contagious HIB bacteria. Most likely exposed to an unvaccinated child, he was one of the exceedingly rare HIB vaccine failures; less than one in a million, I guess. Total herd protection in a more fully vaccinated population would have prevented this nightmare, I think.

The next day, once the antibiotics had worked their magic, he was reaching for me to hold him, whimpering with a charming elfish smile. That was a pivotal moment. Children are typically very resilient and can often recover rapidly from illnesses if the bad illness or cancer is perhaps caught early. In contrast, I did not relish dealing with the much more frequent deaths and dying we witnessed among our nice internal medicine patients at the med center. I liked the happier endings much more. I also realized that I did not have the temperament or steely demeanor to be a surgeon or obstetrician. This group of amazing physicians cannot be appreciated enough.

Subsequently, I took the "suicide" approach again to my residency choices, this time applying to a single pediatric residency: Wake Forest, over other superb programs, such as Vanderbilt, Florida, Virginia, Louisville, and others. Perhaps foolishly, at this point in my career, this was considered blasphemous. But I did it anyway. "Damn the torpedoes, full speed ahead," as some famous admiral (David Farragut during the Civil War) once proclaimed. Fortunately, I was accepted into the program. As Dan Fogelberg reminded me in his song: **"The chance of a lifetime, in a lifetime of chance,"** to describe my plight.

For three decades, our office has accepted monthly medical students and residents from both of the state's medical schools for teaching purposes. Electronic medical records almost completely destroyed that benevolence— we no longer have any extra time.

The toothsome 5'6" blond-haired, 3rd year medical student arrives bright and early on Monday morning. Like so many of our medical students, she is so intelligent. But this student is different for me. She is eager, smiling and ready to take on the pediatric world, albeit with some trepidation, as noted in her nervous questions. I show her the layout of the office, although for some reason it seems like she has been here before (wonder why?)

We descend upon our first patient. She is here for a 6-month well baby checkup with an experienced mother. I introduce Dr. Lindsay to the mother, explaining she is a third-year med student on rotation from the University of Kentucky. I discuss the routine issues, including solid foods, bottles, teeth brushing, car seats, and developmental expectations.

As is my custom on the first few days with a new medical student, I attempt to show them all the nuances and pearls of obtaining the pediatric history and examination, and how it varies from newborn to infant to toddler to preschooler to teenager.

In this case, I demonstrate the gentle touch needed to examine: the ocular muscle balance and red reflex; the pinpoint areas for each valve of the cardiac examination; the 3 cardinal features to check for hip dislocation in the young infant; the TMs without boxing the pinna; neurological "primitive reflexes," and so forth. Normal infant, and yet every patient we see can teach each medical student a few critical points.

"*Wow*," she exclaims. "*No one has yet directly shown me the many subtleties of the infant cardiac and neurological examination.*"

I discuss the vaccination issues with the mother that she has brought up. *Yes, we are down to two or three injections at each checkup with our combo vaccinations. We are finally getting better at limiting the pincushion effects of the past.*

I am in the "med student teaching mode" in the office. I pick a few discussion points for each patient as we go along. After a day or two, I set them free and alone to discuss the history and perform the physical examination on several patients each session. When they deliver their history and physical exam to me, I must invariably remind them to keep the history, the physical, the assessment, and plan in order and separate from each other. For most of the younger patients, wax obscures the ear canal. So, they rely upon me to provide a clear visual gateway to the TM.

Remember, you must always assess the TM for position, color and opacification, and then you must decide whether it is infected or not. This is the ear-mantra for the entire month.

When I am in the teaching mode, I amaze even myself at the multitude of subtle aspects of the physical examination that I perform subconsciously and rapidly all day long, after over 30 years. But for this patient encounter, it is different. I am discovered.

The young mother, whom I have treated since she was a toddler, recognizes the medical student. "*Aren't you…?*" I cut her off. *Yes.*

"I went to high school with her," she responds. "Was she not **Kentucky's Junior Miss** winner that senior year? That was amazing. I saw her!"

Yes, she is my daughter. The third of my four daughters.

The mother says, *"Must be a really nice feeling knowing her many accomplishments. I'll be glad if I can just prevent my own daughter from getting kicked out of kindergarten."* She laughs. Humorously, I wondered the same thing about Lindsay many years ago myself. And then I recalled my own "fond" Kindergarten experience that I described for you earlier???

A prayer for my daughter as she embarks upon her medical career: The following ABCs on how to survive medical clerkships and residency.

"There is no success without hardship."—Sophocles. *So, by god, you are on your way to resounding success!*

I was reminiscing the other day with my medical student daughter about the trials and tribulations in the Training Years of medical school and pediatric residency. Sort of like Potty Training. We all treasure children, but one can only stand so many years of potty talk....

To survive your educational process, I thus advocate for any medical student and resident to learn many of the same things that you learned in kindergarten:

Learn the basic ABCs of each common disease process. You may not need to know all the nuances, but the nuts and the bolts are the keys to saving patients—and on rounds—to avoid being crucified. If you are ever accosted by an apparently mean-spirited attending, remember the following: "How is it that little children are so intelligent and men so stupid? It must be the education that does it" (Dumas. And yes, that was his almost vulgar name, LOL.) Could this apply to your father at home as well, huh? Usually, the mentor's comments are made to help you remember. Be patient, as this, too, will pass.

Some days can be particularly like potty-training: If you don't ask for help, your bottom can get awfully raw. Your attendings are basically there to teach you. It's just that a few use hardball tactics while others will nurse you along.

As can happen rarely in any typical teaching institution, when dealing with an irascible attending, akin to the playground bully: "None are more taken in by flattery than the proud, who wish to be first and are not"—Spinoza. Emulate your mother and Mary Poppins when dealing with this one, dear. A little obsequiousness and a spoonful of sweetness can usually melt even the orneriest of personalities. This is a great training ground, because you will encounter many parents or patients like this in your future, as you have witnessed this firsthand in my office. Practice dealing with them. Usually, these folks have some major underlying stressors. Search for it. And remember, oftentimes, these clinicians may be among the most knowledgeable and best clinicians you will ever encounter. Look beyond their style.

Read a lot and then read some more. This knowledge, if absorbed well like an Ultra-Huggie, will eventually make your difficult diagnoses, your rounds and especially your medical boards like a game of patty-cake. (This, even I understood as an intern. I loved patty-cake.)

Print (or write neatly or type quickly). Messy orders can bring on not only rebukes from the teacher but also visits from hospital executives and barristers.

Get lots of rest on "off-days." If not, nap when appropriate. (Not at Ground Rounds? Bad idea when the chief is watching.)

Try to eat 3 square or round meals daily. At some point in the day, maybe within 1 hour of your Ugh! 15th admission.

Don't whine. Or you'll be put in the corner for time-out.

"A child should always say what's true, and speak when he is spoken to…" Robert Louis Stevens. So never lie. Well, almost never. Be ready to answer and to bail out a fellow colleague if needed. Thus, never, ever, ever sabotage a fellow intern or resident for the sake of roundsman- (woman-)ship. It's OK to respond eagerly, but do not deviously set up your cohorts for a fall or try to make them look silly. It is OK, on the other hand, to make yourself look silly to distract the heat from a cohort who is being blistered ("Tis wisdom sometimes to seem a fool"—Fuller).

"All work and no play make Jack a dull boy." Play hard, when you can. You will/must need a tension reliever. The strain of all this serious illness and near-death is too hard otherwise. Ask your spouse or lover (now a delusional dream, for wannabe still single med school Casanovas!) to be "sym<u>pathetic</u>" as to why you have become such a "<u>pathetic</u>" social moron or walking zombie out of the hospital.

Like mommies, seasoned nurses are always right and best acknowledged for their contributions on rounds. And at the very least, listened to. Say "thanks" frequently to them and always smile and be cordial to them, for they will save your derriere more times than this old boy cares to remember. Never sass them. (My biggest downfall as an intern, but rectified later so as not to get so browbeaten as much as a resident.)

When dealing with pediatric patients, always listen to the mother. She and her clues will help you ascertain whether you have the correct diagnosis on innumerable occasions.

"Hanky-Panky-Half-Well-Done" is a Ne'er do well. So don't you emulate him. You may skip down the hallway, but **neve**r skip a thorough, appropriate examination or skip looking at all lab work/X-rays. You may save a child's life, or more often, for example, save yourself an embarrassing late-night phone call at 3 a.m. for a patient's earache because of your cursory, hurried TM exam due to waxy ear canals.

Wash your hands frequently. You will catch the pediatric viral "crud" otherwise. And you think the stress is bad when you're healthy?

Get all your baby shots, and don't whine. The annual COVID-19 and influenza vaccine—you will soon recognize it as a religious experience each winter when everybody else is getting ill.

And 5 years later, she joined my practice, and in 9 years, she now runs the office here. How cool is that? And we were the only father-daughter practice in Kentucky, I think? I told you my girls love me!

Family Christmas letters–continued

2014.

Dear Friends and Family,

"What d'ya get?" the toys inquire on the Target TV commercial. Well, this summer we got another sweet little grandchild baby girl—Charlotte—from Lindsay/Josh this year. We got another year of good health—mostly—and a roof over our heads, and working plumbing, and good food—if you count hot dogs and canned Ravioli on the alternate weekends with the Frankfort boys, and BK hamburgers on the other weekends with Lydia. Yep, life sure is sweet and delectable at the Bardstown Block household.

We were selected for both home tours for: 1) the Bardstown Garden Club this summer, AND 2) the Stephen Foster Music Society Christmas tour this December. About 200 and 400 people, respectively, local and faraway, toured the Block compound. Been busy decorating and cleaning, especially with our very own omnipresent family dignitaries (babies and toddlers) visiting (wrecking?) all month. Yet, it gave Melinda a chance to show 3 decades worth of Xmas décor! Macy's got nothing on us! Six fully decked out Xmas trees! Deck the halls with "bowels of folly"?

Terrorists everywhere—Sony, Staples, Middle East, Africa—and even wicked little virus terrorists such as Ebola scathing Western Africa. Yet we can't even convince families to get their available life-saving vaccines like Flu and Gardasil? Then there was the huckster election-cacophony of the Republicans' terrorizing the hapless Democrats—making for months of some nauseatingly fictional TV commercials. Whatever happened to civility and good manners of the good old days—I mean c'mon crew.

Mindy/Evan. Frankfort still. Three active, athletic, bright little boys—**Jake, Matt, Ross**. Fun, cute, and whirling dervishes. Still love to visit their Meme and Papa as much as they can. All doing well, and each loves baseball, soccer, swimming, and basketball and NY strip steaks—especially when over at Papa's. Mindy is burning up the highways in Frankfort for their sports activities. Evan's practice is burgeoning. (not burning!) Working on new house plans to build the next Taj Mahal, or U of KY sports complex. Drive you crazy. Probably the best-known couple in Frankfort, and best friends with the soon-to-be KY Governor–Comer?

Misty/Danny. Columbus, Ohio for 3 years now. Great neighborhood, even if it is in Buckeye land—but they will always bleed "big blue." **Wade Parker! and Laina Belle!** (as they are called affectionately by their momma during their mischief) are healthy, prodigies, boisterous (not as much as Frankfort), and they too love to visit their Meme and Poppa. Both are outstanding swimmers too and have apparently developed gills lately. Misty enjoys staying home (shopping a lot) and Danny has made himself an indispensable plant manager at Marathon Oil. We hope a looming transfer will land our babies closer.

Lindsay/Josh. Bardstown 1.5 years. Lindsay has joined the premier peds practice in the U.S. (HERE) and enjoys reminding her father daily how much smarter she really is. She is the ultimate pediatrician, loved by all. **Lydia and newbie Charlotte** are so adorable and sweet and precocious. The maternal clumsy gene is apparently a dominant gene, as Lydia falls out of her chair most meals. They have almost laboriously fully remodeled their historic house in downtown. No shortcuts, either. Josh's dental practice continues to thrive despite the usual hiccups of a new professional practice, which Lindsay was able to circumvent (our practice was 36 years old).

Mollie/Eddie. Fairfax Co., VA. 6 months now. The newlyweds seem more transient than a tribe of Bedouins. But they love their new "digs"—literally next door to Target ("What d'ya get?"), and multiple superb restaurants, and movie theater—in a new pricey condo rental. Mollie became the full-time manager of her pharmacy within 5 miles and just loves bossing everyone around (gets that from momma). Eddie has become "almost" city manager for Fairfax City. Both have found their true niches and excel at their jobs. They visit when they can, but at least now direct flights are available to L-ville and Iceland, er, Rochester.

Melinda. Almost retired from the KY nurse aide program. Still going full-time, helping her kids, grandkids, home, her sisters, and her friends. As timeless, beautiful and as sweet as ever, Papa had hit the winning lottery ticket 39 years ago. More time for travel with hubby. But it seems like every weekend is devoted to all her babies—young and old. She is amazingly always on the go still. Needs a new Lexus—ashtrays dirty.

Papa. Still going full-time, and in addition, busier than ever with medical writing and papers and medical research issues. His practice now has 3 NPs and 7 peds, one of which is the best matriculated (guess who?) Pure joy working with and observing his progeny's progress in the world of peds. Occ. Poppa's thoughts of retiring are still ephemeral. Because Momma needs to boot his arse out of the house for her own sanity. After 3 full years, he just passed the baton on his monthly article for the prestigious national journal, *Pediatric Annals*. Although the love of his life—it became almost like monthly dysmenorrhea for him. He still thinks plaintiff lawyers are the scourge and bane of humanity, like Ebola-for-physicians. He misses his own wonderful Momma and Daddy. But the girls and the grandkids keep him enamored and invigorated. Five years in a row—voted "Nelson Co. Best Pediatrician." Who says the public cannot be bought???

Time's up.

Been a mostly joyous year for our family. Come by if you get a chance—plenty of room. Best hot dogs this side of the Salt River. Swim 365 days a year. The kid's toy Gator is charged and functional.

Merry Xmas—The Bardstown Blocks

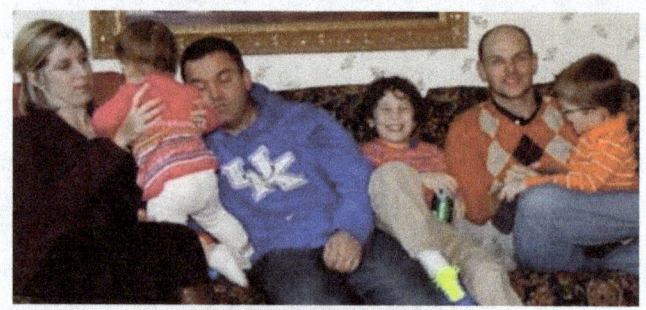

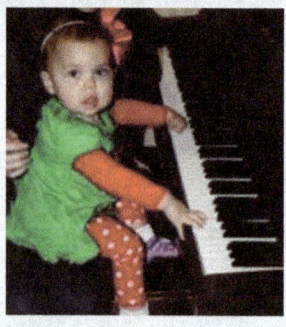

Very happy little boy and little girls—steak-fed.

2017

To all our good friends and curmudgeonly relatives, Merry Christmas 2017.

Fake news spews!

As you may have surmised, this is our annual Xmas tome, encapsulating all the grandiose events, minuscule labors, and picayune peccadilloes of the Bardstown Block family and progeny.

There are things you cannot live without (candy corn, Barbie dolls), and things you should live without (indoor: basketball games, squirt guns, light sabers, drums). Santa has been well-known to provide both. Against his better judgment. The AMEX and Visa are churning out the elves' gifts again. Quite a productive crew. These dudes make all the children happy and their elders lacrimate. Nothing trumps "plastic" though. And nothing we are divulging here is Fake News. And no known Block immigrants are being deported on trumped-up charges. Yet. We, as Alsace-Lorraine and Prussian descendants, do agree with the Robert Frost claim that "fences make good neighbors"—probably for the suburbia. Yet certain "Fences" and "Walls" across certain rough river borders may be delusional aspirations. Money may be better spent keeping good health care and good medicines available, perhaps, rather than thinking that this Wall will keep **bad drugs out**. Even crazy John Candy understood the clandestine transporting used in "Planes, Trains, and Automobiles." Let's not forget about innocents though. "Fruitcakes," you gotta love the fruitcake style of health leadership. Even Hamlet predicted that there was "Something rotten in the state of DC, er, Denmark."

And here is a synopsis of our effort to Make America Great Again (MAGA) **among 4 daughters and 8 grandchildren:**

Mindy (Evan) has just completed the true "McMansion" an amazing architectural behemoth in the style of Frank Lloyd Zappa, er, F.L.

Wright. Years in the making of MAGA in Frankfort, she and her gaggle of 3 boys are all doing wonderfully, loving the wide-open floor plan and indoor court. She burns up the roads daily for basketball, soccer, tennis, swimming, academics, dining, etc., such that her poor old Nissan Armada is being relegated to a similar demise as the Spanish Armada. (Go Brits.) Jake (11), Matt (8), and Ross (5) are each superb students and triathlon athletes. Sweetest little boys. For them, not a ball that does not need to be launched anywhere, anytime, anyplace. Their schedule makes the Tasmanian devil dizzy. Someday, these boys will truly MAGA. And ole Evan is thriving, IM doc and the most popular one in town. Epitome of a good old country doc.

Misty (Danny) is still enjoying her rejoined teaching career (4th grade) and northern Nashville (great shopping and they accept Visa and AMEX too). This is one busy family, too, entertaining a true princess (Laina [5]) and brainiac (Wade (8)) is a full-time job. The little professor knows no topic that he does not have an opinion about, and the teachers are in awe of how to keep him busy. Laina loves her animals, ponies, and dolls. So loveable. Danny still "runs" and manages the Marathon Oil distribution site, and we are in awe as to how much he understands about anything repairs, business, and oil-related. The kids are becoming avid hunters, too.

Lindsay (Josh DMD) now runs the pediatric practice and office in her 4th year here. Beloved by all staff and patients, she is amazing to watch here (no bias here?) She has the "gift", able to sniff out those diagnostic enigmas seen in the office daily [genetics?]. What a joy for a DAD, and the town is lucky to have both her and Josh as healthcare folks. And juggling motherhood too, quite superbly. Her two little lovely ducklings (Lydia (5) and Charlotte (3)) are scintillating, spunky, and active little gals (see how bright in the photo). The family is tremendously integrated into the local community and public school now.

Mollie (Eddie) is a pharmacist who now has received her "own" Rite Aid store in Lexington, KY, and enjoys being a boss of everybody. They have remodeled an old Chevy Chase home in Lexington, which is quite charming. Baby Will (19 months) is growing up so cute. He is ultra quiet and easy going, busy at daycare playing with all the other babies, and is lovable for all. He aspires to MAGA once he graduates from diapers. Some day. Some day. And he will soon have competition for the stinkiest diaper of the house, Mollie tells us. Yes, #9 is on the way. Eddie now manages county planning for Jessamine County, KY, and has assimilated all the attributes of a Mafia Boss from the "Cornbread Mafia" (Joking!) He is a natural for this job—charming, easy-going, soft-spoken, happy, and even-tempered. What? You thought I was talking about county manager—Nope, the husband role.

Melinda (23) or Meme, ageless, is still doing well, driving her Lexus all over, keeping up with all her babes, and enjoying her retirement and free time—lunch with friends, anybody? Though she has not graduated to country-club wife status, like her eldest daughter has. Shop till you drop, eh?

Poppa (old, real old) is still working full-time office pediatrics under Lindsay's tutelage now. And still runs the country's largest pediatric outpatient research group, which is still booming. CDC-sponsored NIH trials, life-saving vaccine research, and numerous other clinical trials continue to pour in. Although his days of whirlwind travel are finally over, he still speaks at some national meetings several times a year. Home landscaping (pool, roses, trees) and 2 Lexington condo rentals keep him occupied and out of the bars. All the patients insist that he never retire. Too many good needy patients he really enjoys.

2017 Merry and happy Christmas to all! The Bardstown Blocks— not the black sheep Blocks of Louisville.

My Sweet Angelic Wife—in the end, a cognitive ghost

It is 4 am. I stare out my bedroom window, the calm before the storm. It will soon be the start of a new full day. I really dreaded Thursday night because it meant that I was on my own with her for the next 3 weekend days without any respite, such as going to work for me, and a caregiver for her.

I see the large white pine trees on my lawn and the mature, stately sycamore tree in the distance. The night weather here in town is calm for now. It is still dark and foreboding outside. Lightning is occasionally flashing in the distance toward the Louisville area, I suppose. A few female deer pass by my sight in the window.

I have been awake for an hour already. Most nights are now like that. Sometimes tears flow. Sometimes I just blankly stare, devoid of any feeling. I had just changed the sheets for the night. They were soaked. She could not help herself. No matter how many "Depends" I even put tape on them. She battled me just to get her out of the bed earlier. In the last two years, every simple functional activity was a struggle and a wrestling match. Most days, I had blood-drawing finger claw marks on my back where I had to restrain her with a "big hug" to prevent her from hitting and kneeing me in a certain strategic spot. My sweet angel, now acting possessed. And unaware. She had been such a dignified, lovely woman. Four decades, we never fought. Never.

It would be 6 a.m. soon. Clock watching. Bad habit of mine. I never took any nursing care courses in medical school; I was slowly learning how to handle the basics with an Alzheimer's dementia patient. In this case, my wife.

I had learned to dress her in a pair of panties and then put loose sweatpants and a loose sweatshirt on her. She was once the epitome of beauty, grace, charm, and fashion sense. Dang, I was once a very lucky guy.

"Form over function" was forever lost on her now. Non-skid slippers cover her feet, as she was very prone to falling over. Her double whammy of dystonic Parkinson's disease now manifested (this occurs in about 20% of Alzheimer's patients) and had nearly wiped out her balance center. She could now barely sit up straight, and her torso was always heavily contorted, leaning to her left side.

Feeding her always required another hour, as I had to spoon-feed small pieces of cereal or waffles into her mouth at a snail's pace. She could no longer efficiently feed herself. Simultaneously, I had to scarf down similar food during this process. I was also losing weight like her, over the last several months, as she continued to deteriorate. For me, stress or lack of time, I did not know.

The Promise

I had promised her decades earlier that I would not ever place her in a nursing home, like her mother had required for the same diagnosis. I kept that promise.

Anyway, not to say that in the last two months of her life that I did not try. When I was at the end, and getting overwhelmed, I inquired about "memory care" rooms or a routine nursing home admission toward her last few months of life after five years. I was weary. They told me that she fell too often, or that she must be able to feed herself, or, most importantly, that she was too complicated for them to handle. Too many medications, too often. And I was supposed to take care of her by myself??? Hospice was unable to help at all, either.

Furthermore, none of the "supposed" Alzheimer's medications ever worked, and they were uniformly fraught with unbearable side effects. We are still in the "Dark Ages" of this treatment. Finally, off-label Abilify seemed to help the aggression a bit. But it was hard to be sure, as she was prone to spitting out her many pills, or worse, hoarding them in her gums, to later clandestinely spit them out and lodge the pill remnants under the pillows, couches, rugs, etc. This hide-and-seek game was apparently fun for her. And then rigorously instilling glaucoma eye drops twice daily! Essential. Imagine a blind Alzheimer's patient.

You Know It When You See It

It subtly started in 2015 when her car scraped the garage door entrance a few times, and lots of key scratches kept appearing on her car door frame. She got lost so easily in our small town, which she was very familiar with, and her forgetfulness was becoming overwhelming.

I knew it for sure when she had trouble remembering the names of her daughters and grandchildren. And now this former social butterfly became more reclusive with her friends. But despite her dementia, until her last year, for 4 years I still drove her down 45 minutes to Louisville one Tuesday each month to "play" Bunco with her old high school friends while I waited in the car. It was one of the two things that she truly enjoyed now. But she eventually became so befuddled and distant around them that even they could not handle her.

One ponders about retiring at the end of one's career, enjoying the accumulated wealth, and traveling with your sweetheart whenever and wherever. Wham! We were both 62 years old when life became ultra complex and totally isolating. Who knew?

But I had been unwittingly prepped for this total care decades earlier. I had raised 4 lovely daughters from infancy to childhood, and this would be no different. I would just not get beyond the infancy stage this time.

I instead became her nurse, her daycare worker, her cook, her laundromat, her housecleaner, her total caregiver, her protector, her CNA, her personal physician adjusting all her interacting multiple medications, and her guardian for her safety—she would often try to run out the back door. In fact, a few kind teachers at the elementary school two blocks away walked her back home when she had surreptitiously snuck out several times. Who knew?

As Charles Dickens stated: "It was the worst of times..." So, my goal each day was just to survive. Numbness had settled in. Not pain. The future was bleak. No time to think, to worry, or to enjoy. Never really depressed, I just existed to keep the status quo. Mostly alone. No conversations in the day or night. I told my daughters not to come around for anything but a quick visit, but any time, bring the grandchildren—my major source of joy. I told them that they had to raise their own families and perform their own jobs. I would take care of Melinda—for the full five years, as it turned out. Earlier, I had a caregiver come in while I was still able to work a truncated 2 to 3 days a week. One day a week, one of those caregivers was her compassionate older sister, Suzie, who had ironically first introduced her to me 4 decades ago. But my work schedule, which kept me sane, became too complex to juggle with her daily needs. I loved my job, my patients, my enigmas, my babies, and my complex teenagers. But I promised...

At the start of the illness, I had to stop all travel, speaking, and research investigator meetings. Vacations would become a nightmare. I could no longer take office "call" coverage, including the nursery on call. I had no one to watch her if I was urgently called out, which was frequent. I had to start simplifying everything in my life. Walmart's "Quick Click" grocery shopping was even problematic—I had to haul her in the truck to pick up the groceries still, then in 20 minutes, literally run into the store to select my own fruits and meats. She also fought the truck door as if it was Satan himself sitting there. I had to head-first hoist her onto the seat.

In 2019, she was hospitalized twice—for complete heart block (pulse=30) with insertion of a pacemaker after 18 hours in the ICU; and three weeks later for an iatrogenic 800 cc chronic pericardial effusion with severe hypotension needing a pericardial drain placement. Three days each time in the ICU. Near death each time, shocky and disoriented. And then, her "Sundowning" each night never became more of a nightmare for the nursing staff. I could never leave her side, even in the ICU, once they experienced that issue. I was the only thing in the world that could calm her down at night. And she lost even more function after these catastrophes.

COVID-19 had just hit the U.S. in early 2020—further exacerbating our isolation. Our wonderful, sweet standard poodle of 17 years died in August; something was amiss—even she knew that much. In November 2020, the seizures became intractable. Her dementia ordeal was finally over with her 4 daughters by her bedside vigil. With some help from "above," her funeral home visitation was the last day before COVID-19 shut down the entire country for the year. The number of her visitors was overwhelming, and welcomed.

My PTSD was just starting. For two months, I was completely numb after the funeral. But I had already mourned for five years, while she had continued to be a true "cognitive ghost." Five years of the mourning process after caring for a chronically dying loved one is quite different from that of the abrupt death of a loved one. Quite. I have experienced both painful versions.

In a few months, I also finally tried to enter the world of social networking and Facebook. My internet social page was a total blank page prior to her death. What a Luddite I was.

But, small-town gossip and opinions afterwards became intrusive with any social excursions for such a public figure as myself. So, those events needed to happen out of town from now on. Remember my earlier discussion of small-town doctoring. Too many office entanglements. Hanging out at the local bar or gym was taboo for a prominent local pediatrician. Plus, I had steered clear of alcohol totally during this five-year vigil. Too easy to get entrapped with this soporific.

I would soon re-enter the world of the "living" again. Although I will be forever in love with Melinda, I have had two relationships since then. One taught my vulnerable self (40+ years with only one amazing woman) about my dating naivete. The other has been a pleasantly ongoing joy for a few years with a likewise widow.

M and I had both agreed upon a quick renewed next phase of companionship for each other, way before either of our deaths. No guilt ever, once you are ready to engage.

Spouses should discuss this issue early in their marriages to help prevent the later accompanying guilt feelings, as I have learned from my new fiancé.

I later experienced my own painful "widow-maker" heart attack in May 2023. I survived with two coronary artery stents and a slow full recovery from the subsequent CHF. Life is fragile.

CHAPTER 10

More Pediatric Conundrums, Part 2

Deeply Hidden Agendas

It seemed like any ordinary day in the Sylvan community of Bardstown, KY. The office schedule was full, a surprising occurrence in the early summer when school is not in session. Glancing at the schedule, the usual potpourri of respiratory illnesses, rashes and checkups beckoned me.

I started by looking at my email, which contained a note about the need for a repeat skeletal survey in a 19-month-old child from Shepherdsville, KY. I had referred the child to the "Mecca" hospital for a spiral fracture of the humeral shaft. The case "spiraled" downward when I had also spotted a missed incidental healing buckle fracture of the radius that was only partially visible as an oblique radius view displayed within the humeral radiograph. This confirmed that the child had been physically abused.

Thus, once again, confirming my age-old proselytizing that clinicians should review their own radiographs of all extremities and chests, in addition to the radiologist's review.

"It's academic, my dear Watson." *Sherlock Holmes*

The afternoon session started nearly as badly.

The seventeen-year-old biracial female from Mount Washington, KY, had been experiencing nosebleeds for the last two weeks. No other alarming details in her history had been divulged so far. She even had normal menses, except for miserable menstrual cramps. Her thorough examination revealed only a friable anterior nasal septum on the right side.

Engaging her with my usual screening repertoire, I queried, "So, how is school, Watson?"

"Ds and Cs."

(Red lights began flashing in my brain.)

"So how did you do the previous year?"

"As and Bs."

No history of drugs, alcohol, rape, molestation, physical abuse, or severe mood problems was uncovered. But, Watson explained how she had been left basically homeless during this school year, as her mother drifted in and out of several relationships with allegedly inhospitable and unsavory males. This had fractured the mother-daughter relationship. Watson had then moved in with her disabled father, who was so impoverished that he could not afford to provide for his two teenage daughters and himself. So, she had resided with "a friend" for several months, while her sister had been domiciled with an aunt. Stressed, and without a family and sometimes no roof, this young lady was a survivor.

Watson recounted how, later in the school year, her father had formed a beneficial relationship with a new woman, who subsequently took the teenage girls under her wing.

Her mood and outlook had improved notably since then. She alleged she had never "cut" and fostered no suicidal or constantly depressed thoughts.

With a normal CBC and platelets in hand, I proceeded to make one or two aspects of her life more tolerable. She received a prescription for a brand of contraceptive pills, which would incidentally improve her dysmenorrhea, along with her acne, over the long term as well. I recommended petroleum jelly 2x daily for her anterior nasal septum. She agreed to return in two months or sooner if any catastrophes, depression, or major dilemmas occurred again.

I remarked at how well she had survived the school year, complimenting her progress in other major areas. I told her my door was open if she ever needed any help.

Fertile and Phantom pain

The pleasant, dark-haired 15-year-old girl, Kit, was complaining of a sore finger, which, after a thorough examination, revealed a completely normal hand. Kit looked fidgety and nervous. Then I asked her how things were going in her life. She hemmed and hawed and finally came forth with her real purpose: She had missed over two months of menstruation.

Kit was wondering whether she could possibly be pregnant, since she had engaged in unprotected sexual intercourse over the last three months. For some magical reason, with Peter Pan-type thinking, she thought she would not get pregnant. After all, she did not believe that could actually happen to her. We discussed the high likelihood that she was pregnant today.

"But I never had sex when I ovulated."

"And when was that?"

"You know, the day just after my period."

I proceeded to explain the calculation of ovulation by counting 14 days backward from the start of her period to predict her ovulation and the maximum days of fertility.

"I guess I shoulda listened more in health class, huh?"

Oh yeah.

We discussed the possible choices for her future. Kit did not want her mother to find out until she had a chance to cogitate. I explained that, regardless, she needed to start folate-enriched multivitamins immediately.

The urine pregnancy test (along with Chlamydia and Gonococcus DNA probes) was performed. We reconvened a few minutes later, and she watched my fingers paginate the computer screen to the final screen, which would determine the remainder of her future.

I asked her if she was ready for the results.

And by some magical twist of fate...

The test was negative. We both sighed with relief.

Now the choice was which contraceptive method to use for the future, and Kit's reminder that condoms were still essential for disease prevention. I could not give her the HPV9 vaccine today because her mother was not available, but it was a top priority for the next visit. She did agree to return in a month to update her menstrual and emotional progress, along with adherence issues. She agreed that sex was not that important to her, but she was proud that she had a steady older boyfriend, unlike her peers!

This brought to mind the lyrics from a seventies song by the musical group "10cc."
"The things we do for love...
You lay down your bets, and then you pay the price."
Kit had a winning lottery ticket this month.

Enigmatic adolescent acute abdomen: Rarer diagnosis than a winning lottery ticket

(Adapted in part from Block, SL in *J of Pediatr Surg*. Sept 1998)

Dr Block, do you remember when...?

Speaking of lottery tickets: Her illness that she is referring to may be the only case that has occurred in over millions of teenagers in the U.S. in 40 years.

On a cold autumn day over 20 years ago, the current mother had presented as a pleasant, sweet 13-year-old teenager from Lebanon, KY, who was writhing on the exam table with significant generalized abdominal pain.

The pain was mostly centered around her umbilicus and of four days' duration. She had also had many episodes of diarrhea and severe bilious (yellow) vomitus multiple times. She denied any respiratory symptoms, sexual activity or vaginal discharge or pain. The tearful, sexually mature young teen was febrile to 103°F, with normal BP, and some mild tachycardia and tachypnea, although with clear lungs. Her abdomen was very tender, and she had major guarding, whereby her abdomen tensed up totally upon any light palpating or touching of it. Her abdominal pain even radiated badly all over when I let go of her belly wall. This "Rebound Tenderness" typically indicates a serious intra-abdominal surgical condition, or an "acute abdomen."

Her blood work showed that her white blood count was 25000 (very high) and her ESR (erythrocyte sedimentation rate) was 126, very high and extremely alarming. ESR is a generic test for acute inflammation. An elevated ESR is what I term a red flag "worry factor," as it does not give a diagnosis. But when it is notably elevated, it tells me to search diligently until I find an answer. Thus, I began searching for the cause of her acute abdominal pain. With my nurse and her mother by her side, I began hunting for right lower abdominal pain indicative of appendicitis.

Her chest radiograph was normal now, but her abdominal radiograph showed many swollen air-filled loops of bowel, indicating that their normal peristalsis function was completely paralyzed (such as an ileus or bowel paralysis). With her major diarrhea, I presumed she had peritonitis that may be caused by bacterial dysentery from Salmonella or Shigella, but this was a bit less likely with no blood in the stool. We had observed several bacterial cases this year in my office. Additional abdominal ultrasounds and a CT scan revealed only an ileus as well, and no appendicitis. However, she was allergic to all the customary intravenous antibiotics to treat bacterial dysentery, thus I was left with trying an empiric trial of IV ciprofloxacin to cover for possible dysentery.

After a lack of much response to 48 hours of antibiotics and IV fluids, the gifted general surgeon and I both decided she needed surgical laparoscopic abdominal exploration for possible atypical ruptured appendicitis or other intra-abdominal catastrophes. This exploration revealed a normal appendix, but with multiple extra luminal (outside the bowel wall) abscesses and pus pockets and debris all over her bowels without any obvious source of bowel rupture. She was indeed very sick. But why?

Her tests on her cervix (under anesthesia) were also negative. Two days later, her intra-abdominal cultures grew the bacteria, pneumococcus, from her surgically-obtained peritoneal pus without any obvious source. I could tell from her initial slide specimens of the pus that the bacteria recovered were classic in appearance for pneumococcus (a gram+ diplococci, for you fluent in microbiology-speak). These respiratory bacteria had no business whatsoever being in the intra-abdominal fluid. None. I was dumbfounded.

(Her illness occurred way before the routine use of the pneumococcal vaccine in infants and children.)

Pneumococcus is a very common bacteria that resides peacefully in the nasopharynx most of the time in most people. However, when a virus invades the respiratory tract, then this opportunistic bacteria also becomes the number one secondary bacterial invader, causing ear infections (acute otitis media), sinusitis, severe pneumonia, and, rarely, meningitis. (We now have a 3rd-generation pneumococcal vaccine, which provides protection against most of these pneumococcal strains.)

This type of pneumococcal infection was a totally extraordinary case of **primary** (without a source) **spontaneous pneumococcal peritonitis in a teenager.** In my literature search, this form of infection had not been reported in a previously healthy adolescent female over the last 40 years in the U.S. In pediatric patients, this specific spontaneous pneumococcal infection has been reported only to occur in much younger children, most of whom were afflicted with underlying specific disorders such as nephrotic syndrome (kidney disorder), cirrhosis (liver disease) or some blood immune disorders. She had none of these disorders.

In the operating room, the internal abdomen was opened up and thoroughly irrigated by the surgeon. Postoperatively, she was then switched to IV clindamycin, which provides good coverage of pneumococcus, based on her Gram stain of the pus. She slowly recovered after a week in the hospital with concomitant abdominal drains for a few days.

As usual, the story does not end here.

After four days at home while recovering, she next developed new onset fevers to 102°F, shortness of breath and left-side chest pain. When I examined her in the office that day, she had markedly decreased breath sounds on her left lung—a finding mostly observed when a large collection of fluid accumulates between the chest wall and the lung, which is another serious infection in itself. Although her first chest X-ray during her earlier hospitalization was normal (I rechecked this), her repeat chest radiograph now showed a large left pleural (lung fluid) effusion and pneumonia. She also had developed a mildly elevated white blood count. With both mom and the young lady in tears as they left the office, I then referred her to the children's hospital, where a chest tube was inserted to drain off the large amount of pleural fluid. IV vancomycin (only used in the most life-threatening cases of pneumococcus or MRSA) was started to provide coverage for any potential resistant pneumococcus in her pneumonia. It may arguably also provide better penetration into the infected fluid. After four days of IV vancomycin, she had finally recovered fully.

I saw her in the office many more times during her adolescent years, but only for mundane illnesses and checkups. Thank goodness.

The reticent 4-year-old

She said, "Do you remember when you saw me for …?"

On a bright, sunny day in my pediatric office during late summer checkup season, the pleasant 30+ year-old White mother greets me along with her reticent, minimally verbal 4-year-old daughter. *I am so glad to see you,* she says. *I have been waiting months to make an appointment with you.* She glances at the daughter, whose interaction seems to be totally self-absorbed in her own world. She is a taller, well-developed, somewhat athletic-looking little girl who is growing appropriately. She has no dysmorphic features and is really cute. But she has a very flat affect. No interactions with me bring her out of her verbal turtle shell.

We exchange pleasantries, and then she describes how her daughter at home has only a rudimentary vocabulary and poor fine motor skills. We discussed the need for a more formal educational evaluation that should be sought as soon as she enters the school system in the next few weeks. Her physical examination, hearing and vision are each normal. However, she cannot name any colors, numbers, or personal body parts.

It seems likely that she may fall in the educational category some euphemistically consider "a slow learner," which comprises about 3% of the general population. (A term which I personally use very carefully for obvious personal reasons.) I tell her that she needs an IEP, or an individualized education plan, to be developed by the school psychologist very soon. Alternatively, I could send her to the developmental specialist center for evaluation, but it would take nearly a year for her to be seen there. But mom is a pragmatist, and also a worrier (like her own mother, whom I have known for decades). She says, Dr. Block, *I really trust your opinion only. What do you think?*

Mom is an intelligent, single, working mother who lives in a nearby small town, whom I have not seen as a patient for over 10 years. But first, I remember something very scary in her past medical history when I was the mom's pediatrician.

Why is she so dedicated to getting my opinion? Because...

She is now, decades later, a devoted follower of Dr. Block because of my attention to detail and swift management of her own past life-threatening illness. Besides, I was always very nice to her.

We discussed the potential diagnosis and prognosis for the 4-year-old girl. She had her diagnosis confirmed later, and she began attending special education classes for her age, which she really enjoyed.

She has a wonderful mother.

Listen to the mother

Five years ago, a precocious, very verbal, dark-haired, well-dressed two-year-old little boy from Greenville, KY, was smiling and talking to me, but he looked very scared and worried. Ten minutes later, he began writhing in pain on his mother's lap, screaming out, "*Dr. Block, help me.*" He had been seen a few hours earlier by one of our pediatricians in the nearby community satellite office for his abdominal pain. While there, he had just displayed a pattern of feeling fine for 10 to 20 minutes, then went into apparent abdominal spasms and intense pain for 5 to 10 minutes, crying out vociferously for help. This pain pattern can rarely be seen in cases of severe constipation. She was instructed to give him several doses of Miralax, and told to return promptly to the clinic if he worsened.

The well-dressed, articulate mother and I had a long history of me taking care of John's recurrent, painful, acute otitis media infections. No better, within an hour, she traveled over to our main office, requesting to see me to figure out John's problem. Good rapport goes a long way. Without an appointment, she was told she would likely have to wait. However, our seasoned office staff recognized this case was different after just a few minutes in the waiting room. They called me to his office exam room urgently.

Listening carefully to her description of his illness, he had a distinct bowel spasm pattern. I then examined his abdomen, which at this moment appeared soft and only mildly distended. His abdominal right lower quadrant appeared a bit tender on palpation with my fingertips. Nothing alarming.

Then, while I was asking more questions about his condition, he went into one of his screaming, writhing fits for 10 minutes again. Thus, I obtained a complete blood count by finger stick to check for possible infection and appendicitis, and then sent him over to get an X-ray in our office, checking specifically with an abdominal upright film, not just a laying down radiograph. I knew what I was hunting for. I had seen this serious condition several times in my career. It occurs in approximately 1 in 10,000 young children, mostly around the age of two.

After about 20 minutes of obtaining these two tests, the abdominal upright (the essential position) radiograph confirmed my suspicion. It showed multiple air fluid levels, but specifically only in the right lower abdominal quadrant (RLQ), and nowhere else. The flat or lying down X-ray showed no pathology. Like my other similar cases, the air fluid levels typically indicate a generalized abdominal ileus—or non-functioning or paralyzed portion of the bowel for whatever reason. However, in my experience, when the ileus is relegated to the RLQ, the odds are extremely high with this symptomatic pattern that I am dealing with a case of **intussusception.** This condition occurs mostly in the RLQ when the small intestine gets sucked into the large intestine at the cecum, or the juncture point of the small intestine to the proximal large intestine. Most of the time, we do not find a reason for the lead point or a cause for this condition. But scarily, lymphomas and dysenteric infections (see my other "currant jelly" case) can trigger it.

I told the mother about my strong suspicion (although I was actually certain in my mind) and that it would need to be confirmed by a barium enema at the tertiary care hospital, just in case. Interestingly, this diagnostic barium enema, when done early, is usually curative for the intussusception itself when it forces the lead point of the small intestine out of the large intestine. Occasionally, emergency surgery is required to alleviate the obstruction. Rarely, this condition can be deadly if not treated in a timely manner (we have seen this happen in our practice once before).

As usual in pediatrics, earlier diagnosis and treatment are better.

I explained to the mother in detail, with the X-ray handed to her to take down to the children's hospital emergency department, that we needed to send him to the tertiary care hospital for diagnosis and management as rapidly as possible. I sent my chart notes with her, showing my suspected diagnosis clearly under the *Impression* section. She drove him down there in the usual 30 minutes, faster than an ambulance could typically perform.

We local practitioners have a superb symbiotic life-saving relationship with our savvy tertiary care cohorts. But sometimes—well??? We must listen to the mothers of our patients, as well as to the referral doctors, even if they are simple country doctors like myself.

They were having an exceptionally busy night. Thus it took the ER staff longer than usual to attend to him. His paroxysms of pain had not abated, and he was deteriorating.

The abdominal findings were worsening severely, as can sometimes happen rapidly with intussusception. He had now evolved into full-blown continuous findings of an "acute" abdomen. The pediatric surgeon was called down to the ER around midnight, and then one foot of bowel was resected shortly afterwards in the operating room. The incarcerated, or stuck bowel portion, had lost its blood supply for too long. That portion was dead. He spent 8 days in the hospital on IV fluids and antibiotics. He recovered totally.

The parents and referral docs are often an underestimated vital diagnostic source for the healthcare team early in severe pediatric illnesses.

Mom's letter

> "It's still mind-blowing that we were one of the rare cases you've seen in 30 years, and you caught it so easily! Words cannot express the respect and gratitude we have for you! Thank you for being the best physician we could ever ask for to care for our children. We love you to the moon and back! Doctor Block! Thanks for being such an amazing doctor!"

> Signed, H. Janes

The preacher's daughter

A few years after I had moved to town, I was trimming my bushes around my front driveway. I am a DIY handyman for most small household chores and repairs. An older station wagon had pulled into the driveway, and out popped this stocky, close-trimmed-haired young man, energetic in his stride, gregarious in his demeanor. *Doc, I've been meaning to come by and introduce myself. I am Pastor Goodlet, the minister of the Highway 245 Baptist Church. I would like to discuss my ministry and the significance of God in our lives. I conduct a church service every Sunday, and you, your wife, and your kids are welcome to attend. I would love to have you there.*

"Well, Reverend, I am sorry to tell you, but I was born and raised Catholic, and I still attend service there most Sundays. I really enjoy Father Clarence... Unless, when I am on call and happen to be summoned to my office, the emergency room, or the hospital. I am on call every 3rd weekend, and most of the time I am busy on those Sundays. Attending to these calls of my own patient flock has to suffice as my way of honoring God."

I certainly understand how important that is, Doc, he replied. We chatted some more, and he told me about his family and his expectant wife. He was so excited. So, I invited him to be a future member of "my flock," and I would welcome his family gladly and take care of any of his children in my office. (Little did I suspect, I would later be a part of the "greater plan.") We parted on amiable terms and with a respect for each other's goals in life: His was the souls of his congregation, mine was the physical and mental health of my patients in the office.

<u>Fast-forward:</u> A few months (2025) ago, I had just finished my BLS and PALS re-certification course and test, when I looked at the instructor's name tag. It was Goodlett. OMG. Yes, it was "her sister." Wait until you read her sister's following story.

I said, Beth, it is so good to see you. You realize your sister is one of my "stolen angels."

She said, *Yes, my dad talks about you all the time at his church.*

The story, as I reminisced:

Ten months later, after my initial encounter with the Reverend, I had just finished seeing my 5th case of RSV bronchiolitis during a busy morning office session, when I walked into treatment room #13. The nurse had warned me. This tearful, fretful, kind-hearted mother was holding her 8-month-old baby in her arms, with a blanket totally encompassing the baby. *Do you mind if I have a look*, as I peeled down the blanket.

In our line of work as a pediatrician, you just know.

This was a toxic (bad sick), infected baby. The soft spot (anterior fontanelle) was bulging. The baby had a mottled, ashen skin coloring. The baby was poorly responsive to any stimuli. The neck was stiff and could not be bent. The bloodstream perfusion (circulation) of the skin/nails was poor. I knew I had no time to spare at all. A possible innocent death was staring at me. I quickly assessed her ears, lungs, and abdomen—all normal. With precious few minutes to spare, I further cursorily explained to the mother that I thought the baby had meningitis, and that I must immediately perform a spinal tap (needle in the lower spine to draw off a few cc's of fluid), a blood culture, CBC, urine culture by a bladder tap, and most difficult—start an IV to administer life-saving antibiotics and IV fluids. This was the standard of care for any very ill baby who probably had a very serious infection. We must know about the spinal fluid before antibiotics are started, if possible.

So, I beckoned my nurse to assist me and restrain the baby, and another one to take the mother out to the waiting room. All this baby procedural stuff was too much visual trauma for any parent to observe. Fortunately, I was well-trained in my residency, evaluating numerous cases of toxic children (before the development of effective bacterial vaccines) so I could perform all these procedures in about 20 minutes flat with a good nurse to restrain the baby, and with all the necessary tools at the tableside. Baby in position, needle was inserted; once I felt the pop of the spinal canal dura (covering) and saw the cloudy (purulent) fluid, I knew.

Time was so critical. The ambulance was being called for immediate transport to the children's hospital. IV fluids were bolused (large intravenous volumes for a baby) to keep the blood pressure up and prevent shock, and the ceftriaxone was injected into the IV for the baby. I brought the mother back into the room to explain that I did everything humanly possible to save her baby's life, and to save her brain and other vital organs. She had tearfully resigned herself to passively watching over her deathly ill child for the foreseeable future. The baby was still poorly responsive.

Now it was up to the good Lord to see her through, I said. Then I recognized the name; this was the pastor's wife and daughter!! Maybe they could use religious advocacy to help pull her through. To be sure that everything went as well as possible, as in this case, I often would ride in the back of the ambulance to monitor my sickest patients in case they deteriorated. Decades ago, our rural EMTs were not well-trained in pediatric airways or resuscitation of the critically ill child. It was hell on the office schedule, but all of our other parents intuitively understood—if this was your critically ill child, where would you want me to be?

I loaded the ET tubes and laryngoscope, as well as the mannitol, the valium, epinephrine, and atropine, into my emergency bag. We finally arrived at the children's hospital emergency room, and my superbly skilled ER colleagues took over her care from there. She was in their optimal hands. They rolled her up to the ICU. They would save her.

As I rode home in the back of the ambulance from this crisis, I pondered, my heart still racing... I was mentally exhausted. The stress of having this baby's life entirely in one's hands... is daunting.

She had HIB meningitis. She pulled through unscathed by seizures, brain damage, hearing loss, etc., after seven days of IV antibiotics. No complications. Totally recovered. Another life saved. But it is not always the case, I knew. Before our wonderful HIB vaccine, the HIB bacteria would seriously infect 1 in 200 children. 1 in 200! Awful!! And numerous children died in the past.

As for the Reverend, he has done an amazing service for the community. He has amassed an incredible amount of parishioners, growing from a tiny Baptist church into a sprawling, almost mega-church. He personally drives his church van each Sunday to pick up those less fortunate, including former drug addicts, felons, and immigrants; welcoming, like Jesus, all comers into his ministry. We share the same philosophy in that regard. Neither of us turns our back on the less fortunate. Our flock needs us. Politics has little role in medical care.

And to really bring home the family dynamics, my former patient now brings her baby to our practice and talks about how her father "sings the praises" of Dr. Block to his congregation, she relayed to me a few years ago. I just blush, as I am not very good at one-on-one accolades.

Interestingly, the Reverend's brother also spent several months training with our practice, first as a 4th-year medical student and later as a family practice resident. He shares his brother's approach to humanity as well: Take care of the patients first, worry about the bills later. A kind, smart doctor.

And the patient's brother married one of our current, talented nurse practitioners as well. Small world. Welcome to rural Kentucky.

Dad's letter to the newspaper, *Kentucky Standard*:

> "...Dr. Block and a team of nurses worked relentlessly to save our daughter's life. They demonstrated concern, composure and great skill as they ministered to her physical need. Dr. Block even accompanied her in the ambulance to Norton's Children's Hospital. The head pediatrician at Norton's Hospital later informed us that it was the effort by Dr. Block and the Flaget staff that saved her life..."

Reverend Goodlett

The berating

I have to admit that not all my encounters with patients, nor with all their parents, are pleasant or even tolerable.

The patient was the 21 y.o. daughter of a well-known community human-relations mother from nearby Bullitt County, with whom I was acquainted for years. I had taken care of the mother's four children for decades. The pleasant young lady presented on this spring-like morning in 1999 with no fever and was not very ill. She was alone in the office. She reported experiencing a runny nose and mild headache for a few days, as well as a slight fever and cough. Basically, not very sick from what I could tell. However, I have been burned a few times before, so I am cautious, and never insinuate that a patient should not have come to the office for such a minor problem. Her hidden agenda may just smack you hard in the face.

My examination, although conducted with total modesty, was completely unremarkable, except for some mild nasal congestion. No sinus tenderness was palpated. The lungs were totally clear. *I think you just have a run-of-the-mill cold. You can just take some decongestants like Afrin, some Aleve, and some Delsym twice a day for your symptoms. However, please return if the condition worsens, or call back in 5 to 7 days if you experience worsening symptoms, including a persistent runny nose, fever, malaise, and/or headache. This may indicate that you have graduated to a sinus infection, I clearly stated. She understood, smiled, and said, Thank you, doc.*

This was a common everyday discussion with teens and parents in my office. But after lunch, I was summoned into the office manager's room. She said that Mrs. Smith was very upset that *I DID NOT treat her daughter.* For what, I asked? Incredulous. She merely had a simple, uncomplicated URI today.

She had yelled at the manager that I was not a good doctor, that I should have given her antibiotics, and that she was not sure that she would ever let her come back to our office. I was flabbergasted. Where in the heck did all this vitriol come from? Wow.

I lost sleep that night, and for days I was terribly worried that I might have missed something. My phone call to her the next day to inquire about what happened was stonewalled.

Left in limbo, I finally suppressed and compartmentalized this upsetting matter after a few days.

Four months later, Mrs. Smith's obituary was in the local paper. She was only in her late 40s. Some of my office staff knew her from their church. She had died of heart failure and had been very sick for the last 6 months. One could only speculate on the cause.

On that bad day, I guess that she was overwhelmingly acutely concerned about her "baby girl" and that she would shortly no longer be able to support or care for her, as she faced her impending demise. I was just the most accessible target for venting about her cruel fate.

And I had better take good care of her daughter in the future, was my hidden warning. Sometimes the "hidden agenda" is deeply buried.

I have added her to my list of unfortunate souls that I pray for.

The real tension in tension pneumothorax.

(Adapted from Block SL in *Infectious Diseases in Children,* July 2008)

One square centimeter.

I can feel the perspiration accumulating on my brow. Or at least I think I can. I stand ready to save a life. I stare at the pink 1 cm area of the human anatomy; the isosceles triangular gateway of this life starts and stops here. I know that this is the only thing that matters to me in the universe today.

Been there, done that so many times in my earlier life while training. Still, few things are more daunting in pediatrics than to intubate an awake, full-term, vigorous infant who is too sick to realize the extent of his illness and too robust to let anyone restrain him. He is still self-ventilating, just not efficiently enough to sustain his life too much longer—his pCO_2 is now 56. This high value shows he is in respiratory failure.

The tongue is slimy, and it slides off the ET blade with ease. He is still struggling with me, not aware that I am trying to save his life. Some days are like that.

The mother in the office baby story minutes earlier, before this respiratory crisis:

The circle will be unbroken.

I was prompt for my 11:30 a.m. appointment with a 4-month-old infant and his mother, Sheila.

I had also been the former pediatrician for the 24-year-old mother. We were reminiscing about the good old days when she visited me, always happy and smiling as a child and a teenager. She was a marvelous cheerleader, even good enough to succeed on our nationally awarded collegiate team. Of course, I had nothing to do with her achievements, for she was so talented. Or did I?

Yes, she remembered the story, and OMG!* the scar on her abdomen! When she was just 8 months old, she had presented to the office with vomiting and even some hematemesis without diarrhea or fever. The bloody vomitus had persisted for half a day, so I had admitted her to the hospital. While there, she developed worsening hematemesis, and I had started her on ice saline water and Maalox lavages, along with cimetidine intravenously. (This was a long time ago, crew.) It quickly became apparent that her predicament was more than a simple gastritis or esophageal tear from forceful vomiting. She was still bleeding. So, she was sent for immediate abdominal surgical exploration at the tertiary care hospital, who would likely decipher her problem.

Diagnosis: Gastric hamartoma with ulcerations. Surgically removed. Another of a plethora of rare diagnostic oddities in rural KY. And, another life saved—thank goodness for superb pediatric surgeons at our referral hospital.

Back to the present day at the office, we were discussing her mundane baby issues—the importance of introducing solids, in what order, and limiting formula intake to a reasonable daily amount. The examination of the smiling infant by me was progressing nicely, including heart sounds, HEENT, neck, and lungs. And then the rap on the door!

My nurses have strict orders NOT to interrupt me during an office visit unless it is really important or another physician is calling.

It was important.

The hospital nurses told me that the 3-hour-old healthy 8-pound infant born by Caesarean-section was tachypneic and having dusky spells. The results of the "capillary" blood gas were not very good—remember this is a 35-bed hospital in central rural Kentucky with a rudimentary level 1 nursery. We take what information we can get. And a neonatologist? Forget it. He/she is me and my talented pediatric partners. On call every night and weekend, too.

The chest radiograph showed a pneumothorax (a deadly collection of air between the chest wall and the lung, sometimes from increasingly vigorous resuscitation). The nurse read from the radiologist's report. My partner had inconveniently overlooked relaying to me that a hospital newborn was having some respiratory difficulties this morning.

So, I needed to apologize to my new mother here in the office.

...*Love to talk further, but you understand.*

And Sheila, the mother of the 4-month-old, truly did.

I rushed to grab my keys, phone, and make sure my glasses were still tied around my neck. (One of the several ravages of old age—presbyopia.) I phone ahead to the nurses—get a Pleurevac (suction device), chest tube, 25-gauge butterfly needle, 3-way stopcock, and 10 cc syringe.

I arrived at the hospital 10 minutes later, which is 6 miles away—the wonders of small towns. Yet, everything seems to take an eternity—from getting behind a truck going the speed limit (OMG!) to parking the car to waiting for the world's slowest elevator. With all the security clamps, stairs are off-limits for accessing the hospital wards.

Off the elevator, I gallop to the nursery.

Where's the X-ray?

The chest radiograph showed a very large tension pneumothorax. Speed dial my synapses for how to fix that problem. The oximeter is hovering around 82 to 85 with nasal cannula oxygen flowing at 4 liters per minute.

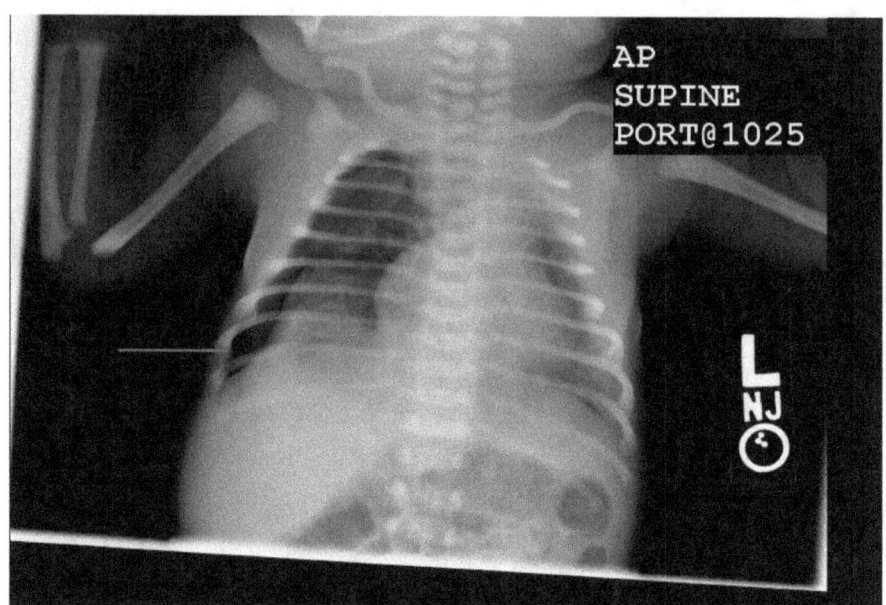

Figure 40. Tension pneumothorax in a newborn with mediastinal shifting.

Nurse, please quickly hand me the 25-gauge butterfly needle, a 3-way stopcock, and a 10 cc syringe.

She looked at me like I had gone mad, but she retrieved it readily.

...After that, have someone else retrieve the small chest trocar and a Pleurovac device. We'll need that as soon as I am finished here.

No. We do not have those up here.

...Yes, we have done this before. Lots of times. Myself, I know.

...I guess I am just much older than you.

...Just set up for a UAC** tray, which you can see is in the cabinet.

...If you dig deep enough, you will also find the sterile trocar buried deeply somewhere in there as well.

...Betadine lotion.

...Alcohol on cotton swabs.

...Now you just twist the stopcock toward me when I tell you to.

I swiftly insert the Butterfly needle in the midline of the subclavicular area of the second rib.

Nothing. I then aim a bit inferiorly.

...Voila.

The air is rapidly evacuated 10 ccs at a time. The nurse and I have become a well-oiled machine now. Even she is impressed. The air stops flowing into the syringe as she pulls on the plunger.

... OK, that makes 55 cc's we have evacuated.

The oximeter is now reading in the 90s.

...Time for the curative chest tube and trocar, please. The transport ambulance often takes 1 to 3 hours to arrive. We cannot wait.

As I sterilely prepare the side chest—palpating the mid-anterior axillary line, the 5th intercostal space, and locating the horizontal nipple line—I will walk the trocar over the superior aspect of the lateral rib, avoiding the inferior aspect (nerves and blood vessels). The mantra from residency is retrieved. I mentally thank neonatologists, Drs. Boyle and Dillard, and ex-residents, Drs. Luther Beasley, Val Wynne, and Sue Harris, among others. They indelibly instilled this into my now pea brain.

The force to penetrate the lung pleura can sometimes be notable. This procedure is life-saving, regardless. Lidocaine was injected into the skin, an incision of the skin was made, and the subcutaneous fat was separated with the clamp. A small opening was made into the chest with the smallest forceps and was covered by my finger on the gauze. I had the nurse stabilize the opposite chest wall, then I exerted some force into the tiny opening I had already made, as I had performed over 30 times before. I used my fingers and a forceps clamp to create a 2cm measured depth for maximum tube insertion. I encountered some resistance with the pointed instrument.

Just a little more force. Then, that unmistakable "curative" pop was discerned. I slide the chest tubing in a few more centimeters. Suction was hooked up.

I breathed more easily now. So did the infant!

NO MEDICAL PROCEDURE IS SIMPLE, HALF THE TIME!

His Oximeter now read in the 80s, so I had the nasal cannula removed, which was set at 4 liters of oxygen, and replaced it with an oxygen mask for the baby. The oximeter moved into the 90s again immediately after the mask was placed on the face. Another perceived deep breath by me.

The repeat chest radiograph now showed near resolution of the pneumothorax. One more step toward saving this baby's life.

Next, I delicately drew the arterial blood gas from his tiny radial artery. Years of practice came into play.

Even before I received the results in five minutes, I instructed the nurses to set up for intubation. His oximeter reading had dropped again. His CO_2 results confirmed my suspicion; it was high.

...*Number 3.5 ET tube.*

...The usual size "0" laryngoscope blade.

...Stylet to the tip of the ET tube.

...Tape.

...The Ambu bag and mask during setup.

...Towel roll under the shoulders.

...Mouth Suction.

It is not working. Why? The Pleurevac plastic suction container is cracked. Scrounging for a new one. Finally, the new Pleurevac is functioning again and bubbling.

...Please, press gently on the trachea when I ask for it.

I have always had trepidation about giving an already respiratory depressed newborn any medication to snow him for this procedure. Besides, the IV was out now.

After some struggling, the supine baby and I get into synchronization. I lifted the mandible firmly with the blade.

With some suctioning, he finally "allowed" me to see the mystical one-centimeter triangular opening. Nothing else in the universe is happening...to me.

The epiglottis had been moved out of the way with the ET blade. I again suctioned the copious secretions. I had the ET tube positioned next to the vocal cords, ready to insert as soon as he inspired and opened his vocal cords. There. Then, I see the ET tube glance off the cords, as the epiglottis flipped down, partially obscuring the cords. This happened during both attempts. We started bagging again.

Could it be? Why was I missing? Why did the cords always seem to flip downwards? I had never experienced this—was the ET blade too short? The baby was only 8 pounds. Blade too short, I guessed?

... Nurse, please hand me a longer number one ET blade.

She found it instantly.

I snapped it on. Twenty seconds later, success! We were ventilating the baby with the Ambu bag attached to the ET tube, and I began happily requesting ventilator settings. The oximeter was now stable in the high 90s.

I drew another radial arterial gas. His pCO_2 was 35, with a pO_2 of 200. Yes!

The tertiary care center's transport team was finally arriving. They took over his care.

Drained and catecholamine-depleted, I proceed to the mother's room to discuss the great progress and good prognosis of her very sick infant.

OMG! I know her well.

She says, "I am glad it was you, Dr. Block. You took such good care of me when I was your patient."

I blush. And say thanks.

I proceed back to the office—to the mundane—where the babies giggle at my big nose and little girls politely tell me I am not so ugly after all.

To all of you neonatal specialists and residents, my deepest appreciation for all you do so willingly and gracefully.

As for me, I have once again experienced the real "tension" in pneumothorax. It will go to the grave with me.

*OMG= oh my gosh!
**UAC= umbilical artery catheter
ET= endotracheal

CHAPTER 11

Peer-Reviewed Breakthrough Research Articles

Simple Country Doctoring While Planting the Seeds for World-Class Pediatric Research

Actually, I am just a "simple country doctor." I initially began as a hayseed in the pediatric research world. Although Jerome Klein, MD, head of the pediatric infectious diseases department at Boston Children's, and the godfather of modern-day ear infections, says, "You should protect your wallet each time someone declares themselves as such." For over four decades, I have practiced full-time office-based general pediatrics "in the country." The small town of Bardstown, KY, with a population of 14,000, is located in central rural Kentucky and is primarily an agricultural community. For those of you who saw the delightful movie *Elizabethtown* by Cameron Crowe, our similar but smaller community is located 25 miles east down the highway. In fact, a "forest" of eight huge grain silos lines the back of our parking lot. And for decades, I have driven a pickup truck. You should try it.

Aside from agriculture/farming, the other major industry here is the production of **bourbon whiskey**. As an article in *USA Today* exclaimed: "*Now that is something to toast about.*" This is the bourbon capital of the world, with over 100 rickhouses or large warehouses for aging bourbon whiskey for up to a decade. For example, we have Jim Beam, Maker's Mark, Heaven Hill, Bardstown Bourbon, Willeits, and Barton distilleries within a 20-mile radius of Bardstown. Bardstown was also noted as one of the Catholic centers of the Eastern U.S., and was formerly one of the five original archdioceses in the U.S. Unlike Boston and New York City, some of these archdiocese cities grew a bit more than others, obviously!

And, my late wife and four lovely daughters always reminded me who the "bosses" are. I am considered the simple boy in the family hierarchy: "You just don't understand, you are just a boy."

In my office practice, even all four-month-old babies giggle at my big nose and silly-looking face; and my teenage female patients too readily agree with my self-disparaging comments about being "big, dumb, and ugly." In discussions with the families, I try to avoid using highfalutin terms (like, what kind of cheese is in hematochezia, anyway?) unless I also use the plain English counterpart. What kind of wood is used to build a "stool" specimen, eh?

More to the Rube than meets the eye, eh?

By contrast, I am asked to review and critique complex articles almost monthly by one of the "top" pediatric journals (*Pediatric Infectious Disease Journal, Pediatrics, Journal of Pediatrics, Vaccine*, etc.) in my spare time. Why? Because of my numerous medical peer-reviewed publications (browse *PubMed* or Google: Advanced search: Authors–Block SL, totaling over 170), my renowned expertise in outpatient care and vaccines, and my willingness to provide high-caliber journals with the real-life perspective of an everyday doctor in the trenches. Very few doctors have the time, expertise, or willingness to spend an extra 4 to 6 hours for FREE, several times a month, while giving their written opinion and recommendations to an erudite medical journal.

I have been fortunate to have been selected to the editorial boards of several prestigious pediatric journals, including *Pediatric Annals, the Pediatric Infectious Disease Journal, Infectious Diseases in Children*, and *Pediatric Drugs*. (For free.) The American Academy of Pediatrics has recognized my invaluable contributions to national pediatric care and research by awarding me the AAP **Practitioner Researcher of the Year i**n 1998. I had also been selected to serve multiple terms on several vital American Academy of Pediatrics national subsection boards. (For free.) Those included the Committee on Pediatric Research; the Section on Pediatric Infectious Diseases; and as executive committee planning member for the **PREP: Infectious Diseases CME** course for 2003, 2005, and 2007. In 2004, among thousands of their graduated physicians, I was awarded the "Distinguished Medical Alumnus" by the University of Kentucky College of Medicine. And recently, in August 2025, I was awarded the prestigious **"Dr. Don Cantley" 2025 Kentucky pediatrician of the year award** by my own peers of the KY chapter of the AAP for "devoting (his) life to improving physical and mental health of children in the local community, and for his passion for the practice of pediatrics" in Kentucky.

Amazingly, for the last 13 years, I have been requested annually by Greg Anderson, PhD, leader of the CDC/NIH national grants committee, to meticulously review three multi-million-dollar grant proposals (100 to 150+ pages of dense, complex issues regarding microbiology surveillance and standard vaccine uptake) which have been submitted to them. This process requires about 40 to 50+ hours of my time to read these complex medical large-scale proposals, to assimilate the details, to write up a thorough assessment on at least three of them, and then to participate in a day-long conference to rate each proposal. They tell me they value the only "in the trenches" practitioner's opinion on the entire committee, which is composed of otherwise elite medical scientists in the U.S. This boy is not afraid to speak up, though. Of course, I get paid next to nothing. I do it because it is a true honor and a part of the thankful reciprocation for all that pediatrics has allowed me to do. Been a busy boy, eh? Financially foolish, though.

In the country: beyond office general pediatrics

Over the past 40 years, our pediatric practice has grown from a quaint two-person group to its present-day bustling 12-practitioner general pediatric practice, along with three retiring older general pediatricians (me too) who had practiced over 40 years each in the same busy outpatient general pediatric group. We had added a new practitioner about every 5 years over the decades. In addition to making an office visit friendly and receptive, this stability and longevity have been a major key to our success. We have also, over the last 30 years, **become arguably the most prolific ambulatory pediatric research group in the United States.** Since the mid-1990s, my partners and I have conducted a plethora of clinical trials annually and have been involved in clinical research for the majority of new vaccines, antibiotics, or ADHD medications available to pediatricians and clinicians.

Thus, a friendly, ambitious, smart private practice office can possibly engender an environment quite suitable for prolific office-based research. Family rapport, great office staff, and stellar reputation have been additional keys to this success. And one foolish person to lead it all.

Now, as for medical writing by a practitioner, that signals a need for a straitjacket. Just like above, when I review articles for medical journals, I have never been paid a dime for the work on any of these over 170 manuscripts, either as a first author or co-author. Imagine your worst college term paper! See, I told you I was a kookie nerd. And a financial genius, eh!!!

Nonetheless, for example, by compiling our own in-office data or working jointly with the NIH or pharmaceutical companies, I have been able to painstakingly write several articles, as first or as co-author, showing changes in microbiology, epidemiology, and treatment of acute otitis media, pneumonia, acute conjunctivitis, ADHD, vaccines, etc. Thus, how does a rube of a country doctor become a principal investigator and author for numerous landmark papers on childhood vaccines and antibiotics, which have been both life-saving and also major morbidity-sparing as well? Let's dig into a bit of it.

Importantly, our philanthropic research patients often may have access to these amazing health discoveries or improvements, 4 to 7 years before anyone else in the world. Of course, some only receive the inert placebo or a non-study "standard of care" vaccine. But they then derive much satisfaction in knowing that they played a key role in furthering the medical knowledge and healthcare for children, teens, and even adults, oftentimes around the world, along with benefiting all future generations as well.

Think of the critical importance of the successes of rotavirus vaccine, pneumococcal vaccines, COVID-19 vaccines, and HPV cancer-preventing vaccines, which several of our patients were able to receive many years earlier than the rest of the world. These were spectacularly successful health-improving projects that I, my partners, and our patients were instrumental in their development.

Working Fool?

And yet, daily, I have been concomitantly working full-time in the office, and see as many or more regular patients than each of my dedicated and superb partners. We identify medical "zebras" or "fascinomas" every other day in this "barn" of daily, mundane illnesses in rural Kentucky. So, one's clinical acumen had better be real sharp here in the country. I also still perform all basic pediatric procedures: circumcisions, tympanocentesis (not for a while), toenail removals, and the alphabet soup of other pediatric procedures such as UACs, IVs, I&Ds, LPs, ABGs, and ET tubes (mostly in neonates).

Our group's philosophy is to take care of any child or adolescent who enters the door, regardless of parental limitations or payment plans, including patients with low-pay (Medicaid, 50%) and no-pay plans (uninsured, 5%). "Take care of the child first, and (usually) the payment will hopefully come later." On the other hand, most private general pediatricians practice in metropolitan or suburban areas, where families are generally more fortunate, affluent, and more likely to be insured. But this is small-town U.S., and one may create ill will and negative gossip by being hoity-toity or by turning a sick child or very anxious parent away. Remember, "listen to the mother." We try to continue our "old school ways." With a wonderful pediatric group also comes a true responsibility to the children and teens of our communities.

And as for one of my crowning achievements, my 3rd daughter (Lindsay Blackmon, MD) has also become a brilliant general pediatrician, and now is the executive director for the entire group of 70 employees and partners. Perhaps another "Chip off the old Block?"

On a realistic note, we really only have four office requirements for patients here: 1) one must be at least minimally respectful and courteous, and not curse or assault our office staff; 2) one must receive all the standard "infant" vaccines in some timely manner. (This is the heart and soul of all preventive pediatric care. See above passages) 3) one cannot threaten our group with assault, lawsuits,, or legal action; 4) one cannot miss more than 3 appointments unexcused (So disrespectful of our time.) In any of those instances, a 30-day notice will be requested for one to seek care elsewhere.

But let's start with a huge ancillary component of our practice, which makes our office truly unique from any other full-time, general pediatric practice in the U.S. For decades, this mega-research component has been directed, spearheaded, and almost entirely run by myself, along with help from Dr. Hedrick. This has required countless unpaid hours/days of extra work and management, along with travel to faraway investigator meetings. I presented intricate, detailed medical abstracts at multiple prestigious national meetings several times a year. I also helped maintain the financing of the hard-working staff of about 15 research folks, along with our head nurse coordinator, Marti Osborne, even during months when no projects were going on. Maintaining this infrastructure was too important.

In summary, I was paid nothing extra by the office for my extra research efforts—ever. To me, the goal was too lofty and too important to quibble about or to jeopardize.

Office-Based Research

I advocate two basic ways to begin planting the NUCLEUS for office-based research:

1. For the more ambitious, the group can apply for a research grant from sources such as the AAP or even a pharmaceutical company. Usually, the grant needs to be sufficient to cover the basic costs of the project. As I have done over the years, it will also involve writing a complete protocol about the project, including the purpose, methods, patient consent, statistical analysis, timeline, and plans to publish, etc. After all, what good is the research data if it merely sits in your file cabinet? This involves a key lead person or investigator (me), who must be truly group-philanthropic and who either enjoys it or is not bothered by the enormous work involved initially and later. But beware, learning the craft is quite time-consuming and requires a true keen sense of intellectual curiosity. Remember, your partners will be MOST encouraging for YOU to do the work.

Example: What If?

In 1985, with our very first grant originating from the American Academy of Pediatrics, within Block and Hedrick's practice (with Chris Harrison, MD, as our mentor and advisor), we examined the following: whether or not the common secondary acute otitis media could be prevented in the young child who initially presented with acute conjunctivitis. All children were treated with topical antibiotic eye ointment, and half of them were randomized to either a placebo or amoxicillin. (Remember, this is an old study.) We found that early treatment with amoxicillin reduced the subsequent rates of AOM by 25% in children with acute conjunctivitis. My first publication was born.

2. For the more economically motivated, participation in pharmaceutically sponsored drug or vaccine trials can both generate

practice prestige, some income, and philanthropic enthusiasm. Breaking into the ranks can be very difficult and risky, though. Thorough, typed charts are recommended. Major unguaranteed capital outlays for hiring personnel to complete case report forms and organize patient flow, and acquiring additional office space are required. Meticulous attention must be given to the following: knowledge of your patient population, understanding your patient's capacity to do the study, careful consent forms, case report forms, follow-up, and all the hidden costs of participating—and there are so many. One can easily lose money without careful consideration of all these factors, which we also found out occasionally, especially when a sponsor went "belly up." Nearly all of these trials are strictly Food and Drug Administration or NIH-monitored, so all aspects of the protocol must be meticulously adhered to. (Prison at Fort Leavenworth is not pretty in the winter, I am told! Unlike the summer???) We have been routinely audited by the FDA over 10 times and have remained unscathed. Their pinpoint checking really does a great service to ensure the integrity of the data for each FDA approval.

Patients/families often appreciate the new or more advanced free medications/vaccines available before anyone else in the world has access to them, along with free medical care, and some modest reimbursement for their time and travel involved with research studies.

Always ask the following before agreeing to the study: "Would I allow my child/teen/spouse to enroll in this study?" If the answer is negative, then the practice should not participate in the study. Furthermore, all physicians and ancillary staff must understand the risks and the benefits of the study. Otherwise, a negative comment can torpedo any research that you are trying to accomplish.

Medical Writing

I entered the world of medical writing when my left ACL blew out. My orthopedic surgeon said I was too old to be acting like a lunatic on the basketball court, my one outlet passion. Creative energies then needed to be displaced elsewhere. For an average doc like me, medical/scientific writing is an art form only achieved with constant practice and repetitive editing.

I liken it to a novice sculptor ("to 'chip' off the old block"), requiring many revisions to achieve the final polished artsy effect. One must be relentless and brain "absCessed," er, obsessed, with the goal of completing the paper. Too many distractions exist out there. I highly recommend having a very seasoned, very smart, and trusted academic cohort (my mentor is often Christopher Harrison, MD) to review and freely comment on your paper, but who also will not ridicule your initial and continued ineptitude.

Several wise books have been published that can help the novice practitioner get started with this process of scientific writing. They provide invaluable ideas about the scientific paper's organization and style. Note: We are not talking about using the iambic pentameter of Shakespeare or the stream of consciousness of James Joyce! Those poetic licenses will never work here. Rather, first consult the Zinsser or *JAMA Textbook of Style* or any number of other textbooks on medical writing.

Clarity, cohesiveness, and simplicity are crucial. (So, someone's simple nature like mine thus becomes an asset.)

Sentences longer than four lines drive me nuts. Emulating and studying the style and works of previous authors on your topic is important. For example, mimic the style of *New England Journal of Medicine* articles. Stick to the facts, and state that your speculations are such—speculations, as these are usually edited anyway. (Thank you, brutal chief editor and friend, George McCracken, MD. Imagine, his review once called me "bombastic.") As you may soon see, one of my personal goals has been to attempt to provide a personal, practical, practice-oriented insight into the implications and applicability of the research results for the practitioner.

1989. Dr. Block Receives National Award for Research (SIDE BAR) article from the Kentucky Standard newspaper

(By Mitchell Douglas, with corrections and edits for accuracy by me.)

Chalk Up a Big Win for a Small-Town Doctor on a Worldwide Scale

Dr. Stan Block, one of five partners who owns the Physicians to Children & Adolescents practice in Bardstown, KY, received the prestigious 1998 Practitioner Researcher Award from the American Academy of Pediatrics last Tuesday.

The annual award, presented at the academy's 1998 annual meeting in San Francisco, recognizes one full-time pediatrician among 100,000 across the United States who has made outstanding and significant advances in the field of pediatrics.

"I look at it as a simple country doctor making important contributions to the everyday care of children throughout the United States and also the world," said Dr. Block...

The academy acknowledged Dr. Block for 16 years of clinically relevant and high-quality research. Block's groundbreaking 1995 article on drug-resistant pneumococcus, published in *the Pediatric Infectious Disease Journal*, was hailed as a "landmark paper." Pneumococcus is a leading cause of acute bacterial respiratory disease, such as ear infections and pneumonia, and kills 40,000 Americans of all ages annually.

In the landmark paper on ear infections, Dr. Block and his own office team were the first in the U.S. and the world to report that the drug-resistant form of *Streptococcus pneumoniae* was very common in children's ear infections.

Dr. Block's practice operates as a research team, compiling data and contributing significantly to the field of pediatric infectious diseases. The research projects are major undertakings, requiring up to two years of research, followed by three to six months of data analysis and an equivalent amount of time for writing. Each paper typically spans six to 12 pages. ("Think of your lengthiest, worst, most complex term paper in college! Yep, that was me help writing it.")

"This is quite an honor. Because of that data we've published over the years, our group is not only nationally but internationally recognized in the world of pediatric and infectious diseases," Block said...

Warp Speed: The COVID-19 Vaccine

Before we move on to my most outstanding publications, I wanted to update you on the role our practice played in the COVID-19 mRNA vaccine development. As you know, COVID-19 killed nearly 1.2 million adults in the U.S. over a two-year period. We had several families where the remaining surviving children were left as orphans when both parents succumbed to infection. Some did not have the vaccine available, but some declined the available vaccine due to internet gossip. (Despite solid medical opinion and science available then.) The fabulous research has been done for you. (We were a key part of it.) And safety issues were actually rare, and much milder, and did not kill like the COVID-19 infection itself.

The deadly, highly contagious epidemic was only halted by the incredibly fast ("warp speed," great job, President Trump!) massive introduction of the two new major COVID-19 vaccines, by Moderna and by Pfizer. They used an older but not previously widely used, highly efficient, life-saving technology known as (Messenger) mRNA. This technology allows a new vaccine to be amazingly produced in less than 1 month– a process which normally takes at least 12 months.

The mRNA technology is fast becoming the best-ever invention in medicine lately (vaccines for TB, HIV, Ebola, medulloblastoma—brain cancer, etc.)

Furthermore, to get vaccines disseminated to the entire population and through the rigorous, tedious FDA process for safety, it required the companies, the FDA workers, and all of us investigator sites to work almost 16-hour days and weekends incessantly, as people were dying overwhelmingly throughout our communities. The hospitals and ICUs were being totally overrun. Makeshift morgues had to house the plethora of dead, nearly all unvaccinated people. Hospital staff were exhausted and terrified at the same time. Brave nurses and doctors at the hospitals often sacrificed not only their entire free time, but often their lives and health as well to care for these critically ill patients. God bless their souls. We were exposed all day long in our offices, too. The medical community was, undeniably, truly heroic.

How did I get involved? All of my voluminous published papers and investigative vaccine work, along with the extremely efficient and accurate research nurses of Kentucky Pediatric and Adult Research, Inc., here in Central Kentucky, came to fruition this decade. Due to my prolific work, a few years earlier, we were selected as one of 7 sites in the world to be granted Pfizer's "golden status." Thus, they priority offered any of their new vaccine projects to our site.

Enter the world of the new COVID-19 mRNA vaccine. This COVID-19 plague was otherwise overwhelming the adult world until the two mRNA vaccines were used.

The COVID-19 mRNA vaccine will be one of the most important medical achievements ever!

It would save so many lives. So, we were chosen as one of 50 worldwide sites to initially enroll adults into the new world-saving vaccine study. Fortunately, as I have stated, our community is very other-oriented and philanthropic in general. And our rapport and stellar reputation were integral. So, in a feverish pitch and with long overtime days and weekends, we were able to enroll over 450 adults in just a few months. We may have saved the lives or health of up to half of the initial enrollees (225). It was an impeccably performed **randomized, placebo-controlled, double-blinded study.** In fact, in this amazing trial of about 43400 adults (FP Polack, *New England Journal of Medicine,* December 2020), this mRNA vaccine showed over 95+% effectiveness in preventing infection, complications, and hospitalizations as well. Crew, it does not get much better than this for any vaccine's protection!

Furthermore, in the first wave of infections, COVID-19 mortality was as high as 20% in unvaccinated older high-risk adults. Thus, with enough data, once the vaccine was given emergency approval within 9 months, we were able to actively vaccinate the other 225 placebo patients immediately, almost before most people could receive it.

In our office, we observed almost no major adverse side effects in any of the study recipients. Much of the confusion about anecdotal side effects of the COVID-19 vaccines stem from 2 things: 1) the single dose Johnson and Johnson vaccine version had some infrequent but very problematic blood clot side effects; and 2) most of the other "reported "major side effects in practices were due to getting infected with the COVID-19 virus within the same time frame as receiving the vaccine. Although it was easy to prove this point, as it could be done through either a nasal swab for COVID-19 (it can often be detected in an asymptomatic or low-grade infection) or a simple antibody test on the blood. The COVID-19 **vaccine** resulted in high "spike protein" antibodies, and **infection** resulted in high "nucleoprotein" antibodies, meaning simultaneous or recent infection. Most of the time, these latter virus-specific nucleoprotein antibodies would disappear in just a week or two, just like the nasal recovery of the COVID-19 virus in acute infection. Wait too long, and one would never know for sure. And <u>much unlike the actual COVID-19 infection,</u> the COVID-19 vaccine heart side effects in mostly young adult males occurred at an exponentially lower rate, and rarely ever required hospitalization, or ever a funeral.

Once again, this example explains why I, our office doctors/NPs, and research staff sacrificed so much, and felt so adamantly about the invaluable contribution that our legendary office research arm continued to make to both patients and science across our own community and the world. And to add to our humanitarian efforts, we were major enrollers of the adolescent group in the world, likely due to our continued earlier efforts to build rapport and to cater to this unique age group. Interestingly, this age niche was my lifelong dream at the start of our practice 40+ years ago in the restaurant with Dr. James Hedrick, my partner. It continues to be so rewarding.

✸ The Pneumococcal Resistance Story: Antibiotic Armageddon?

And the Development of Pediatric Versions of the Pneumococcal Vaccine.

It was the early morning of January 18th, 1992. A cold, dreary day. But a day that would change my life, our practice, and the pediatric world forever. I had perceived that the rate of antibiotic failures of AOM lately had recently been increasing in our practice.

That day, I wandered into our office laboratory and saw that the ear culture on the blood agar plate was growing the most common ear bacteria– pneumococcus– that we recover from a very painful, bad, pus-filled eardrum. It had the typical greenish discoloration and "green" alpha hemolysis (a partial clearing) of the red blood cells on the blood agar plate. Just hold it up to the background lamp. But this one culture plate was different. We had been dropping oxacillin antibiotic disks on these plates for decades to monitor for penicillin resistance of the pneumococcus. (A foolish idea?) In fact, the university lab had called me a few days earlier, and for three consecutive years, they had asked me if I still wanted to survey our pneumococcal ear isolates for **penicillin resistance** using the more expensive and sophisticated MIC method (hinting that it was a waste of my money).

I replied, "Humor the old fool here, because someday I am going to be vindicated for wasting my own practice's research dollars on this Don Quixote venture." (Call me Chicken Little: the sky is falling!)

That was this day. (Don Quixote's "windmill" was actually real in the lab today.) This pneumococcus strain had exhibited absolutely no inhibition of growth right up to the oxacillin disk. That meant I had recovered our first high-level penicillin-resistant (PRSP) strain of pneumococcus, one of the most difficult bacteria to eradicate from any site (bloodstream, meningitis, pneumonia) with customary antibiotics. No customary oral antibiotics for acute otitis media would likely work either, like in this case.

It was time to think outside the "antibiotic box."

Arguably, almost no one in the world had seen this resistant pneumococcal strain in a case of acute otitis media before. No one was looking, actually! The race was on. After a few more cases, the first step was to notify the world-class CDC experts. The next step was to devise a treatment algorithm to treat this incredibly refractory bacterium, which also had the potential to invade as pneumonia and meningitis if it should turn more aggressive and virulent in children.

At this point, no one could actually predict whether it would do so when standard antibiotics did not eradicate it from the middle ear. (As we discovered a few years later, these resistant strains did not tend to invade more, nor were they more pathogenic and destructive than any other pneumococcal strain.) They just did not respond to customary treatments, which could be really problematic and particularly deadly in invasive disease. Thus, high-level esoteric, very narrow-spectrum IV antibiotics like clindamycin, vancomycin, and linezolid had to be used in currently rare invasive diseases with these strains at this point.

And then, vaccine experts/pharmaceutical companies must configure a new version of the infant pneumococcal vaccine to provide protection against these major strains. There are over 90 serotypes (strains) of pneumococcus, which complicates the selection process for a vaccine. In addition, the older "sugar-attached" polysaccharide 23-valent version just did not work in children under the age of 24 months, and it did not prevent the key nasal carriage of bacteria. This was a similar problem we had with the HIB (*Haemophilus influenzae* B vaccine), until brilliant academic and pharmaceutical scientists discovered the way to hook (conjugate) the antigen (inactive bacterial part) onto a protein in the shot. Thank goodness for the diligence and persistence of the pharmaceutical companies—children's best friends.

In 1999, the vaccine manufacturer had just begun convening the world's leading pediatric infectious disease experts in Chicago to discuss the new pneumococcal vaccine formulation. Strangely, this erudite group happened to include me? They needed an ear infection expert that they had worked with. (More story shortly.)

Back to the current pressing office matters.

From this day on, in our office, we continued to sporadically recover several high-level and intermediate-level resistant strains from severe ear infections over the next 6 to 24 months. No current FDA-approved oral antibiotic for AOM was likely to work.

But the good news was that since 1988, I was still continuing to send all my pneumococcal ear isolates to the world-famous pneumococcal expert, Robert Austrian, MD, in Philadelphia for "serotyping." I had to pay for this work out of my own "research pocket," which my partners allowed me to do. But this information would be so critical for picking the most important and most frequent strains, or **serotypes, in vaccine development**. No one else in the world had this window of pneumococcal information open to them–both **antibiotic sensitivities (MICs) AND**

serotypes from the outpatient cases of acute otitis media (AOM). AOM also happens to be by far and away the most common reason for antibiotic prescriptions and office visits in children. Concerns of anti-bacterial resistance from increasing regular usage and overuse were growing exponentially.

I decided to contact the CDC again to report my findings to their respiratory division. When I talked with the chief of the division, Robert Brieman, MD, he was quite nice but also very skeptical at first. After all, where in the heck is Bardstown, and who in the heck is this Block character? (The bourbon imbibing excuse again, eh?)

This report was not from Boston, or Chicago, or UCLA, for that matter. This place was a tiny speck on the map in the midst of farm land. But my persistent science-fiction-like story gained momentum after a while, when I later showed him some more of my MIC data (antibiotic-resistant patterns). I had done my homework thoroughly, it now appeared to him. But in rural Kentucky??? Who is this rube?

In a leap of faith, he subsequently dispatched one of his superb EIS (epidemiologic investigators) officers, Jeff Duchin, MD, to look into additionally working with and surveying the two largest local daycares and the local health department through our office. While stationed here for 2 months, he obtained multitudinous nasal bacterial specimens along with the child's background data to submit to the main CDC lab in Atlanta. I continued my own ongoing bacteriological data analysis on bad ear infections.

Over two years, both the CDC group and I were working in parallel on publishing our findings. My data were perpetually continuing, though. However, once their data was collected after a few months, they wanted to include my preliminary ear infection data as a backdrop to the nasal data without any further elaboration. I had to say no to this suboptimal colossal dilution of my alarming ear findings.

The ear infection data was definitely the most important aspect of either of our observations. I know, because I had to make decisions each day based on the MIC data on an earache when a pneumococcal strain was recovered from that particular patient. Patient care comes first, I explained. These data showed that a lot of shots of Rocephin were essential for the care of our children.

So we separated out each set of data (meaning, I actually just kept my own ear data to write up), and *voila*! The award-winning landmark paper on resistant pneumococcus in ear infections was hatched. I spent weeks tabulating and writing up our ear data. (Like all my freebie scientific articles, no payment was received at any time. What a nerd! Get a hobby!) Both articles were published in the same 1995 issue of *the Pediatric Infectious Disease Journal*.[34]

In addition to the serotypes, my MIC data showed several critical findings on how to treat this highly resistant bacterium, which was heretofore unknown, in an outpatient setting. My thinking outside the box and monitoring daily patient progress were essential here, as you will see.

I went back to my "antibiotic toolbox" and noticed **clindamycin was active against PRSP.** But it was never used for ear infections because it did not cover the other common "gram-negative" bacteria of *Haemophilus or Moraxella*. So, in refractory cases of AOM, one could blindly try clindamycin in anticipation of a resistant strain of pneumococcus. A true gamble, as those other two Gram-negative bacteria can frequently result in antibiotic failure as well.

I also got creative. Perhaps if we doubled the dose of amoxicillin to provide higher concentrations of amoxicillin, we could overwhelm the pneumococcal resistance? And thus by adding standard doses of amoxicillin to the already available amoxicillin-clavulanate (old Augmentin formula), we could empirically treat both groups of bacteria that cause ear infections– the

---

[34] Block SL, et al. Pediatric Infectious Disease Journal. 1995; 14:751-9.

pneumococcus and the *Haemophilus/Moraxella* bacteria. This would later lead to the development of the eventual standard of care antibiotic, **Augmentin-ES**, or high-dose "amox-clav."[35] My concoction seemed to work fairly well, as seen in my papers on this topic. At least we now had one reasonable overall oral antibiotic choice to empirically start treatment. (See article below on amox-clav versus cefdinir.)

Another option I thought worth exploring was treatment with 5-7 consecutive days of intramuscular (IM) or IV ceftriaxone. These children were very ill and feverish with their ear infections, and we were worried about these particular pneumococcal strains escalating to deadly invasive disease. A very scary unknown at this time.

Eventually, over several years, I settled on 3 days consecutively of IM ceftriaxone, which seemed to eradicate the refractory infection most of the time.

(This was the theoretical best guess for that era. However, as effective pneumococcal vaccines became routine over the next 2 decades, I have changed the algorithm for **refractory AOM.** I now recommended starting with a single IM ceftriaxone dose, recheck the ears 5-7 days later, then repeat the second dose only if the ear still appeared infected. The era of resistant pneumococcus was mostly defeated by our ongoing and improving multivalent (13 or more serotypes) newer vaccines.

This latter approach would not be advisable for the unvaccinated or under-vaccinated child! That would often be another fool's errand for them and us. Two or preferably three consecutive IM antibiotic doses, minimum, are needed for this group.

In the meantime, I was trying to disseminate my groundbreaking discovery. So I elected to submit and present my ear infection data for the very first

---

[35] Casey JR, **Block SL**, Hedrick J, Almudevar A, Pichichero ME. Drugs. 2012 Oct 22;72(15):1991-7.

time at the *Society for Pediatric Research* in Washington, DC, in May 1993. My data was selected for a prestigious slide presentation at their largest plenary session. The big time. This was one of my earliest national slide presentations in my career.

So to say I was a bit nervous, yeah, you could say that. I was allowed 9 minutes for data slides and 3 minutes for follow-up audience questions and answers. An eternity on the stage! The latter question portion of the talk was frequently to allow all the ultra-smart and catty doctors and scientists a chance to challenge your data. The room was packed. Dead silence ensued as I strode to the podium.

Sweating a bit, and my heart really thumping.

At this meeting in Washington, DC, over 2000 physicians and scientists from across the U.S. and the world were extremely curious to hear what this unknown hayseed from rural KY had to tell them about the changing resistance patterns of acute otitis media. This resistance phenomenon in outpatient infections had never been seen or reported before. No one was looking for it. Previously, just like in my reference laboratory, we all "knew" that pneumococcus was "always susceptible" to penicillin-like drugs in outpatient settings. Not any more, as I had something no one else in the large audience had.

As my slides would soon point out, I had AOM data identified by our practice's validated real **ear experts**, in cases of **bona fide acute otitis media** outpatients in our rural community practice, many of whom had **failed prior antibiotics**. All the earlier antibiotic clinical trials for acute otitis media in the past had included only pristine ear infections, which I called "virgin" or untreated ear infections as part of the ear clinical trials. And, their study entry requirements often allowed for just including uninfected fluid-filled eardrums and no recoverable bacteria as well, thus terribly skewing the data toward "cure" with some weak antibiotics. Plus, our ear study population was mostly under the age of 24 months, White, in daycare, and again, **many were prior antibiotic failures.** Each of these was a risk factor for failure, and now a high risk for recovering a pneumococcal resistant strain... And almost no centers were testing their pneumococcal isolates for bacterial resistance. (Perhaps only a fool would do that, eh?)

I put up my first two slides.

My laser pointer hand was trembling badly as I tried to control my anxiety. The pointer had now become the infamous "mad moth," bouncing around crazily on the screen, usually missing the PowerPoint target/bullet. "Nerves" and heart pounding still. The audience was loaded with, and intimidating to me, top infectious disease and pediatric experts. So on the next slide #3, I stuck my right forearm under my contralateral armpit and clamped down. Aha! The shakiness disappeared, but I could not turn my body at all toward the audience, unless I rotated it in unison, becoming the comical awkward wooden man syndrome.

Well, my 15 slides passed through clearly and loudly over 9 minutes, and I had announced the new world of pneumococcal antibiotic resistance in AOM was here. First seen in a small rural community and observed by a no-name rube in general pediatrics. Me, the veritable "canary in the coal mine," was a prescient window of what was to affect the rest of the U.S. and the world shortly.

The new pneumococcal protein conjugated vaccine, which we were now concomitantly studying in our office, could not be available soon enough. That would still be another 5 or so years (2000) for the availability of this new, amazing, life-changing pediatric vaccine, which was just now undergoing **placebo-controlled, randomized, double-blinded trials**. (What does it take for a non-medical cabinet head to realize their utter lack of routine vaccine protocol knowledge?)

Oh yeah, about that "question and answer" session—or "goose" the speaker, I call it.

Well, the soft-spoken, kind-hearted Dr. Sam Katz, chief of pediatrics at Duke University, and one of the founding fathers of pediatric infectious diseases and vaccines, stood up before anyone else had a chance. He hogged the microphone, and he lobbed some softball, lofty, homey questions at me. Where did I train? Who was my former chief of staff (Jimmy Simon, MD at Wake Forest—they were good friends)? How big is Bardstown? How many years in practice? How long had I been doing research? How did I get my ear specimens, and so forth? Three minutes were up, and so I returned to my seat—unscathed—with my pulse rate returning to normal in about 30 minutes. No one else had a chance to "disparage" (or pounce on) my talk.

This lecture would be the start of one of my many national presentations on the resistant pneumococcal bacteria in ears, and later lectures about the new pneumococcal conjugate vaccine for young children over the decade.

Now, back to the **pneumococcal vaccine** development story.

It was a snowy, cold wintery day in Bardstown, KY, but Wyeth Lederle vaccine company had convened a "Global advisory board meeting" on "Meeting the challenges of pneumococcal disease prevention" in sunny Jacksonville, FL, in January 1998. Welcome sunshine! Here, the world and the U.S. experts on pneumococcal disease discussed the risks and benefits and approaches to a new vaccine for invasive disease in children. Yes, I was invited to consult, as the only general pediatrician there. Ear infections were not a primary focus– yet.

But then I was invited to the third Wyeth International Global Advisory Board meeting in Washington, DC, in October 1999. This is where my input changed the ✷ trajectory for this new life-saving vaccine.

Sitting around a large round table on this sunny day were the world's premier pneumococcal pediatric infectious disease academic experts, like Drs. George McCracken, John Nelson, Steve Pelton, Steve Black, Colin Marchant, and several other power players. And my supportive colleague,

Dr. Frank Malinoski from Wyeth. I was especially honored to sit directly next to the renowned guru, Boston Children's Dr. Jerome Klein, who was the author of several books and articles on the topic. Like the other doctors, despite their erudite stature, they were all also true gentlemen and mentors to me—the self-deprecating, humorous, humble country doc from the hills.

The Wyeth vaccine company had initially settled on 5 serotypes, or strains, for their new pneumococcal conjugate vaccine. (The new "conjugated" formulation was the only way to make it effective for infants at 2,4,6, and 12 months old.)

By contrast, their simultaneous pneumococcal vaccine competitor, Merck, led by another new colleague, Dr. Paul Mendelman, had selected 7 serotypes. But they were having some difficulty with some modest serotype antibody interference issues and lower antibody serotype levels **in infants** as we were testing their vaccine. (Drs. Mendelman and Malinoski would later co-chair the worldwide development of the Flumist vaccine.) Eventually, Merck decided to stop further testing **in infants** due to these marginal possible vaccine issues **in infants**. The marketplace for vaccines can be quite brutal. However, a new pneumococcal vaccine reformulation was approved by the FDA for individuals over 65 years old.

At this meeting, being the only practicing general pediatrician there, and loaded with my preliminary early ear data, which few in the world had seen, I presented my suggestions.

I showed the experts and the company that serotype 9V specifically was wreaking havoc in younger children's ear infections. We were recovering it fairly commonly (in about 25% of cases), and it was nearly universally moderately resistant to multiple antibiotics, thus causing failure many times.

Although the vaccine was being primarily developed to prevent pneumonia, blood stream infections (bacteremia) and meningitis, I stressed that ear infections were not only often the precursor to serious invasive disease, but they also were the most common reason to prescribe antibiotics (10000+ fold more commonly), thus feeding the increasing antibiotic resistance patterns and the need for more surgical ear tube insertions. Consequently, the costs were escalating as well.

So, Wyeth went back to the production engineers, and their initial five serotype Prevnar vaccine was bolstered to include 7-valent serotypes by adding two more serotypes (4 and 9v) based on my insistence for more outpatient infection coverage. (Note that this protection would also definitely extend to other common infections like acute sinusitis and conjunctivitis.) We in the trenches desperately needed all the childhood protection we could muster against bad ear infections. The routine pediatric use of Prevnar 7 was finally launched in 2000.

My later ear data also continued to have an influence on the next generation of Prevnar, which jumped to a 13-valent vaccine. Because once again, as the "canary in the coal mine" of acute otitis media, I showed them at the 2006 global advisory board meeting, we had observed that 2 new highly resistant serotypes seemed to be not only very increasingly recovered, but were not cross-protected by cousin strains as expected. These were the 6A and 19A serotypes, which were expected to be covered by 6B and 19F in the vaccine, respectively. That did not occur.

Because of the sheer higher volume of outpatient ear infections, this modest "replacement" phenomenon was more noticeable in ear infections than in invasive disease. And additional ear data from the *avant-garde* great scientist-physician, Dr. Pichichero in Rochester, NY, further corroborated our findings. Thus, Prevnar 13 for infants was developed, which we also heavily and gladly tested in our office. It launched in 2010. Newer additional serotype formulations of pneumococcal vaccines are being developed by more companies every year, recently, from 15 to 21 serotypes so far.

🏵 1995. Penicillin-resistant *Streptococcus pneumoniae* in acute otitis media: risk factors, susceptibility patterns, and antimicrobial management

Block SL, et al. *Pediatric Infectious Disease Journal.* 1995; 14:751-9.

From January 1992 to January 1994, penicillin-resistant *Streptococcus pneumoniae* (PRSP) isolates accounted for 48 (17%) of 283 isolates from acute otitis media (AOM) or recurrent AOM in 246 ambulatory patients in rural Kentucky. Relatively penicillin-resistant and highly penicillin-resistant strains were detected in 25 (16%) and 23 (15%), respectively, of 157 pneumococcal middle ear isolates. Highly PRSP strains were almost uniformly susceptible to clindamycin and vancomycin. In contrast, highly PRSP strains were resistant to most oral antimicrobials customarily used for AOM, with alarmingly one-third of strains highly resistant to ceftriaxone, **thus the need for several consecutive days of ceftriaxone.** Serotypes 6B, 19F, and 23F accounted for 95% of highly PRSP strains and **serotype 9V** for 48% of relatively PRSP strains. Otitis-prone condition and the number of antibiotic courses before the day of culture were independently predictive of PRSP. Highly PRSP isolates were more commonly isolated from patients recently treated within 3 days (30%) **[the group no one had looked at previously]** versus those who completed therapy more than 3 days earlier (2%)

1995. High prevalence of multidrug-resistant *Streptococcus pneumoniae* among children in a rural Kentucky community

Duchin J, Breiman R, Diamond A, Lipman H, **Block SL**, et al. *Pediatric Infectious Disease Journal.* 1995;14:745.

To determine the prevalence of **carriage** of drug-resistant S. pneumoniae in the community, we obtained nasopharyngeal swabs from 158 (70%) of 227 children attending a child daycare center and from 82 children attending the county health center. S. pneumoniae was isolated from 126 children. Among 123 isolates tested, 65 (53%) were penicillin-resistant, including 41 (33%) strains that were highly resistant; 61 (50%) were multidrug-resistant. Serotypes 19F, 6B, 23F, and 6A comprised 89% of the penicillin-resistant isolates. Surveillance for drug-resistant pneumococci with the use of respiratory secretions obtained by nasopharyngeal swab may provide useful information on the prevalence of drug-resistant strains causing invasive disease and otitis media.

2001. Restricted use of antibiotic prophylaxis for recurrent acute otitis media in the era of penicillin non-susceptible *Streptococcus pneumoniae*

Block SL, et al. *International Journal of Pediatric Otorhinolaryngology.* 2001; 61:47-60.

Population-based sample of all children born consecutively in two different 13-month intervals. Cohort 1 (n=251) was born before, and Cohort 2 (n=274) was born after the restricted use of antibiotic prophylaxis and the documented emergence of widespread penicillin non-susceptible *Streptococcus pneumoniae* (PNSP=PRSP).

Results: Children were mostly White, with the majority (50-65%) enrolled in daycare during each year. The first episode of AOM was experienced by 6 and 12 months of age in 64% and 86%, respectively. Rates of children with recurrent AOM in Cohorts 1 and 2 were 28% and 31% in Year 1, 17% and 23% in Year 2, and 7% and 10% in Year 3, respectively. The number of days of antibiotic prophylaxis was reduced for each year. For each year, a non-significant trend for increased ventilating tube placement from Cohort 1 to Cohort 2, respectively, was observed: 2% versus 2.2%, 4% versus 5.8% [**note parents, peak tube placement is 12-24 months**], and 0.8% versus 2.6%. **Daycare attendance and White race** were consistently significant risk factors for AOM and recurrent AOM.

✺ 2004. Community-wide vaccination with the PCV7 significantly alters the microbiology of acute otitis media

Block SL, et al. *Pediatric Infectious Disease Journal*. 2004; 23:829-833.

Setting: Since Summer 2000, 94% of young children cared for by this 7-clinician, pediatric practice in rural central Kentucky received 3 or 4 doses of pneumococcal conjugate vaccine (7) in the first 18 months of life.

Methods: Among children 7-24 months old with severe or refractory AOM, we compared 336 AOM isolates from 1992-1998 with 83 AOM isolates from 2000-2003 in children who had received 3 or 4 doses of PCV7.

Results: Comparing each cohort (1992-1998 versus 2000-2003), the proportion of S. pneumoniae decreased from 48% to 31%, and nontypable *Haemophilus influenzae* increased from 41% to 56%; (beta-lactamase-positive, 56% versus 64%, not significant). The proportions of intermediate PNSP and resistant PNSP, respectively, were 16% and 9% versus 13% and 6% pre- and post-PCV7, respectively. Vaccine and vaccine-related serotypes, respectively, comprised 70% and 8% versus 36% and 32% of S. pneumoniae strains (P = 0.003). Post-PCV7, Gram-negative bacteria and beta-lactamase-producing organisms accounted for two-thirds and one-half of all AOM isolates, respectively.

Discussion: The overall proportion of S. pneumoniae isolates and vaccine serotypes in AOM was significantly reduced by community-wide use of PCV7 vaccine in our practice.

✺ 2010. Safety and immunogenicity of PCV13

*Bryant KA, **Block SL**, et al. Pediatrics, 2010: 125; 866-875.*

Objective: Invasive pneumococcal disease rates have declined since immunization with the 7-valent pneumococcal conjugate vaccine (PCV7) (Prevnar) became routine. The safety and immunogenicity of PCV7 were compared with those of 13-valent PCV (PCV13), which contains saccharides from serotypes 1, 3, 4, 5, 6A, 6B, 7F, 9V, 14, 18C, 19A, 19F, and 23F conjugated to CRM(197).

Patients and methods: Infants were randomly assigned to receive PCV13 or PCV7 at ages 2, 4, and 6 months with other vaccines.

Results: Subjects received PCV13 (n = 122) or PCV7 (n = 127). All PCV13 serotypes were immunogenic, with 88% to 98% of infants achieving protective antibody concentrations to shared PCV7 serotypes. For the 6 additional serotypes, 97% to 100% of PCV13-vaccinated infants achieved protective antibody concentrations.

Conclusions: PCV13 was well tolerated and immunogenic.

2012. Comparison of amoxicillin/clavulanic acid high dose with cefdinir in the treatment of acute otitis media

[This amox-clav formulation was very first devised and used in our office for AOM caused by PRSP]

Casey JR, **Block SL**, et al. Drugs. 2012 Oct 22;72(15):1991-7.

Methods: This was an investigator-blind trial in young children 6-24 months old with **no history of recurrent AOM** who were randomly assigned to high-dose amoxicillin/clavulanic acid for 10 days or cefdinir but for only 5 days.

Results: In 330 children (average age 13.1 months) with AOM, high-dose amoxicillin/clavulanic acid-treated children had a better cure rate (86.5%) than cefdinir-treated patients (71.0%; p = 0.001).

Conclusion: In children with bona fide non-refractory AOM, **10 days of high-dose amoxicillin/clavulanic** acid is significantly more effective than only **5 days of cefdinir** as therapy for AOM. (**So don't use cefdinir for 5 days—as 10 days is preferred.)**

The Hepatitis A Vaccine Story

Hepatitis A is a wicked viral infection of the liver in humans, particularly in adults who are often hospitalized, and some even die due to the vomiting, fever, and jaundice from the massive liver destruction, which is typically reversible over time. Although children are occasionally severely infected and rarely die from it, they are the main infectious vector for disease transmission. Before our data and the Werzberger trial in New York were published,[36] we had available only limited, poorly effective, and temporary options to control this transmission process.

The Hasidic Jewish population in an upstate community in New York was undergoing an overwhelming epidemic of this viral infection in the late 1980s. They were subsequently willing to undertake a **randomized, blinded, large placebo-controlled trial** to establish whether a brand new hepatitis A vaccine from Merck could provide protection preventively during a community-wide outbreak. The only way to know was to vaccinate all willing children with either vaccine or placebo, and to compare whether infection rates died down in the vaccine group or not in follow-up after 3 weeks post-vaccine.

However, before the Jewish leaders would consider starting the vaccine trial, they wanted reassurance that the new formulation of the vaccine would not cause any immediate problems. They were very comfortable with someone vaccinating an initial group of 10 children. Thus, because of our stellar research reputation, Merck came to my research group to administer the first 10 initial doses of a new, eventual standard formulation in the world to children. We already knew that it was safe and produced wonderful antibodies to hepatitis A in over 1000 adults. Another earlier, different formulation of the same vaccine had produced similar positive results in hundreds of children.

---

[36] Werzberger, A., Mensch, B., Kuter, et al. A Controlled Trial of a Formalin-Inactivated Hepatitis A Vaccine in Healthy Children. *New England Journal of Medicine*, 1992; *327*(7), 453–457.

Thus, the genesis of the following clinical trial in our Kentucky pediatric population was to examine antibody levels of different hepatitis A formulations, each with a slight tweak in cell line production. Once we had established that no immediate reactions occurred (none were really expected), the Jewish population promptly began their vaccine trial.

This pivotal New York clinical effectiveness vaccine, which was a randomized, **double-blinded, placebo-controlled** trial, was a resounding success, with no breakthrough infections in hepatitis A in child vaccinees after 3 weeks post-administration, unlike the placebo control group, which had 25 cases. Thus, our office efforts and this eventual following publication helped to save countless deaths and hospitalizations in adults, and in some children too. And this hepatitis A vaccine (along with the GSK version) would now become the standard of care in young children in both hepatitis A prophylaxis and in routine immunization schedules, likely for decades, across the U.S. and the world. The pediatric hepatitis A Merck version started its "birth" here in rural KY.

🜲 1993. Safety, tolerability, and immunogenicity of a hepatitis A vaccine (VAQTA) in rural Kentucky children

Block SL, et al. *Pediatric Infectious Disease Journal*. 1993;12:976-980.

This study evaluated the immunogenicity and safety/tolerability profile of an investigational formalin-inactivated hepatitis A virus vaccine (VAQTA; Merck Research Laboratories) in 150 seronegative healthy children, 4 to 12 years old. The vaccine was derived from a virus grown in infected MRC-5 cells in either roller bottles or Nunc cell factories (Nunc, Denmark). Subjects were vaccinated intramuscularly in a two-dose regimen initially and at 24 weeks: Seroconversion from < 10 mIU/ml to > or = 10 mIU/ml by modified HAVAB (Abbott Laboratories) was observed in 99% of subjects at week 4 and persisted in 100% of subjects at week 28 (4 weeks after the second dose). The ranges of geometric mean titers of anti-HAV for all subjects at weeks 4, 24, and 28 were 31 to 49, 51 to 79, and 7059 to

29,609 mIU/ml, respectively. The rise in geometric mean titers after **the booster dose was > 120-fold (huge)** and was highest in the recipients of the 25-unit Nunc cell lot. No serious adverse events were observed.

The Evolving Story of Community-Acquired Pneumonia

The following article, which I wrote with my cohorts, helped to elucidate the causes of outpatient pneumonia or community-acquired pneumonia (CAP). This is also considered by lay folks as "walking pneumonia." This CAP version is usually associated with symptoms of a bad, persistent, productive cough for days or weeks, low-grade fevers, no respiratory distress signs, and rarely does the child appear very sick. On physical examination, the child almost always has diagnostic rales or crackles in the lung fields. Low-grade fever is common, as are occasional lung wheezes and rhonchi (bronchitis musical sounds). Typically, it has normal or mild infiltrates (streaky splotches) on chest X-ray.

This antibiotic comparison article confirmed that this form of milder pneumonia is most commonly caused by *Mycoplasma,* a low-grade grade finicky bacterium that is best detected by nasal swab or (+) antibody tests. In addition, this group of children with similar clinical findings is the first to report that *Chlamydia pneumoniae* (not the sexually transmitted version of *Chlamydia trachomatis*) is also fairly commonly detected by nasal swab or blood titers in these milder pneumonias. With either bacteria, the white blood count is usually normal, and the ESR (blood test for generalized inflammation) is only mildly to moderately elevated in children. This type of pneumonia typically responds well to oral macrolides (like the preferred azithromycin), doxycycline, and cipro-type of antibiotics. These data clearly show that amoxicillin is not a preferred initial choice for CAP due to the amoxicillin bio-mechanical resistance of mycoplasma and chlamydia (they lack a cell wall).

Strangely, the current recommendation for CAP is now amoxicillin, based on minimal CAP data. But rather it is based on pneumococci recovered from nasopharyngeal swabs in Scandinavian children with CAP. Nasal swabs of pneumococci reflect either benign carriage or perhaps sinusitis pathogens, not an organism causing a lung infection. Otherwise, we would routinely use nasal swabs to diagnose the bacteria causing ANY pneumonia.

By contrast, perhaps these amoxicillin recommendations are based on the diagnosis of "pneumonia," which often conjures up thoughts of the patient with high fever, sick looking, lobar rales of pneumonia on exam, and a socked-in infiltrate on chest X-ray. This very select, very rare group of pediatric patients is distinctly different from the CAP in our outpatient studies. And its usual cause in pediatric febrile outpatients is pneumococcal bacteria, sometimes associated with bacteremia. But this form of severe pneumonia was very rare in healthy populations in the past, and dramatically even fewer cases have been observed with the routine use of newer pneumococcal vaccines in children. In this earlier study, the population of our 250 children with milder chest X-ray confirmed pneumonia and who were otherwise healthy, no blood cultures were positive for pneumococcus. This lack of pneumococci findings was later verified by the larger, similar azithromycin study of CAP by Harris et al.[37] This other rare type of feverish, sicker patient in the office often has a blood culture obtained (but very infrequently positive for pneumococcus) and typically requires 1 to 3 doses of parenteral ceftriaxone daily and possible hospitalization depending on severity.

----

[37] Harris JA,. Safety and efficacy of azithromycin in the treatment of community-acquired pneumonia in children. *Pediatr Infect Dis J.* 1998 Oct;17(10):865-71.

✵ 1995. *Mycoplasma pneumoniae* and *Chlamydia pneumoniae* in pediatric community-acquired pneumonia: comparative efficacy and safety of clarithromycin vs. erythromycin ethylsuccinate

Block S, et al. *Pediatr Infect Dis J.* 1995 Jun;14(6):471-7.

We evaluated 260 previously healthy children ages 3 through 12 years who had clinical signs and symptoms of pneumonia, radiographically confirmed. Evidence of infection with *Chlamydia pneumoniae* was detected in 28% (74) of patients: 13% (34) by nasopharyngeal culture and 18% (48) by serology. Evidence of infection with *Mycoplasma pneumoniae* was detected in 27% (69) of patients: 20% (53) by nasopharyngeal culture or PCR and 17% (44) by serology (ELISA). For clarithromycin versus erythromycin, respectively, clinical success was 98% (121 of 124) versus 95% (105 of 110); radiologic success 98% (109 of 111) versus 94% (92 of 110). Ten days of clarithromycin or erythromycin were similarly effective and safe for the treatment of radiographically proved, community-acquired pneumonia in children older than 2 years old.

The Early ADHD Story About Management and Testing, and the Use Of Atomoxetine for ADHD

1998. Attention-deficit disorder. A paradigm for psychotropic medication intervention in pediatrics

Block SL. *Pediatr Clin North Am.* 1998 Oct;45(5):1053-83.

Pediatricians frequently encounter patients with behavioral or academic problems in clinical practice. Assessing and managing these patients requires awareness of the numerous physical, emotional, and psychological causes. Because of their limited contact with these patients during a routine visit, pediatricians, as a minimum, should rely on careful parental and social history, teachers' evaluations by checklist, achievement test scores and grades, and the clinicians' own gestalt regarding patients' behavior. This article provides a framework that practitioners can incorporate into their routine office practices. Practitioners must also be knowledgeable about different forms of ADD and learning disabilities, differential diagnosis, and frequently encountered comorbidities. This was a modest armamentarium of psychotropic drugs potentially available, with subtle differences in pharmacokinetics, rates of efficacy, and adverse effects. Appropriate behavioral intervention, educational assessment, and placement when necessary are also essential for optimal management. Enabling the child or adolescent to achieve success in school, to experience positive social interactions, and to regain self-esteem are the more rewarding facets of pediatric care.

Atomoxetine (Strattera)

As part of my ADHD repertoire of clinical studies, this study demonstrates that clinicians should start dosing atomoxetine in the evening for the first 2 weeks for fewer side effects and fewer dropouts, then switch to morning dosing for improved efficacy from there on.

2009. Once-daily atomoxetine for treating pediatric attention-deficit/hyperactivity disorder: comparison of morning and evening dosing

Block SL, et al. *Clinical Pediatrics* 2009:48;723-733.

In this 3-arm, randomized, double-blind trial, once-daily morning-dosed atomoxetine, evening-dosed atomoxetine, and placebo were compared for treating pediatric attention-deficit/hyperactivity disorder (ADHD). Patients received morning atomoxetine (n = 102), evening atomoxetine (n = 93), or placebo (n = 93) for about 6 weeks. Core symptom efficacy was measured at weeks 0, 1, 3, and 6. In the first two weeks, morning-dosed and evening-dosed atomoxetine significantly decreased core ADHD symptoms relative to placebo and produced symptom improvements that were measured up to 24 hours later. Morning dosing was superior to evening dosing on some efficacy measures. But, evening dosing showed greater tolerability with significantly more patients receiving morning atomoxetine reporting at least 1 adverse event than those receiving evening atomoxetine.

The Rotavirus Vaccine Story

For decades, one of the most frustrating (for parents and doctors) and horrible viral illnesses that young children and infants became infected with was the rotavirus. It causes massive diarrhea and usually unrelenting vomiting along with frequent high fevers. The children are absolutely miserable for days, have major problems with drinking fluids, and tolerate no solids for days. It typically can be a prolonged illness for 2-3 weeks as well, especially in babies. And, it can infect children 2 or 3 times a season, due to its multiple sub-strains.

Before the vaccine, **1 in 15 children would wind up in the ER for IV Fluids, and 1 in 75 would need to be hospitalized.** Every child would become infected with it, and there was almost no medical intervention available except for lots of clear liquids (Pedialyte, etc.) at home, either until the symptoms finally receded or the child became too dehydrated to survive without IV fluids. It also killed about 100 children a year in the U.S., and killed millions of children worldwide. Its devastation was legendary in the pediatric medical world.

I am so happy to report that this rotavirus illness has nearly disappeared from the medical world in the U.S. due to the investment, diligence, and perseverance of Merck and GSK vaccine developers. And my research group was a leading enroller in one of the two first clinical trials, which were very integral to its FDA approval. I am myself even the first author on one of the first landmark publications from the Merck vaccine version, as seen below, where we present the data on both the vaccine's superior efficacy and the robust production of rotavirus antibodies in a **double-blinded, placebo-controlled, randomized trial** in American and Finnish children.

(Again, I have no idea where any government health executive cabinet members get the notion that the initial few FDA vaccine studies of any of the newer vaccines did NOT use a placebo control or double blinding in the clinical trials. That is pure mythology on their part, and lacks any credibility on their part.)

✺ 2007. Efficacy, immunogenicity, and safety of a pentavalent human-bovine (WC3) reassortant rotavirus vaccine...

Block SL, et al *Pediatrics*. 2007 Jan;119(1):11-8.

Background: Rotavirus is the leading cause of dehydrating acute gastroenteritis in infants worldwide. Previous studies of a live pentavalent human-bovine reassortant rotavirus vaccine have shown it to be efficacious across a range of potencies.

Patients and methods: During 2002-2004, 1312 healthy infants, approximately 6 to 12 weeks old, from the United States (47%) and Finland (53%) were randomly assigned to receive 3 oral doses of vaccine or placebo approximately 4 to 10 weeks apart. Infants were to be followed for acute gastroenteritis through 1 rotavirus season after vaccination and for adverse events postvaccination.

Results: Three doses of pentavalent rotavirus vaccine at the end of shelf life demonstrated efficacy against rotavirus gastroenteritis caused by human G-serotypes included in the vaccine (G1-G4). **Efficacy against severe rotavirus gastroenteritis was 100%,** and efficacy against any rotavirus gastroenteritis, regardless of severity, was 72.5%. A threefold rise in G1 serum neutralizing was observed in 57% and in anti-rotavirus immunoglobulin A in 96% of pentavalent rotavirus vaccine recipients.

Daunting Practicalities of In-Office Pediatric Influenza, Flu and You: Research and Me

(Adapted from Block SL. The daunting practicalities of in-office pediatric influenza vaccination: 2009-2010. *Pediatric Annals*. 2009)

As I read the summary article on seasonal influenza vaccination in my August 2013 issue of The *Pediatric Infectious Disease Journal* (of which I am an editorial board member), I realized that, yes, colleagues, this annual chore is imminent. For the next several months, you must now attempt to immunize nearly anybody and everybody who comes through your doors older than age 6 months with an influenza vaccine. And even the families of 2- and 4-month-old infants must be reminded and targeted for future "jabs" of the flu vaccine. The Centers for Disease Control and Prevention, the American Academy of Pediatrics, and even the trial lawyers say so. (Yes, litigation might occur for failing to vaccinate!)

So you must beg, cajole, humor, plead, chastise, and castigate about the importance of the influenza vaccine for every not-yet-fully vaccinated pediatric patient. Ironically, you might be held legally accountable even for vaccinating patients whom you will not see during the year or see when no vaccine is available, according to malpractice attorneys. (Wow, extortion at its finest.)

Similar to my earlier discussion about flu vaccines in the December 2009 issue of *Pediatric Annals*, you again are facing the "daunting practicalities" of picking which flu vaccine formulation (plus nasal versus shot) to offer first to each patient. Except for the nasal Flumist vaccine, it will often come down to pricing issues and age limits as to which company's injectable product we select.

For the live intranasal vaccine (Flumist, MedImmune), the transition will be simple, as only a single formulation will be available. (It is also available over the counter now, but not likely to be covered this way.) For each of the pediatric influenza injectables, an option seems to be limited to a three-strain formulation this year.

However, I expect the 4-strain version, which includes the second B strain, to become the preferred option again in the future years. With the constant annual fluctuation of flu strains, aside from the slightly higher cost, insurance coverage issues, and supply issues of quadrivalent vaccines, why would one choose the trivalent shot anymore? But the CDC has dropped the 4th strain of B type at least for this year, 2025.

The two families of B strains (Yamagata and Victoria) together account for up to 25% of circulating influenza strains and cause epidemics every 2 to 4 years. The specific predominant B family "drifts" back and forth. When the trivalent vaccine B strain mismatches, as it has in 6 of the last 12 years, "B" cross-protection is weak to absent. Greenberg et al summarized clearly the possible benefits over a decade of adding an additional B influenza family strain to make a quadrivalent shot formulation: 2.7 million fewer infections, 21,000 fewer hospitalizations, and 1,400 fewer deaths. Yet, the CDC has elected to incorporate only one B strain, at least for this year?

Thus, allow me to share the following with my several reports on influenza and its vaccines, including the newly arrived quadrivalent live attenuated influenza vaccine (QLAIV). In the last decade, I happened to be heavily involved (mostly as first or second author) in these multiple recent, interesting, and important multicenter, peer-reviewed publications on influenza. I hope they will serve as an important resource for practitioners during the upcoming flu seasons. As a typical science nerd, I specifically received no compensation for the large quantities of time and energy involved in the writing and crafting of these manuscripts, which I have summarized here for you.

Finally, no single-dose flu vaccines or other vaccines have contained thimerosal (for two decades), so we can stop beating that dead horse, please. In 2025, the CDC has just banned the use of thimerosal (a mercury sterilizer) in any vaccine.

💥 The Advent of Flumist

As background for the initial, incredibly complex, large-scale Flumist vaccine study, the protocol and study intricacies were developed with the cooperation of the National Institute of Health and the 13 major research sites across the U.S., including Bardstown, KY.[38] (Once again, the big city strikes.) The trial had to start just before the advent of that year's flu season, and we had to enroll and start vaccinating, with most getting two doses in over 1500 children from age 15 months to 5 years at 13 major U.S. centers (1 minor in population) in about a month. The speed and skill of each site was pushed to the limits to get it done correctly and rapidly. Like the COVID-19 vaccine, we all worked overtime, weekends, and nights toward the goal. And then the thorough, detailed illness and follow-up visits promptly started, lasting over half a year (the flu season), requiring nasal flu cultures for any minor or major upper respiratory illness or fever, with some children getting 5 to 10 nasal swabs over the time span. In this study, a single dose of Flumist was highly effective (89%) versus 2 doses (94%) versus placebo. The rates of fever and ear infections were also reduced with the vaccine.

Our site employed over 10 research nurses to obtain these massive amounts of data from our rural patient study population. Once again, nearly all of the over 100 patients were enrolled from our own office site and were not recruited outside the practice. This greatly improved both compliance with the protocol and the follow-up for the visits.

Guess what? Just like all the initial studies on all new vaccines, this study was a **placebo-controlled, double-blinded, randomized study.**

---

[38] Belshe, R. B., Edwards, K. M., Vesikari, T., Black, S. V., Walker, R. E., Hultquist, M., Kemble, G., & Connor, E. M. (2007). Live Attenuated versus Inactivated Influenza Vaccine in Infants and Young Children. *New England Journal of Medicine, 356*(7), 685–696.

2012. Studies of Intranasal QLAIV (Flumist) (some WITH inclusion of 2 B Strains)

Block SL, et al. *Pediatr Infect Dis J. 31:745-751.*

This immunologic bridging study led to the FDA approval of QLAIV (quadrivalent flumist with 4 flu strains) in pediatrics. Using FDA standards, we found that QLAIV was immunologically non-inferior to two different trivalent single B formulations (T-LAIV) for geometric mean titers (GMT). A total of 2,312 healthy patients aged 2 to 17 years were studied: Influenza-vaccine-naïve patients aged 2 to 8 years received two doses; those aged 9 to 17 years received a single dose. Individual adverse events were comparable between vaccines except for fever (5.1% versus 3.1%); no vaccine-related serious adverse events were reported.

2011. A randomized, double-blind, noninferiority study of quadrivalent live attenuated influenza vaccine in adults.

Block SL, et al. *Vaccine.* 2011;29(50):9391-9397.

This additional immunologic bridging study led to the FDA approval of QLAIV (Flumist) in adults. Using FDA standards, we found that QLAIV was immunologically non-inferior to two different trivalent single B formulations (T-LAIV - Flumist) for geometric mean titers (GMT). A total of 1,800 healthy patients aged 18 to 49 years received a single dose of intranasal vaccine.

Pearl for Practice: If needed, the new formulation of QLAIV (including two B strains) could provide important additional protection because of some major chance of encountering a mismatched B strain observed with previous trivalent vaccines.

2013. T-LAIV and Acute Otitis Media (AOM) (an earlier study with inclusion of three flu strains)

Heikkinen T, **Block SL**, et al. *Pediatr Infect Dis J.* 2013;32(6):669-674.

2011. The efficacy of live attenuated influenza vaccine against influenza-associated acute otitis media in children.

Block SL, et al. *Pediatr Infect Dis J.* 2011;30(3):203-207.

Taken together, these two separate meta-analyses of six double-blind, placebo, randomized controlled trials (RCTs) and two double-blind trivalent IIV (T-IIV or flu shot) controlled RCTs in 24,046 children aged 6 to 83 months showed the following:

- Among children with influenza *and* AOM (ear infection), T-LAIV (Flumist) was 85% more effective than placebo and 54% more effective than T-IIV for preventing AOM;
- Among influenza vaccine failures, T-LAIV (Flumist) still reduced rates of secondary AOM by 38% compared with placebo; and
- For an entire 12-month period, T-LAIV reduced rates of all causes of AOM by an estimated 7.5% (12.4% in vaccine-naïve children; 6.2% in the second year) when compared with placebo. This reduction in AOM was comparable to the earliest estimated rates of AOM reduction from PCV7 (Prevnar7).

Pearl for Practice: If you wish to reduce rates of AOM, administer an annual flu vaccine, with a particular preference for Flumist in healthy children older than 24 months.

2008. T-LAIV (Flumist) and Post-Vaccine Virus Shedding.

Block SL, et al. *Vaccine.* 2008;26(38):4940-4946.

This elegant and very labor-intensive open-label trial evaluated the frequency and quantity of viral shedding after an intranasal dose of T-LAIV by obtaining nasal swabs for vaccine virus daily on days 1 to 7, every other day on days 9 to 25, and then on day 28. Three age cohorts ($n = 344$) were studied: 5- to 8-year-olds; 9- to 17-year-olds; and 18- to 49-year-olds. Within these respective cohorts, 44%, 27% and 17% of subjects shed vaccine virus. Maximum shedding occurred on days 2 to 3, but in low quantities

(CFU [colony forming units of flu] of 105, 104, and 103 respectively.) Virus was undetectable after days 10, 6, and 6, respectively.

Pearl for Practice: These data strongly support the current recommendation that LAIV recipients need to only avoid contact with the severely immunosuppressed, and for only 7 days after vaccination.

✶ 2009. Efficacy of T-LAIV (Flumist) Single Dose.

Block SL, et al.C. *Clin Ther.* 2009;31(10):2140-2147.

This post-hoc analysis of the single-dose efficacy of T-LAIV when compared with placebo in three different RCT studies showed a reduction of influenza attack rates by 60%, 72%, and 87%. Also, during the second year after two doses of T-LAIV in the first year only, vaccine effectiveness still remained at 55%. All of the adverse reaction events were reduced with the second dose when compared with the first dose.

Pearl for Practice: The nearly **70% plus efficacy with a single dose of LAIV** should be a vital public health issue. Why? Nearly 50% of vaccine-naïve children never receive their second dose, which renders the injectable flu vaccine nearly useless **as a single first dose only** during that initial first season. Also, most of the mild vaccine reactions with T-LAIV are related to the first dose only in children. Thus, **flu vaccine-naive children** should preferentially receive Flumist, IMHO.

2012. Cell-Culture–Derived TIV (flu shot) for Children and Adults.

Vesikari T, **Block SL**, et al. *Infect Dis J.* 2012;31(5):494-500.

2009. Immunogenicity, safety and reactogenicity of a *mammalian cell–culture–derived* influenza vaccine in healthy children and adolescents three to seventeen years of age.

Reisinger K, **Block S**L, et al. *J Infect Dis.* 2009;200(6):849-857.

In a blinded RCT, more than 3,600 children aged 3 to 8 years and 9 to 17 years were given either cell-culture–derived T-IIV (CC-IIV) or T-IIV (single dose in vaccine-naïve children older than 9 years). CC-IIV was non-inferior. For more than 600 adults (18-50 years old), no difference in immunogenicity was observed in the RCT. Overall, safety and adverse events were comparable in all age groups.

Pearl for Practice: Compared with egg-derived T-IIV, this new "doggy-derived" flu shot vaccine formulation can be mass-produced about twice as fast, allows for the use of a better-matched flu antigen, and finally (Yes!) avoids any hint of a problem for egg-allergic patients.

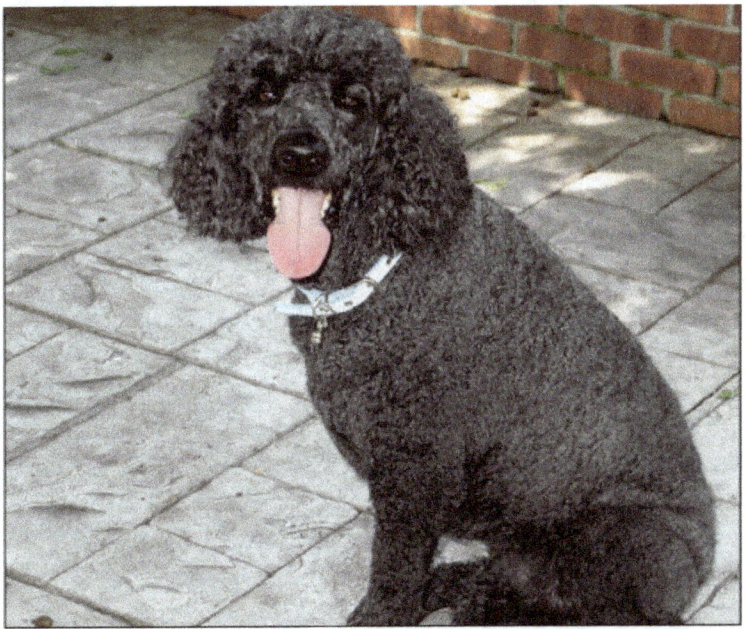

Figure 41. Elle: A happy-to-help (non-literal) representation of a potential source for the canine kidney cells to produce one of the two new non-egg versions of the influenza vaccine—an important scientific development for the faster mass production of influenza vaccines, and for the improved safety in severely egg-allergic children. This method allows a more precise match to the anticipated circulating strains. **And, standard poodles DO NOT SHED. She died just before my wife did. (See earlier chapter.)**
Source: Dr. Block

Vaccine Logistics and Burnout

2011. Timing of the availability and administration of influenza vaccine through the Vaccines for Children Program.

Bhatt P, **Block SL**, et al *Pediatr Infect Dis J*. 2011;30(2):100-106.

2010. A prospective observational study of U.S. in-office pediatric influenza vaccination during the 2007-2009 influenza seasons: use and factors associated with increased vaccination rates.

Bhatt P, **Block SL,** et al. *Clin Pediatr*. 2010;49(10):954-963.

These two studies assessed the effects of office logistics upon flu vaccination in 42 practices during the 2007-2008 season and in 84 practices during the 2008- 2009 season. Shipments of influenza vaccine arrived 4 to 5 weeks later for Vaccine for Children (VFC, mostly Medicaid) recipients than for private insurance recipients. Again, only one-half of all vaccine-naïve children received their second dose, and vaccine rates were 17% to 19% lower in VFC children, probably related to their shorter interval to vaccinate. About 80% of all flu vaccines were administered between October and December, suggesting some type of clinician "vaccine burnout" and "saturation-point" after several months of "begging" by clinicians.

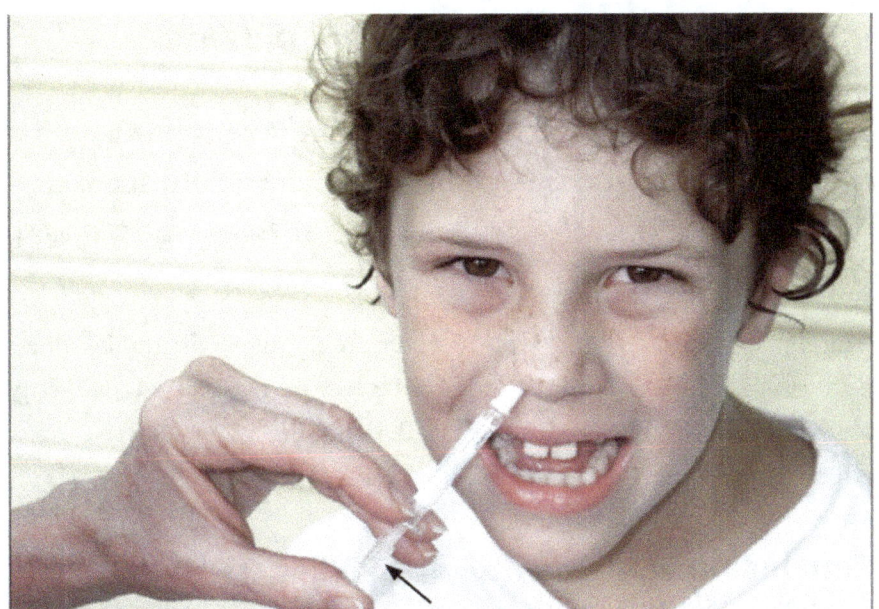

Figure 42. My first grandson, at age 7 (not crying!), while receiving the intranasal live, attenuated influenza vaccination. Note the plastic stopper on the syringe plunger (see arrow), which allows the delivery of the first one-half of the dose to one nostril.
Source: Dr. Block

Children's Vaccine Preferences

2011. Children's perceptions of influenza illness and preferences for influenza vaccine.

Flood EM, **Block SL**, et al. *J Pediatr Health Care.* 2011;25(3):171-179.

A small qualitative survey of 28 children showed that children aged as young as 8 years could understand vaccine rationales, and they would prefer a nasal influenza vaccine over a shot. (Figure 42)

Rates of AOM with Treatment of Influenza

2010. Impact of oseltamivir Tamiflu treatment on the incidence and course of AOM in children with influenza.

Winther B, **Block SL**, et al. *Int J Pediatr Otorhinolaryngol.* 2010;74(6):684-688.

Among 695 children aged 1 to 12 years presenting with flu-like illness during this RCT, **oseltamivir reduced rates of flu-related AOM by almost half** versus placebo recipients (12.4% versus 21.7%), with the largest effect in 1- to 2-year-olds.

Conclusion: A highly PRODUCTIVE 6 YEARS for me and flu vaccines

As a springboard from these papers, more effective flu vaccines—including the addition of a second B strain, the wider use of intranasal LAIV, along with early use of oseltamivir in cases of flu should reduce flu attack rates and rates of AOM, possible flu complications, and antibacterial resistance. Flu vaccine distribution for Medicaid children needs notable improvement.

Clinical Pearl: Tamiflu. The Treatment for Early Acute Influenza

Note that the earlier you start taking Tamiflu, the quicker the abatement of illness is. Thus, starting it within the first 12 to 24 hours will basically stop flu illness within one-half to one day.

As many of my readers may be aware, Oseltamivir on an empty stomach will way too often trigger nausea and vomiting—extremely commonly. I think that it is much higher than the FDA-reported rate of 16% in children. I also think that this higher dosing of Oseltamivir may be worsening the problem, and it was a mistake on the part of the CDC.

Why? How can we prevent the Tamiflu (oseltamivir) GI side effects?

We conducted the original clinical trials in our office with Oseltamivir for flu in the 1990s. Using the higher current dose in the study initially increased the vomiting GI problem. And a few months into the study, if I remember correctly, we started to switch to the lower dose, and most importantly, subjects were told to give orange sherbet (how "British" of Gilead Pharmaceuticals!) just before each dose of the drug. Coating the stomach seemed to alleviate this GI problem immensely. So for years, to improve compliance, I tell all my Tamiflu/Oseltamivir patients to administer the following tastier sweet options pre-dose: sherbet, yogurt, or pudding. I prefer to simplify dosing by using 3mg/kg/dose and 2mg/kg/dose for under 12 months versus older than 12 months respectively (max 75mg/dose).

Also, the fear of increased risk of seizures and delirium with Tamiflu (oseltamivir) was reported mostly in Japanese patients. One must remember that flu itself causes both delirium with high fevers routinely, and that febrile seizures under age 5 years are very commonly triggered by the high fevers of flu as well. No real excess signal for this problem with oseltamivir has been detected in the VAERS reporting or in more recent U.S. analyses that I am aware of, other than baseline or background expectations from flu illness. The only exception is the child with underlying seizure or neuropsychiatric disorders. In my opinion, the benefits of Tamiflu still far exceed the risks here. Thus, Tamiflu is routinely recommended in early cases of flu.

HPV vaccines

2007. Pursuit of Happiness Versus The Reality of HPV

Adapted from Block, SL, in *Infectious Diseases in Children* 2007

A Girl's Declaration of Independence: "Life, liberty, and the pursuit of happiness" —**Thomas Jefferson, 1776**

Every day I learn something new in my office. The following was one of many similar difficult cases that I had seen recently.

The 16-year-old girl from Bullitt County, whom I have seen frequently over the last five years, called the office for a consultation. She had a remarkably troubled background: depression, living with her grandparents, removed from her home because of wayward, drug-using parents, and she had been recently placed in a temporary shelter for out-of-control behavior. She had just returned from living at a girls' shelter for six months.

During the past two years, petulant and rebellious, she had demanded and obtained the freedom to act like an adult—to run around with any boy she chose, to drink whenever, etc. As Patrick Henry cautioned more than two centuries ago, "Suffer not yourselves to be betrayed with a kiss." She wanted all of this by age 13. Such is the exaggerated risk of having no stable parent.

Life Decision

She requested to see me specifically for a discussion—the magnitude of which was astounding.

While in temporary custody, she recently discovered during a routine PAP exam in 1999 that she was afflicted with high-grade 3 cervical precancer (a routine exam for contraception during that decade pre-HPV vaccine). This, in turn, meant she would need a major portion of her cervix removed, which would possibly prevent her from completing a later pregnancy of her own due to the resultant cervical incompetence from the surgery. Less extensive surgery would increase her grave risk for full-blown cervical cancer.

She was asking me, as her pediatrician and her long-time child advocate, for a second opinion. This was not my expertise in any way, but I did tell her that this treatment was very standard for gynecologists and that I would gladly send her to one of my friends in that field for a second opinion. A quite painful and life-altering surgery must be decided quickly. At least three surgical options awaited her, and each must then be interpreted from her teenage perspective.

She was flabbergasted and terribly saddened, to say the least. I could not provide her with any other way out of the trap her lifestyle had laid. Ironically, she had just missed the availability of the new HPV4 vaccination—too late for this young lady who had so many risky behaviors!

The Importance of Self-Care

As her seemingly surrogate father figure in the office, I had befriended her and rationalized with her over the years about the importance of taking care of herself first. I had persuaded her to take her oral contraceptives last year, and I had cajoled her to respect the rules of her home. I explained to her that she would have to sacrifice for her immediate personal well-being first, and extirpate the precancer, or else she would face a potentially deadly silent nemesis. She was finally realizing that this possibly meant no childbearing in her future if she selected the safest surgical option.

This life and death decision at age 16? This kind of devastating decision is not supposed to strike until the adult years. And she had no real parents to guide her.

The Incredulous Rapid Attack of HPV

The truly incredulous part was the rapidity of her HPV's deadly onset—sexual activity at age 13 and ominous cancerous changes within two years—which perhaps should serve as a call to arms for the medical field. According to current guidelines, physicians/providers are not even supposed to obtain PAP smears until age 25. This may need some exceptions to the rule for the highly promiscuous teen.

So why are the younger patients at risk for such severe and rapid disease? Four probable reasons:

- Inadequate production of cervical mucus

- Immature columnar epithelial cells in the transformation zone of the cervix
- Incomplete local cervical immunity
- Increased cervical susceptibility to minor trauma during sexual intercourse

---

"Sir, We Have Done Everything That Could Be Done
to Avert the Storm Which Is Now Coming On."
—Patrick Henry, 1775

Maybe Changes to Office Procedure

This specific case, like several others in this decade, could affect our office procedure for numerous teenage girls, many of whom also happen to be sexually active with multiple partners. But routine HPV9 will have stopped most of this devastation in its tracks for those who choose to receive it. Thus:

First, we must continue to vigorously recruit the young female preadolescents (as young as age 9) and adolescents for the HPV9 vaccine (Gardasil 9, Merck).

Second, we should [perhaps consider initiating the first PAP SELF-screening earlier, by age 21 or within 3 years after sexual debut, particularly for higher-risk teens who have not received the HPV9. A home test self-swab has just become available for HPV/PAP screening! A great alternative.

And note, the current HPV9 vaccine will protect against over 90% of cervical cancers and precancers. We have made amazing strides for our young women. Now, if only we can convince the parents about the critical importance of preventing these deadly associated HPV cancers by getting the HPV9 for their daughters and sons. This would prevent most of the wicked specific 5 cancers in girls and 3 cancers in boys.

"The Pursuit of Happiness"

How monumental are the choices most teenage girls must balance?

- Abstinence and/or pregnancy prevention versus "love" lost?
- Sexually transmitted disease and its prevention versus parental discovery/discipline? (And HPV virus can often circumvent condoms, latex sheaths, and parental commands.)
- Human desire versus tempered restraint?

Each of these dilemmas creates diametrically opposed issues and their own respective dire consequences in the teenage mindset.

She left the office teary-eyed and gave me a hug. She thanked me for taking the time to listen and advise her. Some nights, I don't sleep so well.

✴ The Gardasil Story: HPV Vaccines

One of my most exciting lifetime accomplishments has been my major involvement (13 research studies/articles) in the development of the HPV vaccines for preteen and teen populations. No vaccine, in my opinion, compares to the population benefits of the HPV4 and then the HPV9 Gardasil vaccines, **especially for women.** In the late 1990s and 2000s, it was staggering to learn how many of my older teenagers, younger mothers, and adult women in my own office had been stricken by a cervical precancer/cancer and all of its accompanying biopsies, terror, miscarriages from cervical incompetence, costs, and pain from this virus. Add to that, we were continually observing several women in the community who were either on chemotherapy for cervical cancer, or dying from cervical cancer (Refer to HPV story on good choices: see article above).

To know that I and my research office have been an integral major part of this HPV vaccine incorporation into routine teen care is incredible. What other country doctor can claim that they have been fundamental in helping to save over 40,000 U.S. lives annually from a devastating cancer, and to prevent over three-quarters of a million women from terrifying and disfiguring precancers, with the likelihood that many of these would have become full-blown cancers? **Over 10 years, that amounts to sparing 400,000 women/men from certain cancers' death, and 7.5 million females from precancers in the USA!**

Furthermore, in 2006, I was the **first author** of the very first paper on the **randomized placebo-controlled double-blinded trial** of HPV4 for the intended vaccine target: pre-teens and teens. I was also instrumental in persuading that the 2-dose data on HPV4 were included in the paper after much internal debate. Why? The paper's essential word count for the journal requirements was already borderline. Plus, I was battling another counterargument: the doses were only two months apart in this earliest study. Importantly, we had observed that these antibody levels after two doses were two-thirds of the 3-dose schedule. This was still exponentially better than those antibody levels achieved from natural infection's known lifetime protection. The other concern: Scientifically, the two-dose data were in no way a primary objective as well, but rather an incidental finding. Typically, these data would not be included in the seminal paper as well. "Damn the torpedoes, full speed ahead," eh? So, my suggestion: let's get the medical world to help, not just me, to decide the importance of the 2-dose data.

But my persistence paid off. It led to the next iteration of a simpler dosing change for HPV4 for those under age 15. And thus, it further spawned a 2-dose HPV9 schedule 6 months apart as seen in our later *JAMA* article on HPV9.[39] This would now become the current FDA standard for the population of recipients younger than 15 y.o..

In addition, as a full-time practicing general pediatrician with about a 25% adolescent population, I knew the huge hazards of incomplete vaccine

---

[39] Iversen OE, Miranda MJ, Ulied A, Soerdal T, Lazarus E, Chokephaibulkit K, **Block SL**, et al. Immunogenicity of the 9-Valent HPV Vaccine Using 2-Dose Regimens in Girls and Boys vs a 3-Dose Regimen in Women. *JAMA. 2016 Dec 13;316*(22):2411-2421.

schedules when trying to complete three doses of any vaccine, whether cancer-preventing or not!!! And for any teenager or pre-teen, administering any shot is a battle more often than not! Furthermore, this previously "required" 3-dose schedule often scared off many families of 9 to 15-year-old children.

Parents thought: You mean it will take three shots to fully protect my little angel? That seemed unreasonable for many folks—so why bother with any doses?

If we could only confirm that after two doses, and by testing it instead at six months apart, to show that the antibody levels were still incredibly high, as they were in this first study that I wrote. And yet we knew that these antibody levels we observed earlier after two doses were still way beyond what was considered a protective level, even compared with natural infection's immunity levels. But it was going to take a second FDA-sanctioned study to get FDA approval for the two-dose schedule into routine use.

What about all the recent brouhaha of using even a **single-dose schedule for HPV9**? I say, proceed with great caution. It looks promising, perhaps. And, if that is the only shot one can accomplish, hey, I will accept that. But I have major reservations about any non-live vaccine's **durability** with a single shot. For non-live vaccines, the immune system almost always requires a priming dose, then at least one additional booster dose. That is just how the antibody-producing organs of the immune system work! Especially since the shot is being administered mostly to pre-teens and young teens, whose durability of protection is most essential after age 15 years and beyond, when sexual activity becomes more commonplace. Will single-dose protection last 10 to 20 years? Thus, I say: **stick** with a two-shot HPV9 schedule for the younger patients. Pun intended. This is too deadly a disease to gamble on.

Vexing Vaccination Issues for Adolescents 2007

(Adapted from Block SL in *Infectious Diseases in Children* 2007)

Vaccinating adolescents demands a unique approach for patients and parents.

As I try to fit another vaccination into the already crowded immunization schedule (and this time for adolescents!), I feel obligated to explain why I need to give this mother's pre-adolescent or teenage daughter (son) three shots at the present visit. The tears usually tend to inundate the young daughter's cheeks. How am I going to reassure her and find the time to explain to this mother (or father) and daughter that these vaccines are worthwhile, and that they are safe?

Please note that I have raised four teenage daughters. I thus empathize with facing the trepidation of teenage needle-phobia. I have experienced the exasperation of attempting to rationalize to a daughter the necessity of protecting our family members from strange, rare, and distant "exotic" diseases. After all, who is going to ever personally see pertussis, meningococcal invasive disease, or even cervical cancers or precancers? (Not my angels.)

Unfortunately, these dangerous diseases are still continuously present or floating just beneath the surface.

Why vaccinate for HPV?

The new nine-valent human papillomavirus vaccine (HPV9, Gardasil9, Merck) is recommended with two critical explanations that should always be stated upfront to families:

First, this is a vaccine that can prevent a huge number of cases of common female/male cancer/precancers, venereal warts, abnormal Pap smears, colposcopies, cervical and vaginal surgeries, and tremendous associated cancer anxiety.

Second, most insurance companies or Vaccines For Children (VFC) funds cover most or all of its expensive cost.

Seven high-risk HPV Serotypes account for over 90% of all cervical/genital/(posterior) oral precancers/cancers, and serotypes 6 and 11 account for 90% of all venereal warts. The primary reason for giving this vaccine is its efficacy. Yes, in scientifically sound clinical trials (the first with HPV4 were **randomized, placebo-controlled**), the vaccine is nearly 100% effective in preventing cancer invasion caused by the 7 type-specific strains. Compared with the pre-vaccine era, this would translate overall, for the serotype-naive (that is, most 9- to 15-year-olds and about 85% of 16- to 25-year-olds), to a 90% reduction in all cervical precancers/cancers. Thus, a girl's lifetime risk for a devastating cervical precancer drops from 1 in 20 to 1 in 100 patients. And a lifetime risk for venereal warts likewise drops from 1 in 10 to 1 in 100 of all recipients.

A few decades ago, pre-Gardasil, we had been witnessing similar ominous changes in our practice as well, with a notable number of older adolescent females developing grade-2 or even grade-3 cervical lesions (see above story), and that risk has nearly been eliminated with the HPV9 vaccine.

Other Considerations

Durability

Protection has been documented for 10 years in our now adult women in the long-term clinical trials for HPV9.[40] These established data mean most likely HPV9 will provide lifetime protection, as we know from previous other vaccine data. So the issue remains: when giving the two doses of HPV9 vaccine to a 10- or 12-year-old, can we expect the vaccine to show nearly lifetime longevity? I say yes.

---

[40] Moreira ED, Block SL, et al. Safety Profile of the 9-Valent HPV Vaccine: A Combined Analysis of 7 Phase III Clinical Trials. *Pediatrics. 2016 Aug;138*(2):e20154387.million

REMEMBER adolescents have a higher frequency of cervical HPV acquisition after sexual debut (37% to 55%), higher susceptibility to infection, and higher frequency of <u>severe</u> cervical disease (seven-fold), as our earlier case above demonstrated. Thus, starting vaccination at age 9, 10, or 11 seems like a prudent approach. Especially since 5% of girls have become sexually active by age 13 y.o., and 25% by 15 y.o.

Safety

With several millions of doses already administered across the world, almost no isolated major adverse events—other than background noise or a preventable 10% rate of post-shot syncope—have been reported. Please ensure that patients remain seated for at least 15 minutes after vaccination, which stops this latter problem. We should also warn our patients that minor local reaction rates per dose approximate the following: sore arm (50%), redness (10%), swelling (10%), with severe local reactions in about one in 100.

Morality

I cannot really argue religious beliefs when it comes to giving a vaccine to prevent cancer for one's daughter. My only three questions for those parents who ask about its morality are:

1.   Would I give this vaccine to my daughters? (So, do you believe me, the AAP, and the CDC or not?) Me—**yes, 100%.**
2.   Will giving the tetanus (TDaP) booster promote your daughter's stepping on rusty nails? Me—**no way. Thus, this HPV9 will not promote sexual activity either. Three studies have confirmed this.**
3.   And finally, "You know my daughters (and my sons) are perfect angels too. Isn't it all those other boys (or girls) that you cannot trust?" (OUCH!) She or he is likely going to marry one of "those people" one day and may be exposed to HPV then if they are sadly not vaccine-protected. The vaccine is nearly 100% protective for

over 90% of strains of HPV pre-exposure. Perhaps, jokingly, just like kennels check our dogs for rabies vaccine status, check the dating partner for HPV9 status before they start commingling? (LOL) Remember, HPV status is almost never known in males or young females. It hurts to use the "girls are better than boys" or vice versa argument. But girls do bear the brunt of HPV cancers and precancers overall.

The following is a handout I give to any of my fence sitters or reluctant families regarding Gardasil9 for their child or teenager. It has been published across the U.S. by the national bookstore, *Scholastic Books*.

✸ Pediatrician, Stan L. Block, M.D. Answers Questions about Human Papillomavirus (HPV) Vaccine: A handout for parents

1. What are some of the common misconceptions among parents about the HPV vaccine?

Many parents believe the vaccine can actually cause their child to contract HPV infection. The truth is, there is *no* live HPV virus in the vaccine, just the inactivated virus shell. Thus, **your child *cannot* contract the virus from being vaccinated.**

Parents also tell me they believe the HPV vaccine may be dangerous or that it hasn't been studied long enough. The HPV vaccine has been available and distributed for more than two dozen years. In a recent study of first-generation HPV vaccines published by the Pediatric Infectious Disease Journal, we analyzed worldwide studies of more than three million pre-adolescents, adolescents, and adults from various countries over 10 years. The data showed *no* increase in the incidence of serious adverse events that parents will often bring up, such as autoimmune diseases, blood clots, and neurological conditions.

To date, more than 200 million doses of the HPV vaccine have been given worldwide. In 20 years, I have administered over 20,000 doses in our office without any notable side effects other than the short-lived (1 to 2 days) mild to moderate headaches, sore arms, low-grade fever, or malaise.

2. What do you say to parents who ask: Why does my child need the HPV vaccine? And why do they need it so young?

We have been searching for vaccines to prevent cancer for decades! You now have a specific cancer prevention vaccine at your fingertips with just a small injection (two or three times) for your children and teens. No months or years of radiation, surgery, or chemotherapy to treat these cancers. No more loss of life for a third of these cancer patients.

The HPV9 vaccine is a thoroughly studied cancer-prevention vaccine that can effectively prevent about 90 percent of at least five kinds of cancers and pre-cancers (cervical, vulvar, vaginal, penile, and anal cancers), as well as perhaps up to 50 percent of oropharyngeal cancers—cancer of the back of the throat, including the base of the tongue and tonsils. That means prevention of over 40,000 cancers annually in the U.S., according to the Centers for Disease Control (CDC).

In addition, by administering the HPV9 vaccine, we can now prevent 85-90 percent of high-grade and 50 percent of low-grade cervical pre-cancers in women. These have previously been documented at a terrifying annual rate in the U.S., with over a quarter million high-grade and half a million low-grade pre-cancers.

We know that vaccinating our children—both boys and girls—starting at 9 to 11 years old will provide the best protection possible since it is way before the start of any kind of sexual activity. The vaccine is most effective if it is received *before* they are exposed to HPV infection—preventive measures similar to most other recommended childhood vaccines. And importantly, the rate of worrisome adverse events versus really just background noise is almost zero at this age. (e.g., ovarian failure, arthritis, blood clots, neurologic conditions, etc. They do not typically become an issue until after 15 years old, long after any vaccine-related concerns if HPV9 is given at the younger age.)

3. What do you say to parents who think their child won't get HPV because they are not yet sexually active, or they believe receiving the HPV vaccination is a pass to start having sex?

In my opinion, there is no vaccine that we currently give to our kids that is more important and that prevents more devastating disease and death in this century. But sadly, it's all because of the sexual connotation that we're avoiding the discussion. We must stop this epidemic! Three different studies have shown that receiving this vaccine does *not* promote adolescent sexual relations.

Just to put things into perspective: without the vaccine, <u>25 percent of _all_ people</u> are going to end up infected with a high-risk strain of HPV at some point in their lifetimes. And, they can pass on this risky HPV infection for <u>up to two years</u>.

Half of the unvaccinated girls who have *not* been sexually active and are negative for HPV will wind up with HPV by the time they graduate from college. Without the vaccine, one in 20 girls will develop a surgically treated pre-cancer (cervical, vaginal, or vulvar). But the rate drops to one in 100 in those who receive the HPV9 vaccine before age 15. Those are statistics that speak volumes and should make every parent run to vaccinate their children against HPV.

4. Would you get the vaccine for your children?

Absolutely! And I have four daughters. Who doesn't want to avoid the devastation and mortality of cancer? The HPV9 vaccine is over 99.5 percent effective in preventing the nine strains of virus that it includes. And these nine strains account for over 90 percent of cervical pre-cancers/cancers and from 80 to 90 percent of vulvar, vaginal, anal, and penile cancers, as well as 90 percent of deadly posterior oropharyngeal cancers. That means each year, the HPV9 vaccination will prevent over 40,000 future cancers in boys and girls. Historically, of those 40,000 new cancer patients, one-third would die, and the other two-thirds could develop major complications after radiation, chemotherapy, or surgery. In addition, the vaccine will prevent 90 percent of disfiguring and difficult-to-treat venereal warts in both genders.

5. What do you say to parents who have fears and doubts about the vaccine's effectiveness and/or safety?

An ounce of this prevention is worth over a thousand pounds of cure—radiation, chemotherapy, and surgeries. Physicians have seen too much death, destruction, and devastation during their careers from these specific cancers that can now be prevented with two doses of a simple, effective, and very safe vaccine.

When parents tell me they've seen scary things about the HPV vaccine online or their child shouldn't get the vaccine because they aren't old enough to have sex, or that they will meet the "perfect future spouse" who also has not been exposed to the virus, I implore them to reconsider. We are talking about a vaccine preventing horrific cancers and pre-cancers here. And this is a studied and scientifically documented safe way to prevent many cancers and precancers.

Thus, the HPV vaccine could end up saving your child's life and reproductive health. Do *not* let the sexual inference or internet fear-mongers get in the way of that. Finally, spend a week helping in the gynecologic cancer ward, and then tell me prevention with the vaccine is not worth it.

Stan. L Block M.D. is a pediatrician who has been treating and vaccinating children and teens for more than 4 decades. He was

president of Kentucky Pediatric and Adult Research, Inc., and a member of the Medical Advisory Board for Think About the Link®, an education campaign developed by the Prevent Cancer Foundation® to increase awareness of the connection between certain viruses and cancer.

Landmark paper!!!!!! First HPV4 data comparison ever in the true targeted group for vaccine: pre-teens and teens.

✵ 2006. Comparison of the immunogenicity and reactogenicity of a prophylactic HPV4 vaccine in male and female pre-adolescents, adolescents, and young adult women

(Adapted from **Block SL,** et al. *Pediatrics* 2006; 118:2135-2145.)

Objective: Prophylactic vaccination of 16- to 23-year-old females with HPV4 (types 6, 11, 16, 18) L1 virus-like particle vaccine has been shown to prevent type-specific human papillomavirus infection and associated clinical disease. As a surrogate for effectiveness, we conducted a noninferiority immunogenicity study to **bridge** the previous efficacy findings in young women to preadolescent and adolescent girls and boys, who represent a primary target for human papillomavirus vaccination. There is no way to test for vaccine effectiveness against actual infection in this younger population.

Methods: We enrolled 506 girls and 510 boys (10-15 years of age) and 513 females (16-23 years of age). Participants were vaccinated on day 1, at month 2, and at month 6, and serology testing was performed on day 1 and at months 3 and 7 on blinded samples.

Results: By month 7, seroconversion rates were > or = 99% for all four human papillomavirus types in each group. By month 7, compared with women, anti-human papillomavirus geometric mean titers in girls or boys were noninferior and were 1.7- to 2.7-fold higher. Most (> 97%) injection-site adverse events were mild to moderate in intensity.

Conclusions: Noninferior immunogenic responses to all four human papillomavirus types in the quadrivalent vaccine **permit the bridging of efficacy data that were generated in young women to girls**. The results in boys lend support for the implementation of gender-neutral human papillomavirus vaccination programs. Two-dose data need further investigation. This vaccine was generally well-tolerated.

✸ 2016. Safety Profile of the 9-Valent HPV Vaccine: A Combined Analysis of 7 Phase III Clinical Trials

Moreira ED Jr, **Block SL**, Ferris D, et al. *Pediatrics*. 2016 Aug;138(2):e20154387.

Objectives: The overall safety profile of the 9-valent human papillomavirus (9vHPV) vaccine was evaluated across 7 Phase III studies, conducted in males and females (nonpregnant at entry), 9 to 26 years of age.

Methods: Vaccination was administered as a 3-dose regimen at day 1, and months 2 and 6. More than 15,000 subjects received ≥1 dose of HPV9 vaccine. In two of the studies, >7000 control subjects received ≥1 dose of HPV4 vaccine.

Results: The most common AEs (≥5%) experienced by HPV9 vaccine recipients were injection-site AEs (pain, swelling, erythema) and vaccine-related systemic AEs (headache, pyrexia). Injection-site AEs were more common in HPV9 vaccine than in qHPV vaccine recipients; most were mild-to-moderate in intensity. Discontinuations and vaccine-related serious AEs were rare (0.1% and <0.1%, respectively). Seven deaths were reported; none were considered vaccine-related. The proportions of pregnancies with adverse outcomes were within ranges reported in the general population.

Conclusions: The HPV9 vaccine was generally well tolerated in subjects aged 9 to 26 years with an AE profile similar to that of the HPV4 vaccine; injection-site AEs were more common with the HPV9 vaccine.

The following study is the result of my push to consider a two-dose regimen as a result of our incidental finding in the 2006 pediatric study.

✵ 2016. Immunogenicity of the HPV9 Using 2-Dose Regimens in Girls and Boys Versus a 3-Dose Regimen in Women

Iversen OE, Miranda MJ, Ulied A, Soerdal T, Lazarus E, Chokephaibulkit K, **Block SL**, et al. JAMA. 2016 Dec 13;316(22):2411-2421.

Importance: The HPV9 vaccine protects against 7 high-risk types of HPV responsible for 90% of cervical cancers and two other HPV types accounting for 90% of genital warts.

Design, setting, and participants: Open-label, noninferiority, immunogenicity trial conducted at 52 ambulatory care sites in 15 countries. Five cohorts were enrolled.

Interventions: Two doses of the HPV9 vaccine administered 6 or 12 months apart versus three doses administered over 6 months.

Results: Of the 1518 participants (753 girls [mean age, 11.4 years]; 451 boys [mean age, 11.5 years]; and 314 adolescent girls and young women [mean age, 21.0 years]), data from 1377 were analyzed. At 4 weeks after the last dose, HPV antibody responses in girls and boys given 2 doses were noninferior to HPV antibody responses in adolescent girls and young women given three doses (P < .001 for each HPV type).

Conclusions and relevance: Among girls and boys aged 9 to 14 years receiving 2-dose regimens of a HPV9 vaccine separated by 6 or 12 months, antibody levels 4 weeks after the last dose was noninferior to a 3-dose regimen in a cohort of adolescent girls and young women.

�֎ 2017. Human Papillomavirus (HPV4) Vaccine in Preadolescents and Adolescents After 10 Years

Ferris DG, Samakoses R, **Block SL**, et al. *Pediatrics*. 2017 Dec;140(6):e20163947.

Objectives: We describe the final 10-year data for the long-term follow-up study of the HPV4 vaccine in preadolescents and adolescents.

Results: For HPV types 6, 11, 16, and 18, 89% to 96% of subjects remained seropositive through 10 years postvaccination. The preadolescents had 38% to 65% higher geometric mean titers at month 7, which remained 16% to 42% higher at 10 years compared with adolescents. No cases of HPV type 6, 11, 16, and 18-related diseases were observed. No new serious adverse events were reported through 10 years.

Conclusions: A 3-dose regimen of the HPV4 vaccine was immunogenic, clinically effective, and generally well tolerated in preadolescents and adolescents during 10 years of follow-up.

The following data show that the protection of 2 or 3 doses of the HPV9 vaccine will most likely last a lifetime.

2023. Ten-Year Follow-up of HPV9: Immunogenicity, Effectiveness, and Safety

Restrepo J, Herrera T, Samakoses R, Reina JC, Pitisuttithum P, Ulied A, Bekker LG, Moreira ED, Olsson SE, **Block SL**, et al. *Pediatrics*. 2023 Oct 1;152(4):e2022060993.

Method: Boys (n= 5 301) and girls (n= 5 971) who received three HPV9 vaccine doses in the base study (day 1, months 2 and 6) enrolled in the extension.

Results: Geometric mean antibody titers peaked around month 7, decreased sharply between months 7 and 12, then gradually declined through month 126. Seropositivity rates remained 95% by immunoglobulin G-Luminex immunoassay at month 126 for each HPV9 vaccine type. After a median 10.0 years of follow-up postdose 3, there were no cases of HPV6/11/16/18/31/33/45/52/58-related high-grade intraepithelial neoplasia or condyloma in males or females.

Conclusions: The HPV9 vaccine demonstrated sustained immunogenicity and effectiveness through 10 years post three doses of HPV9 vaccination of boys and girls aged 9 to 15 years.

New Meningococcal Vaccines: Can't be used fast enough for my patients!

As you can surmise from my earlier case studies, I have a particularly keen interest in meningococcal vaccines for children and teenagers. Having personally witnessed and been terrified by 10 cases of this deadly and devastating bacteria in my 40+ year career, I am getting tired of the intense fear and anxiety this rare infection invokes for both my patients, families, and me. It is one of the most horrific diseases that a physician can manage. I have been lucky that my outcomes have all been successful so far (guardian angels, thanks!)

My research group and I have been integrally involved with the development of different formulations and dosing of this superb vaccine by two different companies. Most recently, I am proud to be the first author on the currently just available, most broad-based version, which now includes the five major serotypes, or strains, of the meningococcal vaccine. The alphabet soup including types A, B, C, W, and Y has been an arduous road. The inclusion of very complex serotype B into the five-valent version has been an extremely complicated bioengineering feat, and the companies are to be congratulated for their diligent work. Over time, compared with the pre-vaccine era, we may expect up to a 90% drop in cases of deadly meningococcal invasive disease in all pre-teens and teens. The next step will be figuring out a schedule for younger children. Few diseases are more terrifying for physicians and families than when encountering this disease.

2019. Men ACWY-CRM (MCV4) conjugate vaccine booster dose given 4-6 years after priming in adolescents and adults

Tipton M, Daly W, Senders S, **Block SL**, et al. Vaccine. 2019. 30;37(42):6171-6179.

Background: Vaccination strategies against bacterial meningitis vary across countries. In the United States, a single dose of quadrivalent meningococcal conjugate vaccine (Men ACWY) is recommended at 11-12 years of age, with a booster dose approximately 5 years later.

Methods: In this phase IIIb, multicenter, open-label study, healthy 15-55-year-olds, who received Men ACWY-**CRM** (Sanofi) (N = 301) or Men ACWY-**D** (GSK) (N = 300) 4-6 years earlier or were meningococcal vaccine-naïve (N = 100), received a single Men ACWY-**CRM** vaccine dose.

Results: Percentages of participants with hSBA seroresponse at 28 days post-vaccination were >75% for each serogroup in those primed with either the Men ACWY-CRM or Men ACWY-D vaccine. Seroresponse was observed in ≥93% of primed participants and ≥36% of naïve participants 28 days post-vaccination. At 5 days post-booster, among primed participants, hSBA titers ≥1:8 were achieved in ≥47% of participants for Men A and in ≥86% of participants for Men C, Men W, and Men Y,

Conclusions: A booster dose of the Men ACWY-**CRM** vaccine induced a robust and rapid anamnestic [good immune memory] response in adolescents and adults, irrespective of whether Men ACWY-CRM or Men ACWY-D vaccine was first administered 4-6 years earlier. The safety profile was acceptable.

✴ 2015. A comparative evaluation of two investigational meningococcal ABCWY vaccine formulations

Block SL, et al. *Vaccine*. 2015 May 15;33(21):2500-10.

Background: This 5-valent version will eventually be the only MCV version available, since it includes all five major Men serotypes in a single shot.

Methods: A total of 484 healthy 10–25-year-old participants were randomized to receive two doses, two months apart, of an investigational MCV 5 (Men ABCWY - five serotypes) versus placebo.

Results: Seroresponse rates for serogroups ACWY were significantly higher after two doses of either MCV5 formulations than after one dose of standard MCV4-D (Sanofi), respectively, A: 90–92% versus 73%; C: 93–95% versus 63%; W: 80–84% versus 65%; and Y: 90–92% versus 75%. Both MCV5 formulations induced substantial immune responses against several serogroup B "test" strains. No vaccine-related serious adverse events were reported.

Conclusions: Both investigational Men ABCWY formulations elicited robust immune responses against serogroups ACWY and serogroup B test strains, and had acceptable reactogenicity profiles, with no safety concerns identified.

The New Vaccine to protect the Unborn Child (to be given to pregnant mothers)

Group B beta strep is a far distant cousin to the group A strep of sore throat. Unlike strep throat, its primary target for its attack is the newborn baby and occasionally the genitourinary tract of a mother. Like the meningococcus bacteria, it primarily causes deadly and devastating bloodstream and meningitis infections. Unlike the meningococcus, GBBS has alarmingly common high infection rates, as it used to infect 1 in 200 newborns in the past. Thankfully, obstetricians have notably dampened the frequency of this infection by preventively administering intravenous antibiotics to the high-risk or culture-positive mother prior to delivery. But many babies are still slipping through the cracks of this approach.

GBBS has two age groups for attack: the 0 to 7 days early onset version and the 7 to 60 days late onset version, with typically two slightly different manifestations. When the pediatrician or neonatologist, with very high levels of observation and diligence, encounters this deadly or devastating bacteria, it is worse than a fire drill. We are often looking at shock and life-or-death predicaments for this fragile newborn.

With our recent vaccine work on a GBBS6 vaccine for healthy adults (as reported here), and eventually for use in pregnant mothers, this bacterial infection could become a relic like measles. Oops. To do that, mothers would have to be willing to protect their babies based on our good science and advice, and ignore the perpetual internet naysayers.

I am proud to tell you that we were one of 4 sites in the world to provide the very first testing of this marvelous vaccine to eventually protect the innocent, immunologically fragile newborn.

✖ 2021. Safety and immunogenicity of a novel hexavalent Group B strep conjugate vaccine in healthy, non-pregnant adults

Absalon J, Segall N, **Block SL**, et al. *Lancet Infect Dis.* 2021 Feb;21(2):263-274.

Background: Group B strep (GBS) is a major cause of invasive disease in young infants. Maternal immunization is a potential strategy for prevention. We aimed to assess the safety and immunogenicity of a novel hexavalent (serotypes Ia, Ib, II, III, IV, and V) GBS conjugate vaccine (GBS6).

Methods: This phase 1/2, placebo-controlled, observer-blinded, dose-escalation trial was done at four clinical research centres in the U.S. (Kentucky, Georgia, and two sites in Utah). Healthy, non-pregnant adults aged 18-49 years were randomly assigned.

Findings: 364 patients (52 in each dose group) were vaccinated and included in the safety analysis. Three participants reported at least one serious adverse event during the study; none were considered related to the vaccine. GBS serotype-specific IgG geometric mean antibodies increased by 1 week after vaccination for all GBS6 groups, peaked at 2 weeks, stabilised by 1 month, and declined gradually but remained higher than placebo at 6 months.

Interpretation: GBS6 was well tolerated in healthy adults and elicited robust immune responses for all dose levels and formulations that persisted 6 months after vaccination.

Do Pressure Equalizing Ear Tubes Work?

In this National Institute of Health-sponsored study from Pittsburgh and Bardstown, this "PE tube for ears" study showed only minimal benefit to the insertion of tubes for the child with recurrent and frequent episodes of AOM. Yet, as a practitioner for 40+ years, I have often found that PE tubes will have a major benefit in the real world when careful diagnostic criteria and diligent pediatricians examine ears, like in our own pediatric practice. We often see children from urgent care centers and ERs who do not have a bona fide ear infection upon follow-up examination within a few days. They are busy clinicians and may not often take the time to clean the ear canals, a common problem, or they often use very suboptimal instruments, speculums, and weak batteries for their lights.

I believe that PE tubes can still be a game changer for some young children who are highly prone to ear infections or refractory to medication, even if the effects observed here are very modest. So if you have a child in the higher risk factors group–especially a strong family history, under 24 months old, AOM onset before 6 months old, winter season, day care attendee, male, White race, or smoke exposure, do not be alarmed if we still tell you that the child will likely benefit some from PE tubes for recurrent AOM.

2021 Tympanostomy Tubes or Medical Management for Recurrent Acute Otitis Media

Hoberman A, Preciado D, Paradise JL, Chi DH, Haralam M, **Block SL,** et al. N Engl J Med. 2021 May 13;384(19):1789-1799.

Methods: We randomly assigned children 6 to 35 months of age who had had at least three episodes of acute otitis media within 6 months, or at least four episodes within 12 months with at least one episode within the preceding 6 months, to either undergo tympanostomy-tube placement or receive medical management involving episodic antimicrobial treatment.

Results: The rate (±SE) of episodes of acute otitis media per child-year during a 2-year period was 1.48 ± 0.08 in the tympanostomy-tube group and 1.56 ± 0.08 in the medical-management group (P = 0.66). The frequency distribution of episodes of acute otitis media, the percentage of episodes considered to be severe, and antimicrobial resistance among respiratory isolates were not reduced with tubes.

Conclusions: Among children 6 to 35 months of age with recurrent acute otitis media, the rate of episodes of acute otitis media during a 2-year period was not significantly lower with tympanostomy-tube placement than with medical management.

Acknowledgements

Any mistakes or errors in the book are mine entirely, as I painstakingly crafted and wrote the entire danged thing. Being like one of RFK, Jr.'s telepathically-diagnosed "mitochondrially-challenged" people, what else was I going to do with my free time? (LOL.) I was not thrilled with other options of mall-madness, wrestling rings, fishing, hunting, 4-wheeling, and honky-tonking Jimmy Buffett-style days. Bad knees and a bad back prevailed.

Nearly all the cases here were strenuously de-identified intentionally for privacy reasons, except where obvious, in which case prior consent was obtained.

I would like to give credit to the following major influencers on my life's work:

To my father, Stan Block, Sr., and mother, Camilla Block, who were always supportive, available, and gently guiding me in my formative years. To my lifetime partner in marriage, much-too-good-for-me Melinda, who for 40+ years was my patient, encouraging bedrock at home; and to my 4 wonderful daughters, who really taught me about female behavior and slyly being manipulated. And to my 43-year lifetime partner in work, James Hedrick, MD, who helped me build this incredible, massive rural pediatric practice, as well as being a linchpin for all our world-class research and for my international medical publications. Also, to my partners: Drs. Ron Tyler, Alan Smith, Dan Finn, Rebecca Findlay, and yes, my daughter Lindsay Blackmon.

To (God rest their souls) pediatric chairman Jimmy Simon, MD, and cohort resident Lee Finklea, MD, who taught me so much of the science and humanitarian aspects, respectively, about being the best pediatrician possible. To my best friends from medical school: Drs. Tom Sither and Dave Atcher; college—Dr. Eddie "Too Tall" Tillett and Bob Williams (the original streaker), Wilson Sims, Roy Irwin, and Rick Beardsley; high school—Mike McCarthy; and family friend—Linda Sims.

To the innumerable gracious, talented referral physicians who accepted my complex pediatric patients, you folks are too many to add here. But a few physicians really stood out: ophthalmologist Craig Douglas, surgeons Mickey Anderson (local), H. Nagaraj, and Tom Foley (university); orthopedist Mike Sewell; infectious diseases Gary Marshall and Jerry Rabolais; oncologist Sal Bertolone; Cardiologists Chris Johnsrude and Roddy McDowell.

To some of the many brilliant pharmaceutical clinical directors who allowed me to humbly help publish their data: Peter Paradiso, Paul Mendelman, Frank Malinoski, Doug Kelsey, Pam Polino, Karl Kraft, and Rick Haupt.

To the omniscient journal chief editors who took a chance on me and nursed my many writings along: George McCracken and Stan Shulman; along with the "who's who" of pediatric physician experts—Chris Harrison, Jerome Klein, Jon Bradley, Stephen Pelton, Ken Alexander, Ken Zangwill, and internal medicine experts—Bob Belshe and Kristen Nichols.

To the copy-editors who helped fine-tune my unpolished text: Andaleeb Asghar and Kathleen Sperduti.

And a special thanks to Edna Cook.

www.ingramcontent.com/pod-product-compliance
Lightning Source LLC
Chambersburg PA
CBHW062320120626
46553CB00015B/21